POWER SPEED ENDURANCE

A Skill-Based Approach to Endurance Training

Brian MacKenzie
with Glen Cordoza

First Published in 2012 by Victory Belt Publishing Inc.

ISBN 13: 978-1-936608-61-4

This book is for educational purposes. The publisher and authors of this instructional book are not responsible in any manner whatsoever for any adverse effects arising directly or indirectly as a result of the information provided in this book. If not practiced safely and with caution, working out can be dangerous to you and to others. It is important to consult with a professional fitness instructor before beginning training. It is also very important to consult with a physician prior to training due to the intense and strenuous nature of the techniques in this book.

Printed in the USA

RRD02-13

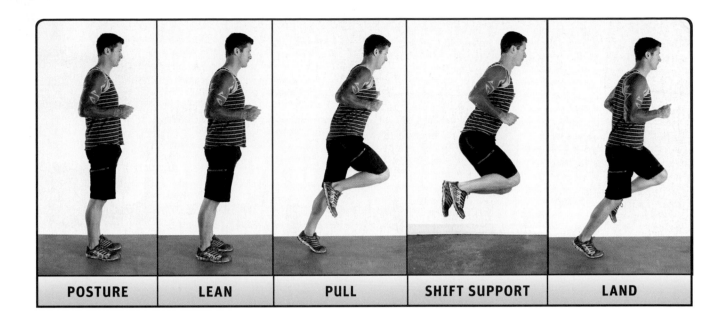

| POSTURE | LEAN | PULL | SHIFT SUPPORT | LAND |

Sweating and running, that was our edge in the evolutionary arms race. Our ability to run at a consistent pace for long distances, and to regulate our temperature through sweating, played a critical role in our survival as a species. Humans—slow, weak, and lacking natural weapons like claws and teeth—could doggedly pursue animals to exhaustion under the merciless African sun. Whether we were escaping predators, tracking down and hunting animals, moving to a new landscape with fresh foraging, relaying a message to a neighboring village, or playing games in the form of sport, we ran. Our ability to run allowed us to not only survive, but also to thrive. So if someone says they are built to run, they are just connecting to a fundamental truth of our species.

Although running is no longer essential to our survival, it doesn't change the fact that our bodies are designed to do it. However, numerous studies indicate that roughly 85 percent of the 44 million recreational and competitive runners in the United States succumb to injury, so if we are designed to run, what's with all the injuries?

A lot of the blame can be attributed to the shoe industry, founded on bad ideas and a victim of its own success. But that isn't the root of the problem. The issue at the heart of all running-related injuries is mechanics. Instead of moving as our bodies are intended to and working with the laws of nature, we work against them. Most of us assume that running is a natural instinct and so requires no training. As a result, athletes rarely consider that improper technique is to blame for their injuries.

People born into running cultures, such as the Tarahumara of Mexico or the high-altitude Ethiopians or Kenyans, get a natural indoctrination. In our own culture, running plays a very small role in daily life; some people might dash across an intersection occasionally or even get on a padded treadmill at the gym, but that's about it. Running needs to be taught to the average person, even, as hard as it may be to hear, to the average runner. Fortunately, there is a very complete and very scientific method of learning this skill that was once so fundamental to our species.

The Pose Method, developed by Dr. Romanov, has allowed us to see running from a different perspective. Through extensive research and personal experimentation, Romanov devised a model for running: fall forward, utilizing gravity; shift supports; and drop the feet directly under the body as you move forward. This changing of supports, or transitioning from one position to the next (one Pose to the next), as you fall is the basis of his method.

Today, running mechanics, as revealed by Romanov, is a worldwide phenomenon. Professional athletes and recreational runners everywhere have embraced this running technique, which seeks to harness the power of gravity. Whether you call it Chi Running, barefoot running, or evolutionary running, it all comes down to treating running as a legitimate skill to be acquired, not an innate human instinct that develops of its own accord.

I subscribe to this school of thought and implement Romanov's running strategies, but my evolution as an athlete and coach didn't stop with Pose. I've continued to experiment with different methods, techniques, drills, and strategies for running. Over the coming pages, I'll shed light on the conventional running lore and present a running method based on Pose principles that will not only help reduce injury, but also get you performing at your full potential. My method isn't all that different from Pose or other running-mechanics systems, but the way in which I layer the positions that comprise the movement is unique. In other words, my intention is not to reinvent the wheel, but make it spin more efficiently.

Running-Stance Checklist

Before I delve into the mechanics of running, it's imperative that you understand how to position your body for movement. My good friend Kelly Starrett, owner of CrossFit San Francisco and creator of the Starrett Movement and Mobility Method, has a saying: "Position is power." Setting athletes up in a strong position (or posture) prior to movement is at the core of everything we do. For example, you wouldn't prepare for a dead lift—a power-lifting exercise that requires you to bend over to pick up a barbell and stand up with it—with a flexed back because it would make you round forward as you pull the weight off the floor, compromising your power and increasing your risk for injury. Instead, you set up for the lift by stabilizing your trunk, tightening your body, and then lifting the weight off the ground while maintaining the integrity of your posture. This increases your leverage, allowing you to lift the weight with less effort, and reduces your susceptibility to injury. Running is the same as a dead lift in that if you set up for a run in a structurally weak position, you compromise the movement by decreasing power, balance, and stability.

To increase your learning curve and put you in the strongest position possible, I've provided a running-stance checklist. As a general rule of thumb, you should check off each step on the checklist before starting to run. Is my midline stabilized? Check. Do I have a neutral posture? Check. Are my arms in the correct position? Check. After you've checked everything off, you're ready to move on to the next step, which is applying motion to that position.

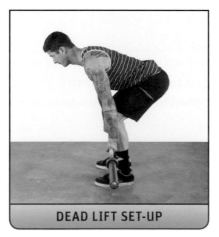

DEAD LIFT SET-UP

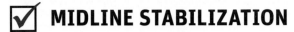

☑ **MIDLINE STABILIZATION**

☑ **HEAD POSITION**

☑ **ARM POSITION**

Midline Stabilization

Throughout this book, you will see the term "midline stabilization" over and over again because all movement begins and ends with it. Our limbs are designed to work around a stable body. It's what allows us to transition from one position to the next without injury.

Running is merely your ability to fall forward under a stable body while shifting supports, that is, falling from one position to the next. If your midline is not stabilized when you fall forward and shift your weight from one foot to the other, the shock wave that gets sent up your body will make your spine compress and flex. This compromise in posture places additional leverage on your extremities, which causes you to overload or misuse the muscles and joints that are in action. The result: You move slower, become fatigued sooner, and invite injury.

To avoid these problems you need to establish a neutral posture (flat back) and stabilize the position by engaging your abs. Don't make the mistake of trying to stand straight up without using your core. Time and again I've seen athletes try to correct forward flexion (rounded back) by pulling their shoulders back and driving their chest forward, causing them to overextend, which is another structurally weak position. In order to run as efficiently as possible and handle the force placed on your body when you land, you have to not only turn on the musculature in your trunk to lengthen and flatten your back, but also understand how to set your hips and ribcage in a stable position.

A neutral posture, or the flat back position, represents the key setup stance for all the forthcoming techniques. To teach this setup, I'll often use the hollow rock exercise because the load order sequence (step-by-step setup) is the same as setting up in the correct running stance: Flatten your low back and set your hips in a good position by squeezing your glutes, brace your trunk by engaging your abs, lengthen your spine by setting your rib cage over your pelvis, and then increase tension in the abs to maintain the position. The hollow rock test also gives you a general idea of the tension required from your midline to achieve and maintain a neutral posture while moving fast, or while handling a heavy load.

Note: the amount of muscle engagement in your core depends on the intensity of the situation. For example, if you're sitting in a chair or standing upright, only 15 to 20 percent tension is required to maintain a stable posture. But if you're sprinting or back-squatting a heavy weight, you have to increase that intensity to match the force being applied to your body, which in this case could be as much as 80 to 100 percent contraction.

Hollow Rock (Finding Midline Stability)

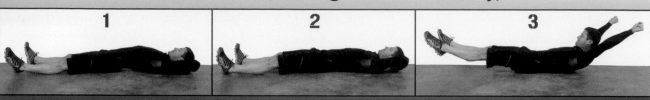

1	2	3

1. To execute the hollow rock, lie on the ground with a relaxed body. Look closely at the photo, and you'll notice that my back is arched. If you take this same position and flip me upright, I'm overextended, which is a broken position.

2. To achieve a stable position, I engage my glutes and contract my core, drawing my belly button toward my spine. Notice that my lumbar spine is now flat on the ground. This position represents roughly the level of tension necessary for standing upright or sitting in a chair. My core is engaged at about 15 to 20 percent tension—just enough to keep my upper body stabilized and my posture straight.

3. To achieve the hollow rock position, I elevate my lower legs, draw my lower ribs in as if I were doing a crunch, and extend my arms overhead. Note that I keep my glutes engaged, which causes my legs to externally rotate, and my shoulders pulled back. When done correctly, this position is extremely difficult to hold. Remember, the purpose of this drill is to illuminate the level of tension that you must achieve before you apply force to your body—whether in the form of running, lifting, swimming, or cycling—as well as teach you the load order sequencing for establishing a neutral posture.

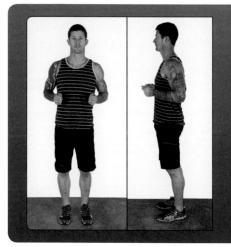

Correct Running Posture

1. I've achieved the correct running posture by squeezing my glutes and engaging my core.

Midline Faults

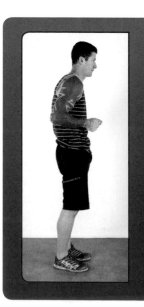

Flexion: Here I'm illustrating a flexion fault. My midline is disengaged, and my shoulders are rounded forward, causing a break in posture.

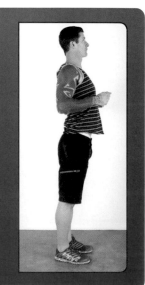

Extension: To avoid a flexion fault, I overcompensate by driving my chest forward, causing me to overextend. Notice the curve in my back. This not only causes a loss in power and efficiency, but also increases my chances of injury.

Head Position

After you've figured out how to stabilize your posture by engaging your midline and glutes, the next step is to establish a neutral head position. In the photos, you'll notice that my head is positioned directly over my shoulders and is centered over my midline. With my head balanced perfectly over my base of support, I can preserve the integrity of my posture while expending very little energy to do so. In addition to being energy-efficient, a neutral head position stabilizes the cervical spine, which helps absorb the shock sent through the body during the striking phase of the run.

Although the notion of keeping your head in line with your trunk seems straightforward enough, a lot of athletes still tilt their heads up or down. The former is common during a hard sprint, and the latter usually during the onset of fatigue or if the athlete looks down at his feet as he runs. In either case, this deviation from neutral creates additional pressure on the cervical spine, which in turn places more stress on the trunk. Over time, this will cause the midline to collapse. And then the dominoes don't stop falling. Once midline stability is lost, mechanics are compromised, fatigue sets in, and risk of injury dramatically increases. It's important to note that a deviation from a neutral head position can also be a result of a broken midline: when your midline collapses, your body searches for stability wherever it can.

To establish a neutral head position, place your thumb and pinky on your collarbones, raise your index finger, and set your chin on top of it (see Neutral-Head Test, below). To avoid asymmetrical muscle loading, which can result in a break of the midline or tension or stiffness in the neck, it's important that you limit flexing, extending, or lateral shifting of your head as you run. The only parts of your head that should move are your eyes.

Neutral-Head Test

1. To find my neutral head position, I lift my left hand to chest level with a hang-loose sign.

2. I place my thumb and pinky on my collarbones.

3. I extend my index finger and rest my chin on it. This roughly centers my head in the correct neutral posture.

4. I've achieved a neutral head position. Notice that I'm focusing my gaze straight ahead, and my head is centered directly between my shoulders.

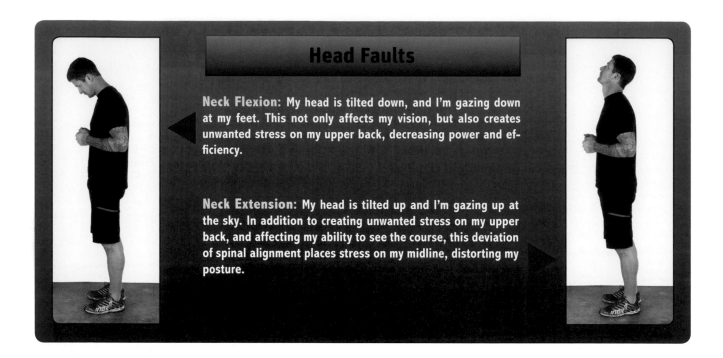

Head Faults

Neck Flexion: My head is tilted down, and I'm gazing down at my feet. This not only affects my vision, but also creates unwanted stress on my upper back, decreasing power and efficiency.

Neck Extension: My head is tilted up and I'm gazing up at the sky. In addition to creating unwanted stress on my upper back, and affecting my ability to see the course, this deviation of spinal alignment places stress on my midline, distorting my posture.

Arm Position

Once you understand how to establish a neutral posture, the next step is to set your arms in the correct position. To accomplish this, bend your arms at a 90-degree angle or more, pull your shoulders back, externally rotate your arms so that your thumbs are facing the sky, and close your hand as if you were holding a piece of paper between your thumbs and outside knuckles of your index finger.

The key is to stay as relaxed as possible. Your arms are not there to work, but to provide balance and stability as your run. For example, if you lift your right foot off the ground, your left arm moves forward to compensate for the weight shift—contralateral motion. The distance the arms move depends on the rate at which you're traveling: if you're sprinting a short distance, your arms need to move more to generate momentum and compensate for the higher foot pull than if you're running a marathon, in which case your arms will move only slightly to keep up with the faster cadence.

Regardless of the running intensity, your arms should be held close to your body—no flaring elbows. If you bow your elbows out or flail your arms from side to side as you run, not only is energy dissipated, but additional torque is also applied to your spine, which compromises the structural integrity of your posture. Another common fault related to arm positioning is an alternating forward and backward movement of the shoulders. Ideally, the shoulders should remain square and fixed. If you're corkscrewing your body, your core is either disengaged or your foot is crossing in front of your opposite hip. When this happens, you have to counterbalance your weight by twisting your shoulders. To remedy this problem, you have to readdress trunk stability and learn proper running mechanics, which I will get to shortly. For now, it's imperative that you spend time mastering the checklist. If your core is not stable, your posture is not neutral, or your arms are not in the correct position, nothing else I teach you will work.

Arm Position
(Upper-Body Mechanics)

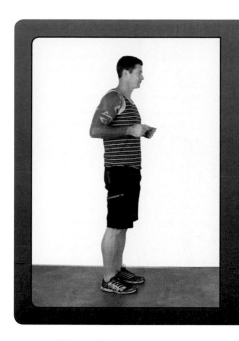

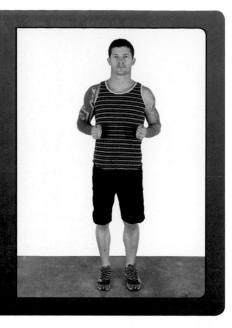

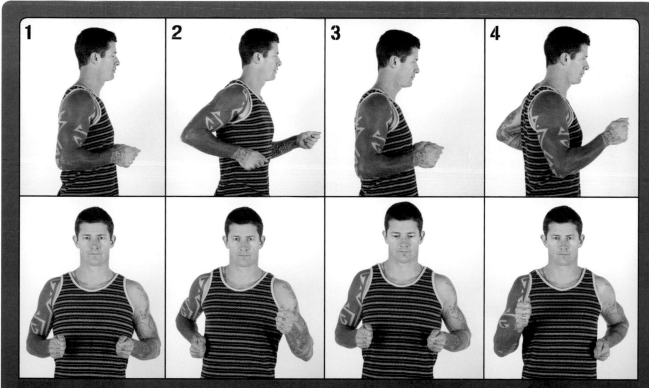

1. To assume the correct arm position, I bend my arms at about 90 degrees, pull my shoulders back (pull shoulder blades toward each other), externally rotate my arms so that my thumbs are pointing upward, and make a soft fist as if I were pinching a piece of paper between my thumbs and knuckles of my index fingers. Note that my arms are in tight to my body, my midline is stabilized, and my head is in a neutral position.

2. Keeping my arms relaxed—there is just enough tension to maintain my position—I pull my right elbow back and swing my left arm forward as if I were landing on my right leg. Notice that my shoulders remain square and pulled back. To avoid internal rotation of the shoulders or to prevent your shoulders from rolling forward, focus on keeping your elbows in tight to your body and your thumbs pointed to the sky.

3. I momentarily return to a neutral running position as if I were shifting supports.

4. I pull my left elbow back and swing my right arm forward as if I were landing on my left leg.

6 FACTORS IN RUNNING

There are six key factors involved in proper running mechanics. Without getting into the minutiae of each category, I've provided a summary of each factor as it relates to running. There are natural laws at work that affect economy of motion. If you abide by these laws, working with them instead of against them, you will make great strides in improving your running efficiency. For a more detailed breakdown of the following concepts, I suggest that you read Dr. Romanov's *Pose Method of Running* or *Pose Method of Triathlon Techniques*.

1 GRAVITY

Gravity affects everybody and everything the same way. As far as gravity is concerned, you are not special or unique. Proper running mechanics allow athletes to use this natural acceleration force to their advantage. Instead of pushing off the ground and using muscular effort to achieve forward motion, if you shift your general center of mass (GCM) over your base of support (i.e., fall), you will use gravity to initiate and maintain forward motion.

2 GROUND-REACTION FORCE

Ground-reaction force corresponds to the striking phase of the run. For example, if you land on the ball of your foot with your leg under your general center of mass, you minimize impact and increase propulsion, allowing you to keep up with your leaning position so that you can maintain forward motion. However, if you extend your leg out in front of your body and land on your heel, you're creating more force than necessary, and to maintain forward motion, you have to shove yourself off the ground. The former technique reduces muscular activation and saves your body from unnecessary punishment, while the latter is more punishing to the body and requires more muscular effort to move forward.

3 MUSCULAR ELASTICITY

Muscular elasticity is the muscles' ability to stretch or contract when forces are applied and then return to their natural state once that force is released. Jumping rope is a prime example of muscle elasticity at work: you have to drive off and land on the ball of your foot to propel your body into the air and absorb your weight as you land. Imagine trying to jump rope off your heels; it's impossible. You have more muscle elasticity below the knee, primarily in the foot, than anywhere else in the body. The muscles in your calf; your Achilles tendon; and all the intricate muscles, ligaments, and tendons in the foot help you absorb the force of your body's impact with the ground.

4 MUSCULAR CONTRAC-TION

Muscular contraction and muscular elasticity work in conjunction with each other. The more muscular elasticity you use, the less muscular contraction you need. For example, if you land on the ball of your foot when you run and allow your heel to kiss the ground, muscle elasticity cushions your impact, reducing muscular contraction. But if you land heel first and roll through the ball of your foot, muscular elasticity is taken out of the equation because you're not cushioning the impact with the muscles of your foot. In this situation, you not only transmit more force through your ankle, knee, and hip, but also need to recruit more muscles to carry out the movement.

5 TORQUE

Torque is created when your GCM passes beyond your base of support. To avoid falling on your face, you need to keep accelerating to maintain forward motion. For example, if I place a baseball bat in the palm of my hand, I have to keep my hand positioned underneath the bat's GCM to keep it from falling out of my hand. The acceleration force being applied to the object is the torque. In other words, I have to compensate for the torque being created on the top of the bat by creating torque on the bottom. The human body works the same way. When we fall forward to run, we create torque at the top end. In order to prevent falling to the ground, we have to maintain the equilibrium of our body by applying an acceleration force with our feet, which is provided by the cycle of shifting from one foot to the other. That acceleration (or deceleration) produced by alternating your feet is the torque that you're applying to your body.

6 MOMENTUM

Think of a car that has to accelerate to 60 miles per hour from a dead stop. While accelerating, RPMs increase and additional gas is required to bring the car up to speed. Once that car hits 60 miles per hour, it shifts into a higher gear, the RPMs drop, and it can maintain that speed using less gas than it did while accelerating. Its momentum helps keep it in motion. It works the same way with running, cycling, and swimming. Once you're in motion, it's easier to maintain that pace because you're using the momentum of your body to your advantage.

Proper Running Mechanics

Traditional running wisdom tells us to push off the ground with a long stride, lift the knee, land the foot in front of the body, strike with the heel, roll through the foot, and repeat. As you will come to understand, this model of running, which is still common even among elite endurance athletes, is highly inefficient. In addition to working against the forces of gravity, you increase muscular contraction, take muscular elasticity out of the picture, reduce torque, and stop the momentum of your body with every step. While running in this fashion for a short distance at a slow pace will probably have little detrimental effect on the body—it's just not enough volume to cause damage—tack on high-intensity training and long-distance runs, and you're asking for trouble.

To run efficiently and reduce your chances of injury, you have to use gravity to your advantage, maximize torque to maintain momentum, and use muscle elasticity to reduce muscular contraction. In short, you have to learn how to run using the forces of nature to your advantage.

Forward Motion

What is the first thing you do when you're trying to move forward? Most of us push off the ground with one foot while stepping forward with the other one. Although this puts us in motion, every time we push our foot away from the ground we wage a momentary battle against gravity: you are using your own energy to propel your body. In addition to exerting unnecessary energy, this is a direct violation of our primary goal, which is to let the forces of nature do as much work as possible.

A much better approach to moving forward is to simply shift your general center of mass over your base of support. The moment you do this, the power of gravity will take hold, forcing you forward.

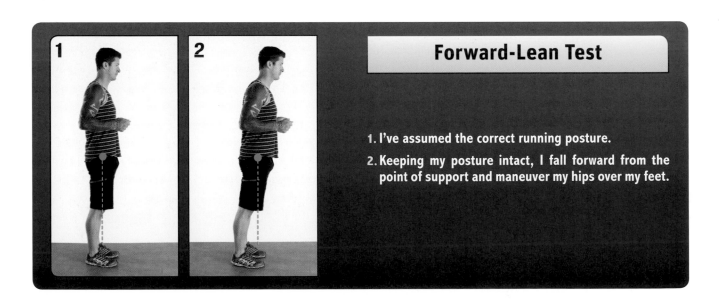

Forward-Lean Test

1. I've assumed the correct running posture.
2. Keeping my posture intact, I fall forward from the point of support and maneuver my hips over my feet.

To help you understand this concept, take a second to perform this test: Assume the proper running stance previously demonstrated and then lean forward from your hips as if you were a tree falling in the woods—see forward-lean test. Make sure to flex over your point of support (ankles) and avoid bending at the hips.

What happened?

If you stepped forward with your dominant foot to keep from falling on your face, you just used gravity to accelerate forward. No pushing off the ground or energy was needed. Nature, in this case, did all the work for you.

Maintaining Forward Motion

Forward motion, as you just experienced, is simply the loss of balance in the form of a fall. Instead of pushing away from the ground and wasting energy to initiate forward movement, you fell forward and then used your leg to prevent a fall. To keep up with the momentum of your fall to maintain forward motion, you have to alternate your feet and land underneath your GCM.

Another way of thinking about this is to imagine a fully inflated ball resting on a perfectly flat surface. Its GCM is located in its center, and its contact point with the ground is positioned directly underneath its GCM. Unless you force the ball into motion with a push, it remains fixed in the same position.

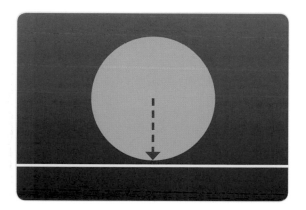 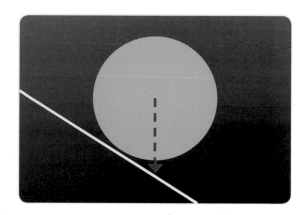

Now take that same fully inflated ball and place it on a slight downward slope. The ball's GCM is still located in its center, but its contact point with the ground is now slightly behind its GCM. Because the GCM is in front of the ball's base of support, the power of gravity pulls it down the slope. No outside force, other than the power of gravity, is needed to get the ball rolling.

Forward motion in running is analogous to that fully inflated ball. The moment you move your hips past your base of support, gravity starts pulling you forward. To prevent falling to the ground and maintaining forward momentum, you have to alternate your feet and place your supporting foot underneath your GCM to keep up with your forward fall. Think of it like this: Your body represents that fully inflated ball, and your fall represents the slope. The steeper the slope, the faster the ball rolls. The same is true with running. The farther you fall, the quicker you have to maneuver your feet to keep up with your GCM, and the faster you run.

If you're still struggling to grasp this concept, find a perfectly straight object, like a baseball bat or broom handle, and balance it in the palm of your hand. If you can keep that object perfectly balanced it will maintain its equilibrium. However, if it begins to fall, which it will do all on its own, you will have to maneuver your hand in the direction it's heading to prevent it from dropping. The greater the degree of the fall, the faster you have to move your hand. This simple test is analogous of your body moving forward when you run, in that the degree of your fall determines how fast you have to move your legs.

Stopping Forward Motion (Motion Faults)

There are several faults associated with falling mechanics, most notably breaking at the hips, leading with the chest, and landing out in front of your body. The first two faults are posture related and should be addressed using the checklist and falling mechanics. The third, however, is usually perceptual in nature. Falling as a means of moving forward is not instinctual to most adults. Unlike children, who seem to breathe, walk, and run naturally, adults change the mechanics of innate movement patterns. We start taking short, choppy breaths through the upper chest instead of long, smooth diaphragmatic breaths. We walk with our feet ducked out instead of keeping them straight. And we run by pushing off the ground and landing on our heels instead of falling forward with a stable body and letting gravity do the work.

To reverse-engineer these motor patterns, you have to spend an ample amount of time training the skill of the movement. For running, that means keeping your feet under your body and shifting supports as if your legs were spinning around an imaginary wheel under your hips. The moment you step out in front of your GCM, you stop the momentum of your forward fall and slow down. To continue moving forward, you have to reaccelerate up to speed, which can be accomplished only by driving your foot off the ground. This is like accelerating a car to 60 miles per hour, slamming on the brakes to slow down, and then repeating the process over and over

PERCEPTION OF FALLING

The fear of falling is innate, just as the actual practice of running is innate. So we have two natural instincts that are competing with each other. When we're just learning how to walk, the fear of falling doesn't prevent us from moving forward because our lack of stability keeps us moving. Hitting the ground is simply part of the learning process. As we grow older, however, experience tells us that hitting the ground won't feel so great. The fall is perceived as a potentially harmful action, so to avoid hitting the ground, we instinctually step out in front of our bodies to prevent a crash. But the quicker you learn to love falling, the quicker you will learn proper running mechanics.

So how to conquer this fear of falling, reverse-engineer the instinctual reaction, and accelerate your learning curve?

It's really quite simple. Remember when you first learned how to ride a bike? If you're like most of us, you started out using training wheels to gain confidence and improve your balance and coordination. Once you could ride without struggle, the training wheels came off and you tested your abilities on two wheels. Although failure was guaranteed in the beginning, you quickly learned how to stabilize your body and use forward momentum to keep yourself upright. With each passing week, you got more skillful and more skillful, and before long, you were jumping off curbs, bombing down hills, and attacking corners.

Running requires a similar progression laden with deep practice to let go of the fear so that we can develop skill. In other words, if you're new to the fall, you may want to put on some training wheels by practicing falling into a wall to get used to the mechanics. Once you can fall forward with a stable body, step away from the wall and practice falling forward and alternating your feet underneath your GCM. You're bound to make some mistakes, just as you did when the training wheels were taken off your first bike. But as you learn the proper mechanics and hone the techniques, your perception of falling will no longer be dictated by fear. Instead, the fall will turn into a useful tool for efficient movement.

Falling Wall Drill

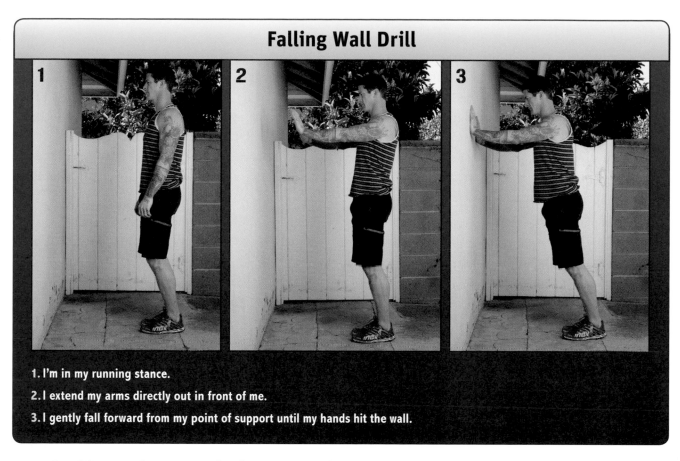

1. I'm in my running stance.
2. I extend my arms directly out in front of me.
3. I gently fall forward from my point of support until my hands hit the wall.

again. In addition to burning a ridiculous amount of gas, you will wear out the car's engine. Your body reacts just like the car in that you burn energy and effectively beat your body into submission. It's an expensive and unforgiving cycle. If you were a ball, you would now be deflated and rolling down a bumpy surface. Your GCM is still centered, but the contact point with the ground is positioned out in front, slowing the momentum of the roll.

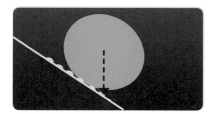

Pulling Mechanics, Shifting Supports, and Landing

- ☐ **Pulling mechanics:** The removal of your foot from the ground.

- ☐ **Shifting supports:** The transition from one foot to the next.

- ☐ **Landing:** The manner in which your foot hits to the ground—otherwise referred to as catching the fall.

Now that you understand how motion is created and maintained, let's examine proper technique and some of the factors that prevent you from running effectively. Remember, your ability to maintain forward motion is predicated not only on your ability to fall forward with a stable body, but also on your ability to pull, shift supports, and land correctly.

The Foot Pull

To execute a correct foot pull, draw your heel toward your butt using the power of your hamstrings while maintaining a neutral foot position. In Figure A, you'll notice that my foot is directly in line with the opposite leg and centered directly under my hips (GCM). Tendencies to avoid are dorsiflexion of the foot (Figure B), lifting the knee up (Figure C), and extending your leg behind your body (Figure D). Flexing your foot creates tension through the support system as well as impedes your ability to land on the ball of your foot. Pulling your knee toward your chest engages the hip flexor and quadriceps and shuts off the glutes and hamstrings, which can not only irritate the knee and hip, but can also cause your foot to end up out in front of your GCM. And swinging your leg out from behind your body indicates a push, which makes it difficult to pull your leg back under your GCM. All of these faults cause you to exert more energy than necessary and dramatically increase your susceptibility to injury. To avoid these common tendencies, pull your heel toward your butt—using the strength of your hamstring. Put simply, don't leave your foot behind your body. In addition to conserving energy, it will be easier for you to land your foot directly under your GCM to catch your fall.

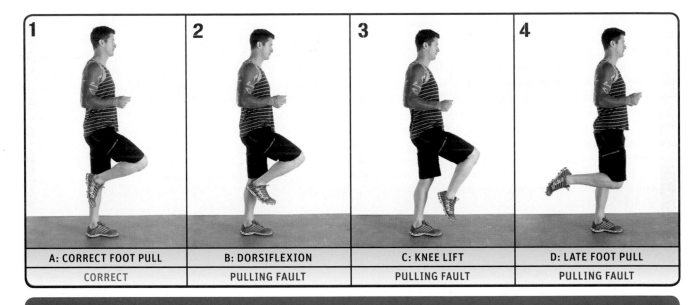

1	2	3	4
A: CORRECT FOOT PULL	**B: DORSIFLEXION**	**C: KNEE LIFT**	**D: LATE FOOT PULL**
CORRECT	PULLING FAULT	PULLING FAULT	PULLING FAULT

1. To execute a correct foot pull, I draw my right leg straight off the ground using the strength of my hamstring. Notice that my right foot is relaxed and in line with my left leg.

2. This is dorsiflexion, which you don't want to do. I've managed to pull my right foot off the ground using my hamstrings, but instead of keeping my foot relaxed, I've flexed it upward, engaging my shin muscles.

3. Using my hip flexor, I've pulled my knee up toward my chest. My foot is now in front of my GCM, increasing my chances of landing with my foot in front of my body.

4. I'm demonstrating a common fault that occurs when you push off the ground with your supporting foot. Notice that my right leg is trailing behind my body. This not only increases my susceptibility to injury, but also makes it difficult to position my foot under my GCM as I continue to move forward.

Pulling Mechanics Changing Under Speed

As I mentioned before, the angle of your fall dictates your speed at which you travel. Your fall also dictates the height of your foot pull (and, as you will learn shortly, the manner in which you land). For example, if you're running a marathon, you only need a slight foot pull—ankle to calf or ankle to knee depending on your fitness—to meet the demand of your slight lean. However, if you're in an all-out sprint with a lean that's 17 degrees or more, you need to pull your heel all the way to your butt. In addition to getting your foot under your GCM faster, a higher foot pull allows you to exert more force off the ground and allows you to cover more distance with your stride.

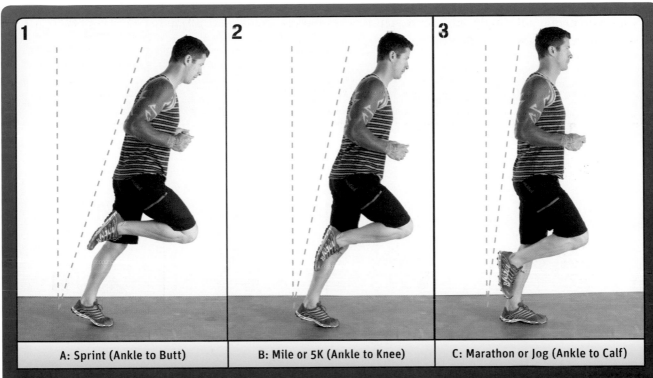

| A: Sprint (Ankle to Butt) | B: Mile or 5K (Ankle to Knee) | C: Marathon or Jog (Ankle to Calf) |

1. To effectively maintain forward momentum and keep up with the degree of my forward fall, I pull my foot up to my butt. Notice that my right foot is relaxed and still in line with my supporting leg despite the high pull. It's also important to notice that I'm on the ball of my left foot.

2. I've pulled my foot up to knee level to represent a moderate/intense speed, which would be characteristic of a hard 5K or mile pace. My right foot is relaxed and in line with my left leg. It's important to note that I still land on the ball of my foot but allow my heel to drop slightly to compensate for the lean.

3. Falling slightly forward to maintain forward momentum, I pull my foot up to my calf, which is characteristic of a slow to moderate jog. Just as in the other foot pulls, my right foot is relaxed and in line with my supporting leg. It's also important to note that although I still land on the ball of my foot, I allow my heel to kiss the ground before shifting supports.

Shifting Supports

When you shift supports there is brief moment when both of your feet leave the ground and you're completely suspended in midair. This airborne stride is what separates running from walking. If you're falling and pulling correctly, your feet should cross paths and your legs should remain under your body as illustrated in the photos. If your catch foot trails out in front of your body or your opposite leg swings out behind your body, you might want to consider readdressing your foot-pulling mechanics.

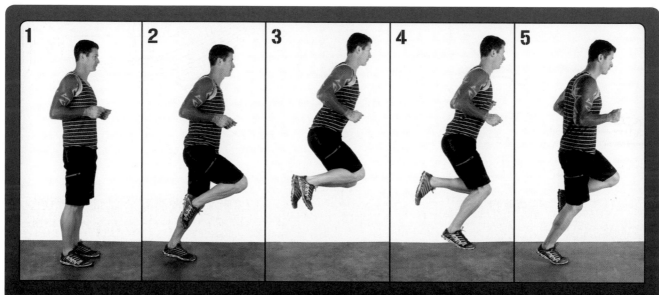

1. I've achieved the correct running stance.

2. Keeping my posture intact, I fall forward from the point of support and pull my right foot straight off the ground using the strength of my hamstrings.

3. As I pull my right foot off the ground, I shift supports by drawing my left foot up to my butt. Notice that my feet are on the same horizontal plane as they cross paths.

4. As I pull my left foot up, I extend my right leg and catch my fall by positioning my right foot under my GCM.

5. Maintaining a forward lean with a straight trunk, I land on the ball of my right foot and continue to travel forward.

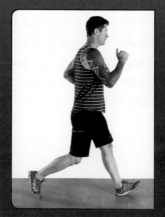

Common Fault: Pushing off with Forward Leg Swing

Here I am pushing off the ground with a forward leg swing. Notice that my left leg is trailing behind my body and that I'm landing on the heel of my left foot. In addition to slowing down my momentum, this faulty mechanic restricts the efficiency of my stride and increases my chances of injury.

Landing (Catching Your Fall)

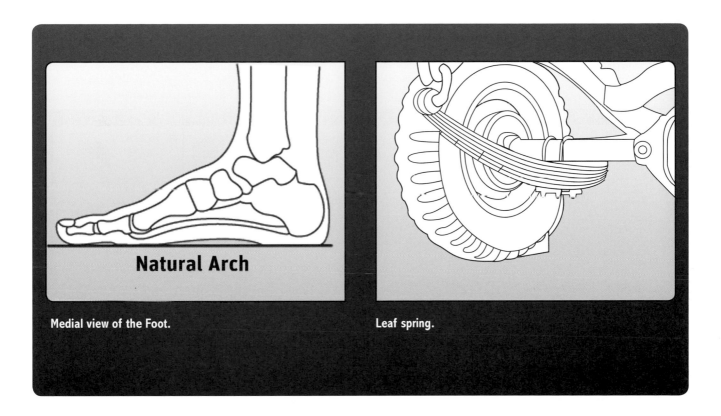

Natural Arch

Medial view of the Foot.

Leaf spring.

The foot is an intricate shock-absorbing system. In addition to having numerous bones, your foot has a series of ligaments (which attach bone to bone), tendons (which attach bone to muscle), and muscles and that give the foot a natural arch. This arch acts just like the leaf spring of a car in that it helps absorb the pressure of your body as you make contact with the ground. However, unlike the suspension of a wheeled vehicle, which centers the arch of the leaf spring directly under the car's axle, the leg (tibia and fibula) is positioned directly over your heel, which displaces the load. This anatomical design allows us to distribute our weight on any point of the foot, depending on where we put it during contact. In other words, we can land on the heel, on the heel and ball of the foot, or on the ball of the foot. As will become clear, in order to use your arch as it was designed, you have to land on the ball of the foot every time you strike the ground. Besides absorbing the shock of your body weight, which can be up to two or three times greater upon impact, landing on the ball of the foot engages the muscular-tendon elastic system, which reduces impact and energy expenditure. In a nutshell, this tightly bound system of bone, ligament, tendon, tissue, joint, and muscle is your body's suspension system. If you land with your heel or with a flat foot, you don't take advantage of your body's shock-absorbing system (arch), which is a formula for injury. This is analogous of driving a car with no suspension in that it affects the speed and efficiency of travel, as well as places unwanted wear and tear on the engine and supporting parts.

Ball of the Foot Landing Mechanics

To maximize the muscle, tendon, and ligament elasticity in your foot, you want to plant the pad of your foot on the ground—otherwise referred to as a ball-of-the-foot landing—so that your arch can absorb the shock of your body hitting the ground. However, just because you land on the ball of your foot, it doesn't mean that you take the rest of your foot out of the equation. Athletes implementing proper running mechanics will often make the mistake of keeping their heel off the ground with a rigid ankle as they run, regardless of speed. If you're running a mile or longer, this can literally destroy your calves, ankles, and feet. Staying on the balls of your feet is necessary only when sprinting a short distance or running up a steep hill. In all other circumstances, your foot should be relaxed and your heel should touch the ground for a fraction of a second before you transition back on to the ball of your foot to shift supports. This "heel kiss" reduces the eccentric load placed on your calf muscles, Achilles tendons, and ankles during the striking phase of the run, which minimizes the injuries associated with a ball-of-the-foot landing. If you have faulty mechanics or your body is not strong enough to handle the new technique, you're asking for trouble. So give your feet time to get stronger, and give your body time to adapt to the new movement patterns before you enter them in a race.

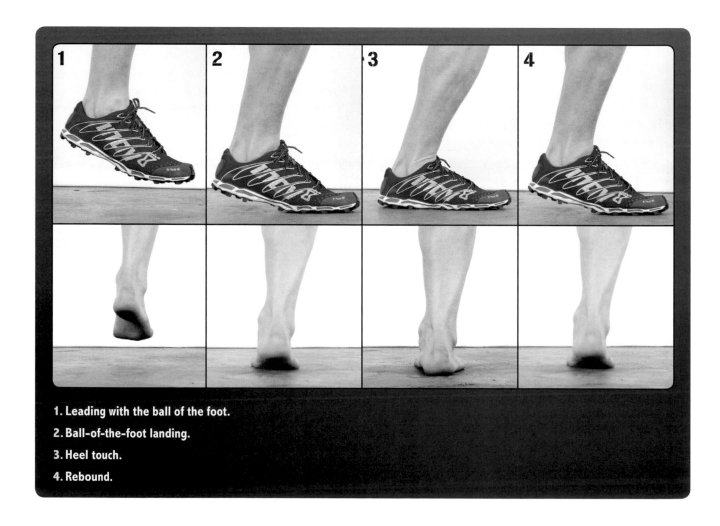

1. Leading with the ball of the foot.
2. Ball-of-the-foot landing.
3. Heel touch.
4. Rebound.

Heel Strike and Midfoot Landing (Landing Faults)

Despite overwhelming evidence that supports ball-of-the-foot landing, runners will still argue until they are blue in the face that a midfoot or heel-strike landing is the way to go. The foot is not structurally designed to absorb the shock of a midfoot single-leg landing. Landing on the heel is also less than ideal. With only a thin layer of fatty tissue and skin to cushion your fall, you take muscular, ligament, and tendon elasticity out of the equation. As a result, the ankle, knee, and hip joints have to take the brunt of your body weight's impact on the ground, which slows you down and can result in injuries.

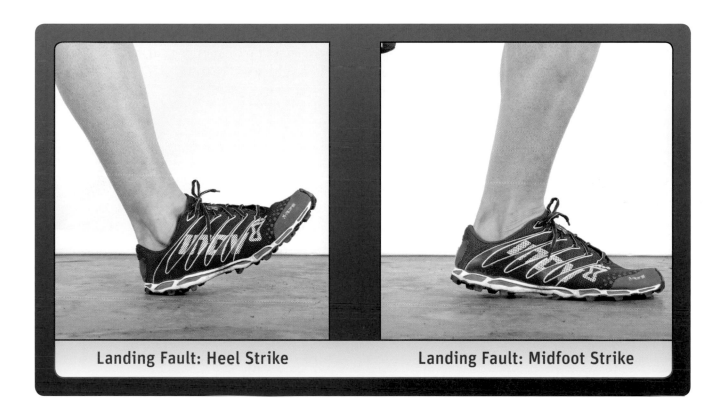

Landing Fault: Heel Strike   Landing Fault: Midfoot Strike

Overpronation (Landing Fault)

Overpronation of the foot is another landing fault that results from poor running mechanics. In this case, the runner lands on the outside of the foot as he heel-strikes (supination), and then transferring his weight to his supporting leg (pronation), his ankle collapses (overpronation) and the knee twists inward—otherwise referred to as a valgus knee bend. While this "technique" has been shown to take a terrible toll on the body, running enthusiasts still argue that this is a natural rolling of the foot that reduces the impact of landing; to avoid injury, all you have to do is buy a shoe with extra padding that compensates for the problem. As I've stated again and again, the best way to prevent injuries is to correct dysfunctional movement patterns. Buying a shoe as a means of solving a mechanical issue will do nothing but put a dent in your bank account. In order to run efficiently and reduce your susceptibility to injury, you have to learn to land on the ball of your foot.

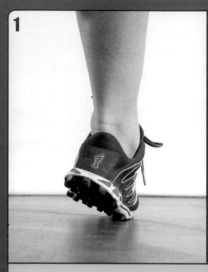
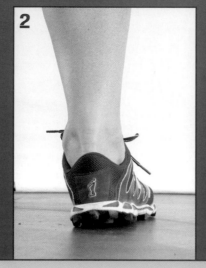
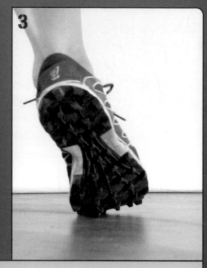

Landing Fault: Over-Pronation

1. I land on the outside of my foot (supination).

2. My ankle collapses as I overpronate, stressing the ankle and compromising the integrity of my knee.

3. As a result of overpronation, my leg is forced into external rotation as I extend my leg to shift supports, and the process is repeated.

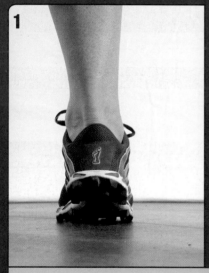
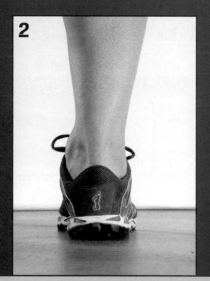
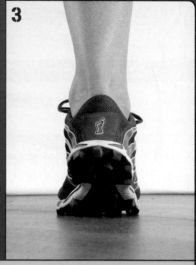

Correct: Neutral Foot Landing

1. I land on the ball of my foot.

2. I allow my heel to kiss the ground. Notice that my ankle is neutral and not collapsing to either side.

3. My heel naturally lifts straight off the ground. From here, I can maintain the integrity of my ankle and knee as I pull my right foot off the ground and shift supports.

Landing Fault: Inside Knee Bend

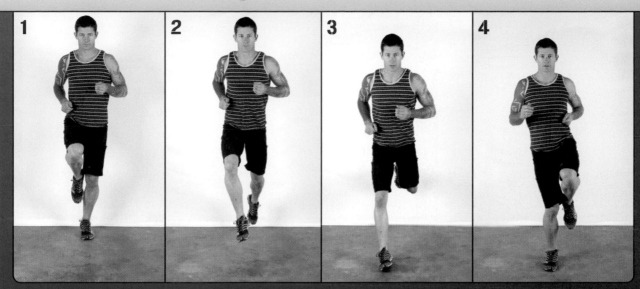

1. I've pulled my right foot off the ground.

2. I shift supports by extending my right leg in front of my body. Notice that my right leg has crossed over my centerline.

3. I land in front of my body and make contact with the outside of my right heel (supination).

4. As I transfer my weight through my foot, my ankle collapses (overpronates), which causes my knee to cave in (valgus knee). In addition to causing stress on both my ankle and knee, which will inevitably lead to injury, I compromise the integrity of my midline, slow down my movement, and expend unnecessary energy.

BAREFOOT RUNNING

There's no doubt that barefoot running is an excellent way to help build proper running mechanics, strengthen your feet, hone proper landing technique, and increase balance and proprioception. But it's not an end-all, cure-all solution. It doesn't address key factors such as posture, gravity, or the foot pull. In fact, if you're an endurance athlete who plans to compete in long-distance events, barefoot running can be detrimental to your running mechanics. For example, most barefoot runners lift the knee up using the hip flexors instead of pulling the heel to their butt. Although a knee lift primes the foot for a ball-of-the-foot landing and is ideal for trail running, in which you have to protect your toes from ramming into rocks, roots, and other objects, it's not the most efficient way to run. In addition to taking more energy— lifting your leg with your hip flexors turns off the hamstrings—the knee lift increases your chances of heel-striking should you decide to put on a pair of shoes to run. My recommendation is to run barefoot to strengthen the ligaments, tendons, and muscles of the foot, but still focus on the mechanics presented in this chapter.

THE PERFECT SHOE

Although modern shoes cause faulty mechanics, such as pushing off the ground and heel striking, they still serve a very important purpose. They protect the bottoms of the feet from glass, jagged rocks, other sharp objects, and the unforgiving surface that asphalt presents. Unless you have ginormous calluses on the bottoms of your feet from years of barefoot running, I suggest that you wear shoes when you run.

However, it's important that you choose a shoe that protects your feet but doesn't try to overcompensate with excess padding or support. A minimalist zero-differential shoe with a flat sole is your best bet. If possible, avoid shoes that try to cover up mechanical issues that should be addressed through skill training. For example, if you land on the outside of your foot—commonly referred to as an underpronation—you shouldn't buy a shoe with cushioning to dampen your impact. Instead, focus on landing with a neutral foot and incorporating barefoot-running drills.

It's important to mention that if you're in a shoe that has a lot of support, or you use arch supports or orthotics, don't jump straight into a zero-differential shoe. This can cause more harm than good. It takes time for your bones, muscles, and joints to adjust to the demand and increased range of motion. If you're in a shoe with a 10 mm heel lift, drop down to one with a 7 mm differential. After a couple of months, drop to 5 mm and then to 3 mm, until you get to zero. Be patient with the progression, keep the volume and intensity low, and listen to your body. It may take up to a year for your joints and tissues to make the adjustment. Once you develop the appropriate neuromuscular patterning to support the foot the way it was intended to be supported, you can reap all of the benefits of barefoot running while still protecting the bottoms of your feet.

INSIDER PERFORMANCE TIPS

PROGRESS SLOWLY

If you're new to this system of running, you may experience soreness and pain, which can ultimately lead to injury. To avoid this, I suggest that you progress slowly. Start out doing short, low-intensity runs, with an emphasis on skill development. It will take time for your body to adapt to the new technique, especially your calves, ankles, and feet, which are probably severely underdeveloped thanks to traditional running mechanics. To develop these muscles, incorporate jump-rope drills into your training and barefoot exercises. Don't push the envelop by throwing yourself into 400-meter intervals at high intensity. Instead, start out doing 50 or 100 meters and gradually work up to longer distances. Use the time to focus on skill and position. If you're patient and progress slowly, your body will adapt to the new motor pattern, you will recover faster, and you will be more efficient.

FOCUS ON QUICK FEET (CADENCE)

A faster stride will reduce the amount of time you spend on the ground and decrease ground-reaction force. This not only reduces the impact of your body hitting the ground—you're not coming down with as much force because of the lower foot pull—but also increases efficiency and thus keeps you going longer. For some runners, this shifted focus also improves other factors, like faster foot pull and ball-of-the-foot landing. Ninety steps per minute per leg is the lowest possible cadence without compromising muscle elasticity.

BE AS QUIET AS POSSIBLE

There's a saying: "You never hear a barefoot runner coming." That's because a barefoot runner lands on the ball of the foot with a bent knee. Muscle elasticity is utilized with each stride and the runner lands as softly as possible to reduce the impact on his foot and leg. The result: absolute silence in his approach. Poor running mechanics can often be heard as well as seen. If you're landing with a loud clunk, you're probably landing with your heel or midfoot and not using muscle elasticity. Sometimes trying to run as quietly as possible will yield a soft, fast, and efficient stride.

MIND THE CHECKLIST

Midline stabilization is always the first thing to go when you set off on a run. For that reason, you must be careful to remember each step in the posture checklist. Make sure your midline is stable, maintain a neutral head posture, and keep your arms bent at 90 degrees with your shoulders externally rotated. Even if your mechanics are not up to par, simply maintaining the integrity of your posture will help reduce the onset of fatigue and keep injuries at bay.

LEAN FROM YOUR POINT OF SUPPORT

The only way to initiate forward movement using the accelerating force of gravity is to fall forward from the ankles with a stable body. A lot of athletes make the mistake of leaning with their chest and breaking forward at the hips. This not only compromises the integrity of the midline but also works against gravity.

LAND UNDER YOUR GCM

It's important that you land as close as possible to the vertical projection of the body's GCM. This not only allows you to maintain the forward momentum of your fall, but also helps to avoid excessive impact on the body's support system.

PULL WITH YOUR HAMSTRINGS

Always engage the hamstrings to execute the foot pull as you alternate your feet and shift supports. In addition to saving energy, pulling your foot up using the power of your hamstrings makes it easier to position your foot under your GCM to maintain forward motion. If you engage the hip flexors by pulling your knee up, you shut off your posterior chain, creating quad burn, and increase the risk of landing in front of your body, which, as you already know, is a recipe for disaster. It's important to note that the hip flexors are involved, but the hamstrings are the prime movers.

To maximize muscle elasticity and reduce muscular contraction, always land on the ball of your foot, no matter what. However, it's important to remember not to stay on the ball of your foot forever. Unless you're in an all-out sprint, your heel should kiss the ground to avoid damaging your Achilles tendon, calf muscles, and foot.

FILM

You have no idea what your running mechanics look like unless you go to the video. Having someone shoot a video of you running, riding, swimming, or even weightlifting gives you the ability to see and understand the mistakes you're making. This is an eye-opening experience for most athletes, who may think or feel as if they are moving perfectly. Video doesn't lie. It checks your ego, and misconceptions, at the door. It sends you back to the drawing board.

To get an accurate reading on how you run, get a friend to film you running for about 10 meters. (You can also use a treadmill.) Do it a couple of times at varying speeds. You may find that you run without fault at slow speeds, but quickly lose it when you ramp up the intensity. It's also helpful to shoot when you're fresh and also when you're fatigued to see where you start to unravel. For example, you can film yourself at the beginning of a 5K, interval workout, or CrossFit WOD, and then at the end. This will give you an idea of what is structurally weak and what mechanic you revert to when stress and fatigue set in. I recommend that you use video to monitor your technique and progression as often as possible. Nothing provides more of a reality check than seeing yourself in action.

RUN UPHILL

Running uphill is a great training practice if you're struggling to grasp lean and landing mechanics. In order to progress up an incline you have to lean forward and strike with the ball of your foot. It's impossible to run up a hill while remaining perpendicular to the ground and landing on the heel of your foot. Not only that, but running uphill forces you to slow down the movement, which helps you understand the mechanics of landing under your GCM to move forward.

VARY TERRAIN

After you've developed the proper running mechanics, it's important for you to constantly vary the terrain you run on—you don't want to limit yourself by doing only your sport-specific interval or distance training on a track or flat road. Obviously, if you're training for an event on asphalt, it makes sense to train on asphalt. If you're training for a trail event, it makes sense to train on a single-track trail. However, to ensure that you're prepared for any scenario, it's a good idea to mix it up by running on single-track, fire roads, asphalt, concrete, grass, dirt, sand, and tracks. This keeps you fresh and engaged by forcing you to adapt to new situations, grades, and obstacles and builds awareness, proprioception, balance, coordination, agility, and control.

RUNNING ON A TREADMILL

I don't have any issues with treadmills, but you don't want to limit yourself to running on a machine all the time. I like to do intervals once a week on a treadmill because I can accurately quantify distance, time, and energy expenditure (calories), which can be used as diagnostic tools for future workouts. Another benefit for a coach is that a treadmill offers a unique opportunity to correct technique and easily identify movement flaws as the athlete runs. The treadmill can also be helpful when filming from a side profile. It's important to mention that when training on a treadmill you always want to increase the incline to one percent or more, to mimic the physics of how your body reacts to the road: if you run on a treadmill with the incline set at zero percent, because of the belt's speed you don't have to lean or strike accurately, which does little to instill proper running mechanics.

RUNNING IN THE SAND

Running on the beach is an excellent way to build strength in your feet and calves. It does, however, require a slight change in cadence. Unlike running on solid ground, which allows you to bounce off the surface using muscle elasticity, the sand absorbs the weight of your body and restricts your ability to transition to the next step. Running in the sand is like having a flat tire in that you're constantly slowing down with every step. To help offset the traction with the ground, a good strategy is to speed up your cadence using short, quick foot pulls. This will make it easier to float on the surface of the sand as well as save you a ton of energy.

TESTIMONIALS

"While writing *The 4-Hour Body*, I conducted thousands of tests and experiments and consulted with more than a hundred scientists, doctors, and world-class athletic coaches. It was a three-year quest to find the smallest inputs that create the largest outputs. On the endurance front, one name came up again and again: Brian MacKenzie. If you want to go from zero to marathon in 12 weeks, or perhaps run 100 miles and dead lift two to three times your body weight without struggle, he's your secret weapon. Listen and learn."

—**Timothy Ferriss,** #1 *New York Times* best-selling author of *The 4-Hour Body*

* * *

"The title of Brian Mackenzie's book, *Power, Speed, Endurance*, calls to mind the famous Olympic motto "Citius, Altius, Fortius" and the author's goal is similarly to attain harmony in athletics, updated to the multifunctional movements that enhance performance today. It has been my pleasure to mentor Brian over the years and to watch his growth as an athlete and now coach. The sincere sharing of knowledge about the latest in sports technology is what the reader needs, and what the author delivers in this book."

—**Nicholas Romanov Ph.D.,** founder of the Pose Method

* * *

"The crew at CrossFit Endurance knows their stuff. Their combination of traditional periodized exercise with CrossFit is spot on. Anybody looking to maximize his or her endurance performance while maintaining, or even improving, fitness must read this book."

—**Josh Everett,** CrossFit Level 1 and O-lift course instructor, NCAA Division 1 strength-and-conditioning coach

* * *

"Simply put, Brian MacKenzie has helped me to evolve into a better athlete. His intuitive thinking, attention to detail, and extensive knowledge make him a very effective coach regardless of your sport or the level you are competing at. He has inspired me to refocus my training by helping me to realize the importance of constantly changing and adapting my goals, both mentally and physically. Brian has been a true coaching asset, keeping me competitive on the world and Olympic stage over the last three years."

—**Erin Cafaro,** five-time US National Rowing Team member, two-time Olympic gold medalist

"I very much respect Brian's work. I was lucky enough to observe him in action working with average people who wanted to learn how to run and be fit. The improvements made in a single morning's teaching were impressive. For those who can't make it to one of his seminars, this book will provide the nuts and bolts of better running and endurance."

—Lon Kilgore Ph.D., Senior Lecturer, Department of Sport, Exercise, and Health, the School of Science, University of the West of Scotland

* * *

"I am so thrilled and excited for Brian's book. During the past several years Brian has had a significant impact on the rapid improvement of our program at San Jose State University. My close relationship with Brian, and the implementation and development of training modalities outlined in this book, have been an integral part of our success. CrossFit and CrossFit Endurance have greatly enhanced the overall competitiveness of our program. Thanks to CFE protocols, San Jose State's women's swim team won its first WAC Conference title, with 11 school records, 2 pool records, 2 WAC championship records, 1 overall WAC record, and WAC Coach of the Year."

—Sage Hopkins, Head Coach, Women's Swimming and Diving, San Jose State University

* * *

"June 18, 2010: I was lying on the pavement in a daze, pain torching the right side of my body, blood spilling onto the street from my face and legs. Unable to move, unable to breathe. All I could see was months—years!—of training spent for nothing. Ten days later, after surgery to fix a broken clavicle, I was told by the top shoulder specialist in the Midwest that he couldn't offer more hope than a possible 75 percent use of my right arm. What he didn't know, what no one knew, was that the most important meeting of my life was a mere five weeks away. On August 12, 2010, I met Brian MacKenzie, and my life, both inside and outside the sport, was revived, but in a much stronger light.

"Since that fateful August day, I, who had been a true believer in the Lydiard method, logging 30 hours a week of training, convinced that I needed to put in at least that much time (without strength work, of course), have been transformed into a stronger, faster, and more durable athlete than I ever could have imagined. By cutting my training hours in half, but making every moment of training purposeful and meaningful, and by eating a clean diet, I not only made a full recovery, with 100 percent use of my right arm, but I did it in half the time. Half. Let that sink in. I took a 20-week PT protocol and completed it in 9 weeks, getting cleared to race in October 2010. It was unheard-of by my doctor or any of his peers.

"As a professional triathlete/duathlete, I can't imagine using any other method of training. It's not just about the faster recovery, it's the fact that I continue to get faster and stronger every day. At 38, I'm able to take on any athlete at any distance, with complete confidence in my abilities. Nothing makes me smile wider than passing a 20-something leg-burner on the run, putting insurmountable distance between us. CFE hasn't just made me a better athlete; it's made me a better person—humble, grateful, and constantly seeking to stretch the bounds of human ability."

—Guy Petruzzelli, professional triathlete, Top 10 internationally ranked professional duathlete

RACE PROGRESSION

If you're new to the sport of running and you're interested in competing in a marathon, it's important for you to start with short distances such as a 5K or 10K and progress accordingly. Use these shorter races as an opportunity to dial in your nutrition and running mechanics and acclimate to the stress brought on by competition. As you get comfortable, increase your distances until you reach your desired goal.

ENVIRONMENT

Each environment requires some adaptability and specific preparation. For example, if you're running a race in the desert, you should know that arid climates suck moisture from your body while leaving you dry, making it difficult to determine the amount of fluid you're actually losing. If you're running at elevation, you need to take into consideration the lack of oxygen and train accordingly. Accounting for morning, evening, and night is also important, as conditions can change rapidly and without warning. The bottom line is that you have be careful to prepare and to subject your body to race conditions so that your body can adapt accordingly.

CLOTHING

Ideally, you want to wear something that you don't need to change. Racing is tough enough as it is. The last thing you need is an annoying rash as result of chafing, which will distract your focus and ultimately slow you down. Just as you need to adjust and adapt to environmental conditions, it's wise to wear clothing that you know is comfortable and won't cause problems.

UPHILL AND DOWNHILL RUNNING MECHANICS

A lot of people wonder whether running mechanics change based on the grade of the slope. The short answer is no. You still use a fall to dictate motion and speed, pull using the power of your hamstrings, and land on the ball of your foot under your GCM. If you're running downhill, you don't need to fall as far forward as you would when running on flat ground. If you're running uphill, you may need to fall forward more to compensate for the steep grade. To improve your efficiency and reduce your energy expenditure, lower your foot pull and increase your cadence. You also have to remain conscious of how fast you're willing to go and direct your speed with your fall. This is especially important when traveling downhill. If you step outside your ability and you pick up unwanted speed, you have to put the brakes on by stepping in front of your GCM, which can cause problems. The moment you feel excessive pounding, change the degree of your fall and shift supports as fast as possible.

Skill Training

To help you develop the mechanics described in this chapter, I've laid out several skill drills in the forthcoming pages. The goal of these drills is to get you back to a time when your training wasn't plagued with injuries. Running should be fun, not something that takes a terrible toll on your body. By utilizing skill-developing drills, this is a real possibility.

As you will notice, there is a considerable amount of overlap with the drills. The reason I've included so many drills is that people have their "Oh, crap" moments with different exercises—so there's something for everyone. You should stick with the drill that highlights your weaknesses and offers the most gains. For example, if you're having problems with the foot pull, and the wall drill doesn't seem to help, you can try the alternating-foot-pulls drill or the elevated foot pulls. You have options.

HOPS WITH FORWARD FALL

The hops with forward fall is one of the first drills I have my athletes perform because it teaches them how to fall correctly and makes them realize how little falling effort is needed to move forward. To perform this drill, jump up and down from your running stance as if you were jumping rope, and then lean forward from your point of support to initiate your fall. The key is to keep your body in a straight line and move your hips over your feet. As your GCM passes over your pivot point, you begin to fall toward the ground like a tree. Rather than stepping forward to break your fall, hop forward and move your feet under your hips to find equilibrium. Repeat until you've completed 10 to 20 falls. It's important to mention that breaking at the hips as you fall forward compromises midline stability. To get the best results from this drill, focus on keeping your core engaged, maintaining a neutral head position, and falling from your point of support.

Key Points:	**Common Faults:**
☐ Fall from your point of support.	☐ Bending from the hips.
☐ Keep your core engaged to keep your spine straight.	☐ Leaning too far forward.
☐ Fall forward only as much as is necessary to initiate movement.	☐ Stepping out in front of your body to stop the momentum of your lean.

The Dose: Perform this drill as needed in the early stages of development. At least 10 to 20 times, or until you can comfortably fall and regain equilibrium without fault.

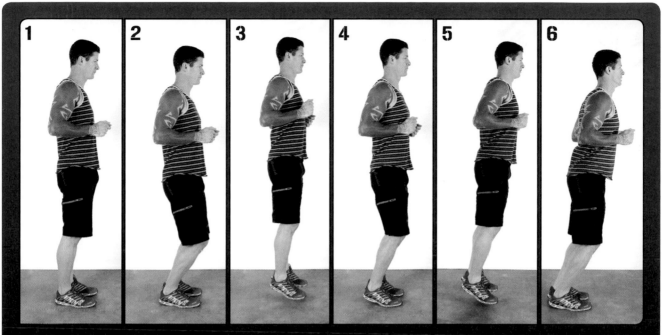

1. I'm in my running stance.

2. Keeping my back straight, I bend my knees slightly.

3. I extend my legs and jump straight into the air.

4. I land on the balls of my feet with my knees slightly bent to reduce impact.

5. As I land, I fall forward from my point of support to initiate forward motion. Note: Hop up and down a couple times to establish a rhythm before you lean forward.

6. Without breaking my rhythm, I hop up again, but because of the degree of my fall, I jump forward. From here, I will level out by pulling my hips back and repeat the drill until I've completed the desired number of repetitions.

PULLING WALL DRILL

Once you understand how little you have to lean to initiate forward movement, the next step is to learn proper pulling mechanics. In this sequence, I demonstrate the pulling wall drill, which is one of the best drills for teaching and ingraining this aspect of running mechanics. To execute this drill, position your heels about three to five inches away from a wall, establish your running stance, and then pull your ankle toward your butt using your hamstrings. To get the best results, do at least 20 pulls with one leg before switching to the opposite leg. This drill will not only teach you how to pull correctly, but also highlight common faults. You may find that when you start doing this drill, you'll kick your heel into the wall or pull your knee up using the hip flexors. The former fault is a result of trying to push off the ground to propel yourself forward; the latter indicates a late pull, which will happen if you lean too far forward, mistime the pull, and engage the hip flexors to lift the knee up to compensate for the distance lost. Although the knee lift allows you to catch up with your forward momentum, it instills inefficient motor patterns and shuts off the hamstrings, which are way more capable of doing the job.

Key Points:

☐ Keep the knee of your supporting leg soft.

☐ Pull your ankle up to knee level.

☐ Maintain a neutral—i.e., relaxed—foot.

☐ Use the power of your hamstring to pull the foot to your butt.

Common Faults:

☐ Kicking the heel into the wall.

☐ Pulling the knee up using the hip flexors.

☐ Flexing the foot.

The Dose:

At least 20 pulls per leg before moving on to the next drill. You should perform this drill until you have embodied proper pulling mechanics. Once proficient, you can incorporate this exercise into your warm-ups before sport-specific training. To increase the demand of this drill, you can hook a resistance band to your ankle and pull against the tension.

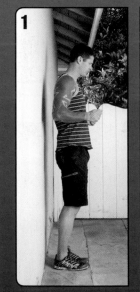 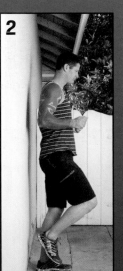 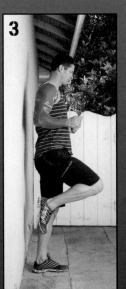 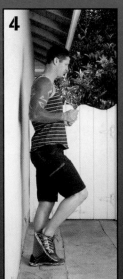 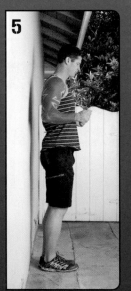

1. I'm in my running stance. Notice that my heels are about three inches from the wall.

2. Keeping my midline stabilized, my spine straight, and my left knee slightly flexed, I pull my right foot toward my butt using the power of my hamstrings.

3. I pull my right foot up to my left knee. Notice that my right foot is relaxed and in line with my supporting leg.

4. Keeping my right foot in a neutral position and in line with my left leg, I ease my foot to the ground.

5. I place my right foot next to my left foot. After completing 20 pulls with my right foot, I will switch legs and repeat the drill on the left side.

RUNNING WALL DRILL

Once you understand how to fall and the fundamental mechanics of the foot pull, the next step is to combine the two principles in the form of a running wall drill. If you look at the photos, you'll notice that I stand a few feet away from the wall, extend my arms out in front of me, and then lean forward with my posture stabilized. With my arms keeping my body positioned at a slight forward angle, I begin to run in place using the same pulling mechanics previously demonstrated. In addition to ingraining proper falling and pulling mechanics, this drill forces you to adjust your pull to the angle your body would be at if you were traveling forward. Once you've done 10 to 20 pulls per leg, turn and take off running alongside the wall, keeping the same lean and pulling mechanics you performed at the wall.

Key Points:

☐ Keep your feet positioned directly under your body.

☐ Maintain a stable body as you turn and take off on a run.

Common Faults:

☐ Disengaging the midline as you lean forward into the wall and when you turn to run.

☐ Kicking your heel back or lifting your knee up.

The Dose:

At least 20 total pulls or until you can complete at least 10 pulls per leg with perfect technique.

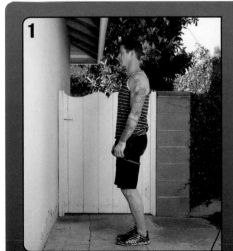
1 I'm in my running stance.

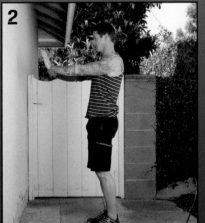
2 I extend my arms directly out in front of me.

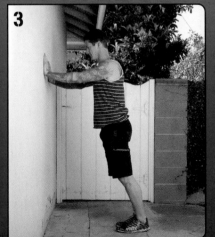
3 I gently fall forward from my point of support until my hands hit the wall. Notice the slight angle of my body.

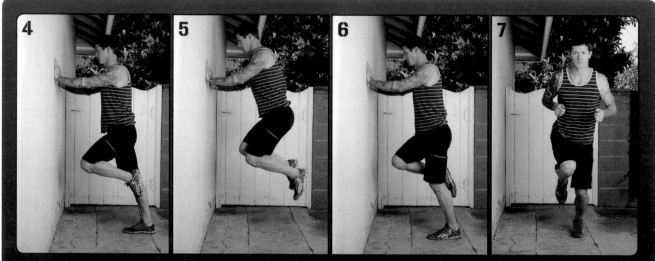

4) Using the power of my hamstrings, I pull my left foot up to my right knee. 5) As I ease my left foot toward the ground, I alternate feet and shift supports by snapping my right foot off the ground. 6) I land on the ball of my left foot. 7) Keeping the same lean, I turn my body counterclockwise and run alongside the wall.

ALTERNATING FOOT PULLS

This drill combines the previous drills into a highly effective skill-training sequence. To perform this drill, begin by hopping back and forth from foot to foot, like a boxer's shuffle. More specifically, you fall forward slightly while alternating your feet and shifting your weight back and forth as if you were going to bust into a light trot or jog. After you develop a rhythm or cadence with your feet, pull your right ankle up to your left knee and then immediately revert back into the forward shuffle. Repeat this 5 to 10 times, then switch legs. After you've completed about 10 pulls with each leg, increase the degree of your lean and run it out as you did in the previous drill. In addition to developing coordination, and ingraining proper leaning and pulling mechanics, this drill teaches you how to absorb and rebound using muscle elasticity.

Key Points:

☐ Shuffle back and forth from foot to foot and develop a strong rhythm before executing the foot pull.

☐ After one pull, revert back to a light trot and regain a consistent rhythm before executing your next pull.

☐ Absorb the shock of your shuffle using the ball of your foot and allow your heel to kiss the ground to maximize muscle elasticity.

Common Faults:

☐ Breaking at the midline and bending from the hips.

☐ Hopping with both feet instead of shuffling back and forth.

☐ Landing with a flat foot.

☐ Performing an incorrect pull by either pushing off the ground or lifting the knee.

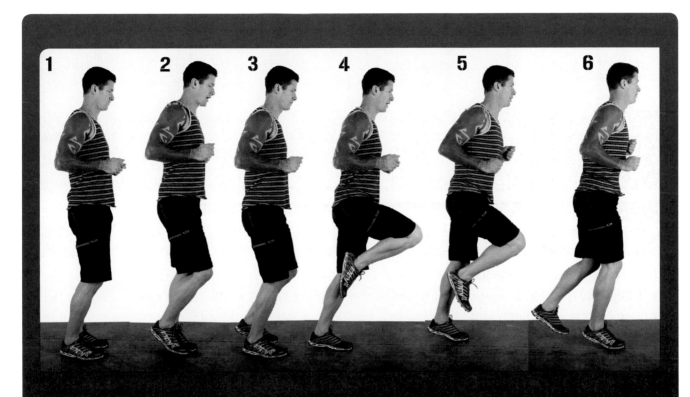

1. I'm in a proper running stance with my knees slightly bent.

2. To start the shuffle, I fall slightly forward and momentarily shift my weight onto my right leg and pull my left foot slightly off the ground.

3. I continue to shuffle forward by shifting my weight onto my right leg.

4. As I transfer my weight to my left foot, I pull my right foot up toward my butt using the power of my hamstrings.

5. Without shifting supports, I extend my right foot toward the ground. Note: You don't want to extend your right leg out in front of your body. Rather, keep it under your GCM and allow the momentum of your fall to carry you forward.

6. I land on the ball of my right foot. From here, I will resume a shuffle, regain a consistent rhythm, and execute another pull with my right leg.

STABLE-ARM DRILL

Runners often master the fall and the pull relatively quickly but immediately forget the most important aspect of proper running mechanics, which is to maintain a stable posture. To test your stability, interlock you hands and extend your arms out in front of you. Begin running in place, and after 10 or 20 foot pulls, fall forward slightly while continuing to run. If your midline is stable, your arms will remain locked straight out in front of you (Sequence A). If your core is not engaged, your arms will swing from side to side, compromising your balance and making it very difficult to run (Sequence B). After you've experimented with the previous drills and you feel comfortable changing supports while in a forward lean, perform the stable-arm drill to see how stable you are. In addition to instilling midline-stabilization mechanics, this drill offers valuable feedback about the level of tension required in running. In other words, the faster you run, the more you'll need to engage your core to maintain balance and maximize energy efficiency.

Key Points:

☐ Stabilize your midline, run in place, and then fall forward to initiate forward motion.

☐ Keep your arms positioned along your centerline as you run.

☐ The faster you run, the more you have to stabilize.

Common Faults:

☐ Swinging your arms back and forth as a result of weak midline stabilization.

The Dose:

Use this drill as a diagnostic tool to test midline stabilization.

Sequence A: Stable-Arm Drill with Engaged Midline

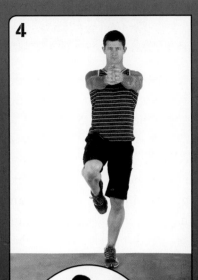

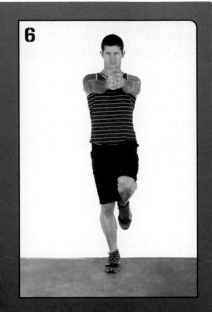

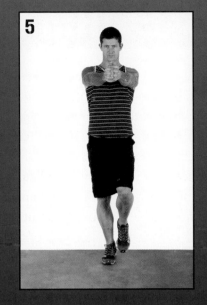

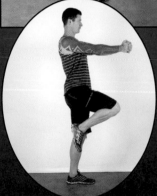

1. I'm standing in a neutral posture.

2. I interlock my fingers in front of my body.

3. Keeping my arms straight, I raise them to chest level.

4. Without falling forward, I pull my right foot off the ground using the power of my hamstrings.

5. I drop my right foot and begin to elevate my left foot.

6. Keeping my midline engaged, I run in place by alternating my feet and shifting supports. Notice that my arms remain locked in line with the center of my body.

Sequence B: Stable-Arm Drill with Midline Disengaged

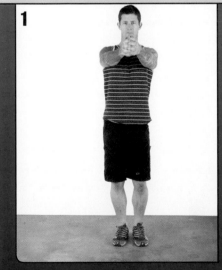

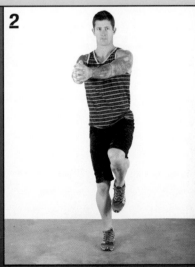

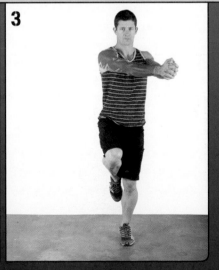

1. I've interlocked my fingers and positioned my arms out in front of me at chest level. Note that my midline is disengaged.

2. As I pull my left foot off the ground to run in place, my arms swing toward my right side to counterbalance my weight.

3. With my midline disengaged, I'm unable to stabilize myself as I alternate my feet and shift supports. As a result, my arms swing to the left side of my body.

COP DRILL

Just like the stable arm drill, the cop drill is another tool for testing midline stabilization and ingraining proper falling mechanics. To perform this drill, interlock your hands behind your back as if they were handcuffed. Although having your hands pinned behind your back is awkward, it allows you to increase your focus on stabilization, the fall, and the shifting of supports. The key to performing this drill correctly is to lead the fall with your hips. A lot of athletes make the mistake of initiating the fall with the chest while bending forward at the hips. Not only does this sacrifice a stable midline, but it also compromises balance. Another common fault is to overextend (Sequence B). If you're unable to comfortably lock your hands behind your back without overextending, you probably need to work on shoulder mobility. In such a situation, you may want to focus on the hops with forward lean or the alternating foot pulls drill.

Key Points:

☐ Keep your shoulders externally rotated (pulled back) and your spine neutral.

☐ Focus on shifting your GCM (hips) over your balance point (ankles).

☐ Change supports the moment your hips pass over your ankles.

Common Faults:

☐ Leaning forward with your chest and bending at the hips.

☐ Overextending as you assume the handcuff position.

☐ Stepping forward with your foot to brace your fall and stop the momentum.

The Dose:

Perform this drill until you develop the proper falling mechanics. I usually suggest falling and then running a few meters, leveling out, and then repeating the process until the athlete feels comfortable with the fall.

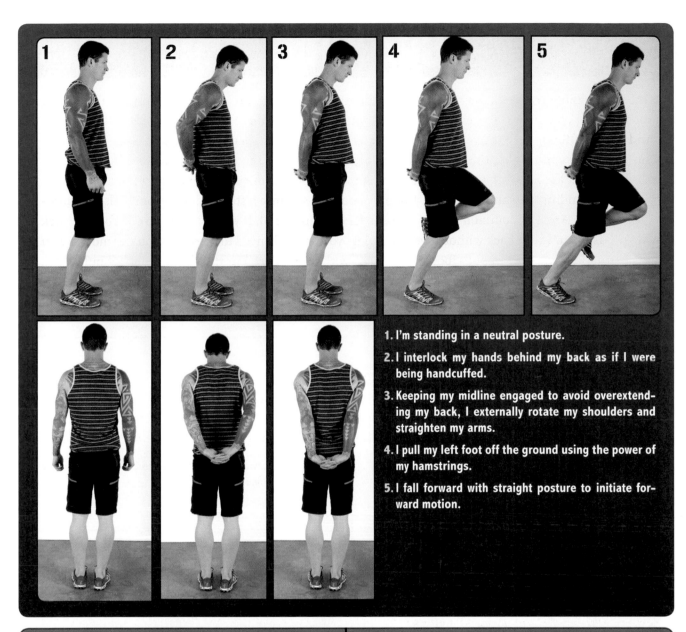

1. I'm standing in a neutral posture.

2. I interlock my hands behind my back as if I were being handcuffed.

3. Keeping my midline engaged to avoid overextending my back, I externally rotate my shoulders and straighten my arms.

4. I pull my left foot off the ground using the power of my hamstrings.

5. I fall forward with straight posture to initiate forward motion.

Common Fault: Flexion

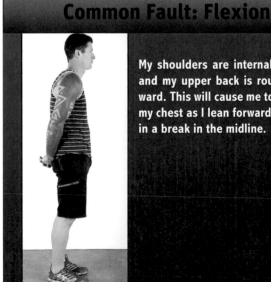

My shoulders are internally rotated and my upper back is rounded forward. This will cause me to lead with my chest as I lean forward, resulting in a break in the midline.

Common Fault: Overextension

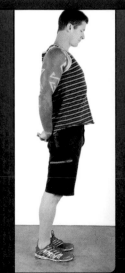

I overextend as I try to straighten my arms and pull my shoulders back into the correct position. This fault is common with athletes who overemphasize this step or lack shoulder mobility. If faced with the former, simply correct the technique by straightening your posture. If faced with the latter, see the mobility chapter.

JUMP ROPE DRILL

The jump rope drill is one of the best exercises for developing rhythm, coordination, and muscle elasticity. To perform this drill correctly, run in place, using proper running mechanics, as you jump rope. If you're new to jumping rope or you're unable to perform this exercise because of a lack of coordination and timing, focus on developing the rhythm and skill necessary by simply hopping up and down. In the meantime, use the other drills in this section to develop proper running mechanics. Once you're able to sequence together multiple repetitions without disruption, start piecing in the running mechanics by pulling your ankle to the opposite knee while shifting supports. The goal is to get the jump rope to successfully pass under your legs as you shift supports. At first the passes will seem choppy and slow, but with a little patience and a lot of practice you'll develop the coordination, timing, and rhythm to run in place just as if you were performing the wall drill.

Once you can run in place without fault, the next step is to add forward motion. All the same principles apply. You want to maintain a stable midline, pull your ankle to your knee, and shift supports as the rope passes under your feet. But now you add a slight fall and begin running forward. If you're pulling correctly, you'll progress forward without restriction. However, if you start to push off the ground, break at the hips, or your foot lands out in front of you, the jump rope will catch your feet as it circles under you, putting you back at square one. To reduce the frequency of this frustrating yet all too common scenario, focus on the mechanics and maintain a consistent cadence. Although the jump rope drill can be extremely disheartening, especially when first starting out, it's an excellent way to teach proper running mechanics and serves as an invaluable tool to correct movement faults.

Key Points:

☐ Learn how to run in place as you jump rope before adding forward motion.

☐ Focus on passing the rope under your feet as you shift supports while maintaining a consistent rhythm. Time, practice, patience, and technique are your keys to success.

☐ When adding forward motion, fall forward from the hips and use correct pulling mechanics.

Common Faults:

☐ It's common for athletes, especially when starting out, to stall with each shift of supports, resulting in a choppy cadence.

☐ When running in place, athletes will elevate the knee instead of pulling ankle to knee.

☐ Breaking at the midline, pushing off the ground, or landing out in front of the body while running forward.

The Dose:

Spend as much time as possible on this drill until you master running in place and can run forward without pause or disruption. Once proficient, you can incorporate this drill into your warm-ups, as a skill-training exercise, or to tune up your rhythm and timing.

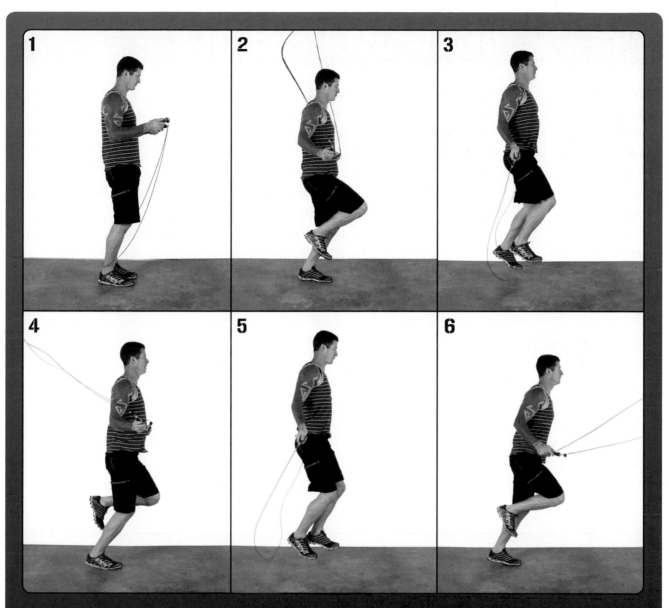

1. I'm standing in a neutral posture with the jump rope positioned behind my feet.

2. As I swing the jump rope over my head, I draw my right heel toward my butt using proper pulling mechanics.

3. I shift supports and alternate my feet as the jump rope passes under me.

4. I catch my body with my right foot and pull my left foot up.

5. I shift supports again as the rope passes under my feet.

6. I alternate my feet and catch myself for the second time. Having successfully run in place and developed a rhythm, I add a slight fall to initiate forward motion.

ELEVATED FOOT PULL DRILL

As I mentioned in the introduction to this chapter, it's important to experiment with as many drills as possible until you find the exercise that clicks. The elevated foot pull drill is another skill-training exercise that ingrains proper pulling mechanics, as well as builds muscles elasticity, strength, and pulling speed. If you get awesome results from this particular drill, stick with it and implement it anytime you're working on your pulling mechanics. While it's good to play around with all of the drills outlined in this chapter, you have to focus on what has the greatest impact on your skill development.

Key Points:

☐ To absorb impact and maximize muscle elasticity, be sure to land on the ball of the foot with a soft knee.

☐ Pull your heel up to your butt.

☐ Focus on speed and efficiency of movement.

Common Faults:

☐ Landing with a flat foot and straight leg.

☐ Executing an inefficient pull by lifting the knee up to your chest instead of drawing your heel up to your butt.

☐ Flexing the foot as you pull.

The Dose:

When incorporating this drill into your skill-training exercises you should perform 10 to 20 repetitions with each leg. Because this is a drill that improves pulling speed and conditions the leg for the repeated impact of running, this is a good one to incorporate into your warm-up whenever possible.

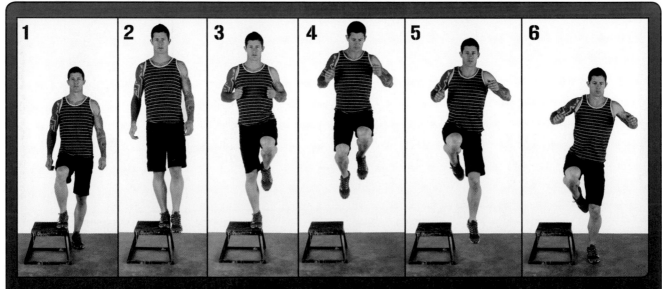

1) I've got my right foot positioned on the edge of a 12-inch box. 2) I extend my right leg and stand upright. 3) Keeping a slight bend in my right leg, I pull my left foot up to my right knee. 4) I jump off the box and pull my right foot toward my butt as if I were shifting supports. Note: You want to pull your right foot up as fast as possible using the power of your hamstrings. 5) As I pull my right foot up, I extend my left leg to find the ground. 6) I land on the ball of my left foot and keep my left leg bent to absorb the impact of my drop.

PIVOTED FOOT PULLS

Like the elevated foot pulls, pivoted foot pulls help teach the proper pulling mechanics, improve muscle elasticity and speed, and build the musculature in the hamstrings. To get the best results from this drill, string together multiple pulls with the supporting leg as fast as possible: the quicker you can pull your foot off the ground as it lands, the better. When done correctly, this drill teaches you how to land on the ball of your foot, react with the ground using muscle elasticity, and pull using the power of your hamstrings.

Key Points:

☐ Execute a full range of motion by pulling your heel up to your butt.

☐ To avoid injury and maximize muscle elasticity, land on the ball of your foot with a soft knee.

☐ Immediately transition into your next pull without hesitation; the less time you spend on the ground the better.

Common Faults:

☐ Landing with a flat foot or straight leg.

☐ Stalling between repetitions.

The Dose:

Perform 10 to 20 pulls with each leg, and include this skill-training exercise in your warm-up routine whenever possible.

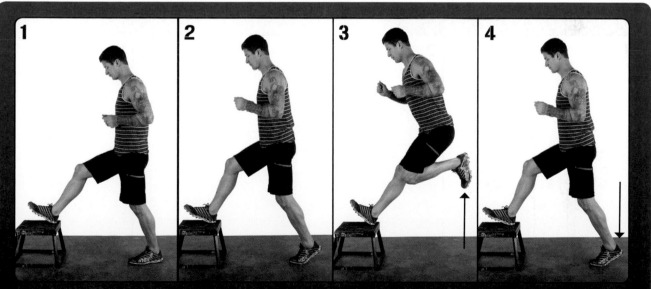

1) I've assumed my running stance and positioned my right heel on the edge of 12-inch box. It's important to notice that my right leg is bent slightly and that my supporting leg is positioned directly under my hips. 2) Keeping my posture straight, I shift my weight slightly forward and rise up on the ball of my left foot. 3) I pull my left heel up to my butt using the power of my hamstrings. 4) I land on the ball of my left foot and absorb the shock of my body weight by bending my knee. The moment my foot hits the ground, I'll snap it right back up as quickly as possible, and repeat this process until I've completed the set amount of repetitions.

CARIOCA

The carioca drill is a lateral-movement exercise that has several benefits. For one, it teaches you how to fall laterally with your body weight, using the forces of gravity to your advantage. Secondly, because landing with the heel is impossible to manage because of the nature of this exercise, it instills proper striking mechanics and builds the muscles of your lower leg, which is essential for those who are not used to running on the ball of the foot. (It also develops the lateral muscles of the legs and hips, which are usually underdeveloped in runners who have neglected strength-and-conditioning training.) Thirdly, the carioca drill helps to develop body and space awareness—that is, coordination. Lastly, it's an excellent warm-up for the muscles and joints and prepares your body for other dynamic movements. If you've played a team sport, chances are you've performed this drill at the beginning of practice, with very good reason.

Key Points:

☐ When initiating motion, fall laterally from the hips, shifting your GCM over your balance point, just as you would when running forward. The key is not to bend at the hips.

☐ Keep your feet directly under your GCM as you move.

Common Faults:

☐ Avoid flexing at the hips and leaning with your chest.

☐ Don't overexaggerate upper-body movement by twisting your shoulders back and forth or swinging your arms from side to side. Instead, keep your arms bent and close to your body as if you were running.

☐ Avoid stepping in front of your body. Just as in running, this will make you push off the ground, compromising your mechanics and slowing you down.

The Dose:

Perform this drill at the beginning of a strength-and-conditioning workout or as a warm-up for sport-specific interval training. To balance the drill, it's important that you execute this exercise on both sides of your body. For example, do the carioca to the left for 10 meters and then to the right for the same distance.

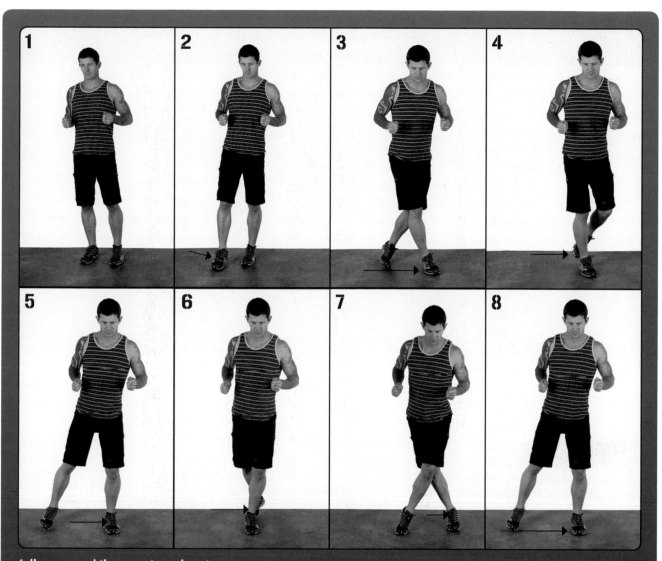

1. I've assumed the correct running stance.

2. Keeping my body straight, I lean to my left, shifting my GCM over my left foot. As I transfer my weight onto my left leg, I begin to cross my right leg in front of my left leg.

3. Using the momentum of my fall to initiate lateral motion, I cross my right foot over my left foot to catch my fall.

4. The moment I plant my left foot on the ground, I swing my left foot behind my right leg.

5. Still falling to the left with my posture intact to maintain momentum, I plant my left foot on the ground directly under my GCM.

6. Keeping my midline engaged to avoid exaggerated twisting of the upper body, I maneuver my right foot behind my left leg.

7. I plant my right foot on the ground directly under my hips to catch my fall.

8. Continuing to use my upper-body fall to move laterally, I land on the ball of my left foot and prepare to repeat the sequence.

PARTNER BAND DRILL

The partner band drill offers two key benefits. It teaches proper falling mechanics and adds resistance to a run, which helps develop speed and explosiveness. With the band momentarily supporting your weight, you can slowly lean forward without having to shift supports to catch your fall (Sequence A, second photo). Although falling forward in such a manner is awkward and seemingly unnatural, it allows you to experience the proper falling mechanics in slow motion. The band also highlights common faults associated with the fall, which include breaking at the hips, pushing off the ground, and stepping out in front of the body (Sequence B). To avoid these tendencies, work on falling forward with a slight lean. After a momentary pause, start shifting supports as if you were going to burst into a light run. Your partner should offer just enough resistance to hold you upright and allow you to keep moving forward. As you get more comfortable with the falling mechanics, you can use the band to add resistance to short-interval sprints. However, it's important to keep technique as your primary focus. If adding speed compromises your running form, slow down and decrease the intensity.

Key Points:

- ☐ Execute a slight forward lean before you initiate a pull and begin shifting supports.

- ☐ Because the band is pulling back on your hips, you have to stabilize your core more than when executing a free or unrestrained run.

Common Faults:

- ☐ When executing the fall, avoid leaning with your chest and bending at the waist.

- ☐ Don't push off the ground or step out in front of your body to stop your fall.

- ☐ Compromising technique as a result of increasing intensity.

The Dose:

To get the best results, set a distance that's 10 to 20 meters. The idea is to keep the distance short to maintain speed and explosiveness. As a rule, the distance should be one at which you can maintain speed and intensity without compromising form. The instant you start to slow down or mechanics break down, stop and shorten the distance.

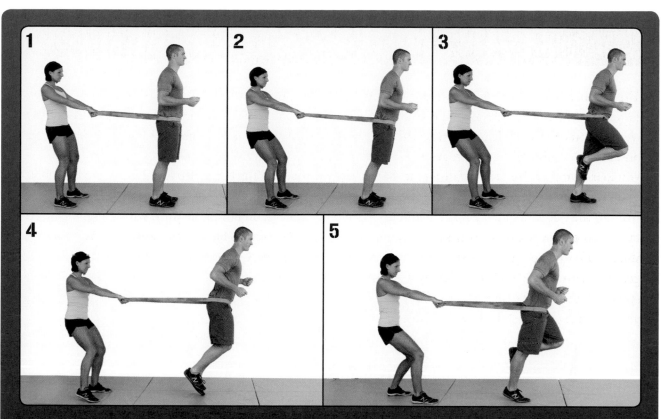

1. Glen is in his running stance. The resistance band is wrapped around his hips, and Katie is creating tension in the band by leaning slightly backward.

2. Glen slowly leans forward from his point of support.

3. As Glen leans forward, he pulls his left foot up.

4. As Glen shift supports, Katie continues to lean back to maintain resistance.

5. Glen accelerates forward using proper running mechanics. To slow his progression, Katie continues to create resistance on the band by keeping her weight back. Note: Katie is not trying to keep Glen in one place. Instead, she shuffles forward as he progress forward while maintaining consistent tension on the band.

Common Fault: Pushing Off

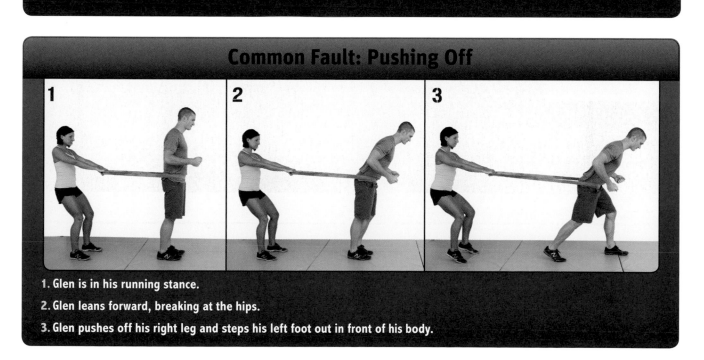

1. Glen is in his running stance.

2. Glen leans forward, breaking at the hips.

3. Glen pushes off his right leg and steps his left foot out in front of his body.

PARTNER FALLING DRILL

Learning how to fall correctly is the most difficult obstacle to conquer when you start recognizing that running is a skill. Although using the forces of gravity to help you move is easy enough to comprehend, your instincts tell you differently. Falling while you shift supports just doesn't click when first learning the skill. In order to rewire your brain and develop the correct instinctive reaction, you must spend time drilling techniques such as the ones demonstrated below. Not only will they instill the correct falling mechanics, they'll also test your reaction.

To perform the following drills correctly, have your partner support your body in a slight lean as you shift supports and run in place. Without telling you, your partner will let go of your hips (Sequence A) or quickly step outside your running path (Sequence B). This will generate one of two reactions. Either you will instinctively step out in front of your body to catch your fall, or you will continue to shift supports and progress forward using the correct running mechanics. If you experience the former, you should start over and repeat the drill until you can carry out the exercise without doing so. If you experience the latter, congratulations, you've successfully reverse-engineered the "I'm going to fall flat on my face if I don't put something out in front of me" instinct.

Key Points:

☐ The focus of this drill is to take your partner by surprise, so if you're supporting his weight, don't present a "tell" that signifies your release of pressure.

☐ Lean forward only slightly, just enough to initiate movement. If you lean too far forward, not only is it difficult for your partner to keep you upright, but it also makes it difficult to shift supports fast enough.

Common Faults:

☐ Breaking in any fashion, pushing off the ground, or stepping out in front of the body to stop your fall.

☐ Avoid an exaggerated lean. Remember, the farther you lean, the faster you have to shift supports.

The Dose:

If you're having trouble with the fall, meaning you instinctively step out in front of your body to counterbalance your weight, you should perform this drill as often as possible, or until you successfully reverse engineer that instinct. If you're already proficient with the fall, executing this drill from time to time to test your reactions is recommended.

Sequence A: Partner Falling Drill with Rear Stabilization

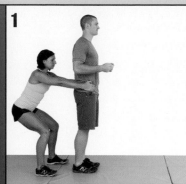

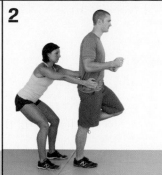

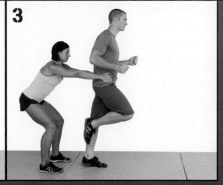

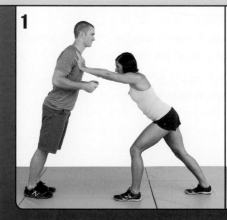

1. Glen is in his running stance with a slight forward lean. Katie is holding his hips to prevent him from falling forward.

2. Glen begins running in place by pulling his left foot up.

3. Glen alternates his feet by shifting supports.

4. Without saying anything, Katie releases her grip on Glen's hips and he accelerates forward using correct running mechanics.

Sequence B: Partner Falling Drill with Front Stabilization

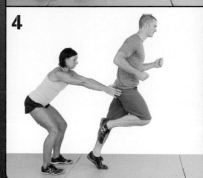

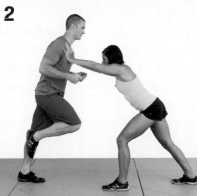

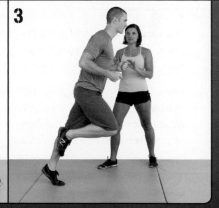

1. Glen is in his running stance with a slight forward lean. Katie is holding his hips to prevent him from falling forward.

2. Glen begins running in place.

3. Without telling him, Katie quickly steps out of his path and he accelerates forward using correct running mechanics.

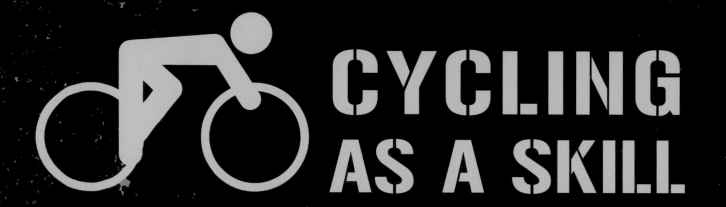

CYCLING AS A SKILL

BY DOUG KATONA

"CROSSFIT ENDURANCE DELIVERS THE BEST OF BOTH STRENGTH AND ENDURANCE."

MICHAEL MYSER
FREELANCE WRITER

TABLE OF CONTENTS

ACKNOWLEDGMENTS

First and foremost, I need to thank my parents for raising and putting up with me. It took about twenty-five years for me to finally clue in to the passion that currently drives me, but it began with you two. Thanks also to my brother and sister for putting up with their big brother and helping me remain the kid I still am at times.

A huge acknowledgment goes out to all the coaches, trainers, and athletes I got to experiment with early on. Genetic Potential, the original experiment—we tested everything under the roof, were told it would never work, and proved otherwise.

Thank you to my mentor and colleague Dr. Nicolas Romanov. You changed the way I think about endurance and running over a decade ago, and you continue to inspire me to this day.

Not a day goes by that I don't thank Greg Glassman. It's the platform you built and allowed us to thrive on that has made this such a great place to be, brother. Dave Castro, most don't understand, thanks for your continued support and for doing what you do.

Thanks to Kelly Starrett (best friend Number 1, J-Star), for co-labeling this world we are in together. I could never have written this book without you.

Thanks to all the coaches within CFE—this is your book as much as mine. Fact.

Thank you to my partner and friend Doug Katona. I could never have done any of this without you, brother. I'm so happy you are here.

A huge thanks to the entire CFE crew: Kaitlin, Eli, and every AC and intern.

Thanks so much to every single person who has attended a CFE seminar.

Thank you to the countless athletes who have shared their training experiences and communicated the pros and cons of the program—every runner, triathlete, CrossFit athlete, and rower. Because of all of you, I continue to learn more every single day.

I know there is someone I forgot to thank because there are so many people who not only helped me complete this book, but also contributed to everything that allowed it to come into being—the seminars, competitions, training partners, etc. None of this would be possible without our combined experience. So thank you!

FOREWORD by T.J. Murphy

When I first began my reporting for a *Triathlete* magazine profile on Brian MacKenzie, I was quick to come in contact with the fact that he was a polarizing figure. On one hand you had the Letsrun.com and Slowtwitch.com crowds raging against him, suggesting that he was an Antichrist, tempting athletes with a gimmicky shortcut to performance that could never possibly work. On the other hand you had an impassioned throng of athletes raving about CrossFit Endurance and about how they were achieving personal records while training only a fraction of the time they used to train.

At the heart of the debate (actually more like a bar fight) is an age-old controversy from the depths of the running world centered on the value (productive or destructive, depending on where you stand) of high-mileage training. The argument has a religious intensity to it, and in years past you would have found me a vociferous proponent of high volume.

I had my reasons. Like most supporters of the high-mileage ethic, the greatest long-distance runners have relied on it. Consistently netting 100 plus miles per week was a signal that you were inarguably serious about running, because that's the way the serious runners trained.

There's no debating the fact that high-mileage training is effective. And what initially ticked me off when I watched CrossFit.com videos was that they discounted "LSD"—long, slow distance—training and attacked traditional methods of running and triathlon training. If you accept that high-mileage, base-strength-speed training plans are all rooted in the thinking and coaching of Arthur Lydiard (1917-2004), then you know that his plan is not based on slow running: it's not a jog-a-thon by any measure. Lydiard's training plan is demanding and rigorous and requires plenty of fast running. If you look at modern representations of Lydiard's work, like that of Joe Vigil—the great Adams State College cross-country coach and one of the most highly respected running coaches in the world—the long- and medium-length recovery runs are expected to get faster and faster as a season develops. Interval and tempo days are ferociously difficult, and in the past, before his retirement, Vigil held his primary camps (in Alamosa, Colorado, and Mammoth Lakes, California) at altitudes well above 7,000 feet. The image of runners being in some sort of blissful Zen state of mind, just taking in the scenery as they loped along at a gentle 8-minute or slower pace, was an insult. So any implication that LSD-type training programs were a lounge in the hammock really pissed off runners, including me.

The emotional connection to any training program is typically tied to some personal success with that program. This was definitely true for me. I got the running bug in 1988 and used a very basic Lydiard training model to run my first marathon in 3:24. Runs longer than 20 miles, steady daily mileage, tempo runs, long intervals, and hill training were all part of the mix. By simply being very consistent with the training and upping my overall mileage, my time dropped to 2:38:47 when I ran the Cal International Marathon in 1991. That is part of the reason I became such a fierce advocate of high-mileage training very early in my career as a distance runner. High mileage became a religion.

As I upped my goals, I upped my mileage. At one point, I was running 90 to 100 miles a week with a 22- to 24-miler on Sundays and a 16-miler on Fridays. The schedule also included two hard 10-mile runs. Again, there was little doubt that my speed was improving. The 10-milers dropped below a 6-minute pace, the long runs below a 7-minute pace. I remember how excited I was to see what I could do in races.

But that's when things started falling apart. Hamstrings, tendons, nerves—everything became vulnerable to injury. I saw physical therapists and chiropractors, I did every "core" or "functional" exercise asked of me, I lifted weights—yet the injuries kept coming and kept getting worse.

When I'd finally had it, like a number of runners before me, I left pure running for triathlon. And while I managed to participate in the sport for 10 years, it was obvious to me that I was somehow compromised in a fundamental way. I was surviving races, but I was slow. I was always just barely getting through training sessions and ironmans. Pain and discomfort of a sinister variety poisoned my love for training. Acute back, knee, and neck pain had become part of not just my training but also my everyday life. I accepted this decline as the simple fact of being an aging endurance athlete.

The three years leading up to my writing about MacKenzie were particularly awful. In addition to waking up each morning feeling like I'd just played noseguard in a Monday Night Football game, my injuries prevented me from training in any meaningful way and I began to put on weight. From late 2009 through October 2010, I sucked up everything I could and forced myself to follow an online running program targeted toward a half-marathon. I ran over and through all aches, pains, and injuries, netting 50 to 60 miles most weeks. In late October 2010, I gingerly raced the half-marathon, crossed the finish line in a disappointing 1:38, and was forced to promptly sit on a curb because my knees were screaming with pain. Two weeks later my right knee shut down in a way I'd never experienced before. This happened to be about the time I first met MacKenzie when he was delivering a CrossFit Endurance certification program in San Diego. As much as I may have initially criticized his (or any other) high-quality, low-volume training program, I finally looked in the mirror and questioned why I wasn't even giving the likes of MacKenzie a chance to make their case.

And when I started listening to what he had to say, I had to admit that, as unorthodox as the approach sounded to me, he made a logical case for CrossFit Endurance. The first piece of advice I took from him was a basic lesson on humility, and I let go of my ego long enough to dig deeper into what he was saying. When I did that, I felt a wonderful sense of freedom and had a simple realization: What the hell did I have to lose? I decided that rather than rant about something I'd never tried, I would give CrossFit Endurance a trial run.

I was so beat to hell that my transition to being an athlete who could fully embrace the CrossFit Endurance program took time. In fact, the way I see it, I still have a ways to go.

But that said, there's no denying that I have gone through a shockingly successful transformation. I can run again, without pain, in a way I haven't been able to run for years. My strength, power, mobility, and stamina are at levels I don't believe I've enjoyed since I was a two-sport high school athlete 30 years ago. While I don't have precise records to prove my case, I'm certain that I'm stronger and more balanced in many ways than when I was 17. When it comes to CrossFit Endurance and supplanting standard aerobic or recovery runs with CrossFit strength training and metabolic conditioning, I can't speak for everyone, of course, but I can speak for myself: I would never go back to the way I used to train. And if I could be a 28-year-old marathoner again—I was 28 when I ran a 2:38—I would use CrossFit Endurance as my training program. Many distance runners—and I once fell blindly into this camp—are far too willing to sacrifice overall health for a performance goal. It's odd that we haven't considered the possibility that health and performance work in concert. And if someone said to me, "But, hey, wasn't it worth taking a beating so that you could run that 2:38?" I'd reply in two ways: One, I now believe I could have achieved that time without enduring the musculoskeletal destruction I did, and two, at the Cal International Marathon in 1991, when I ran 2:38, did I win? Or come in second or third? Not quite. I finished in 81st place. Is finishing 81st in anything worth destroying your health over?

I'm not going to say that Brian MacKenzie has the only answer, or all the answers, or that anyone has all the answers. But MacKenzie is important to listen to. Not only has following his lead changed my life as an athlete, but he's also one of the few coaches I've met who puts everything into it for all the right reasons. The amount of passion, intelligence, and raw, 24/7 effort that he applies to his program and to his athletes is awe-inspiring.

Plus, he has the courage to look at the conventional training wisdom and question it. Like other great coaches—including Lydiard, as a matter of fact—he tests his ideas on himself and then on his athletes. He

also considers every possible ancillary contribution to health and performance and wraps it tightly into his program when it's appropriate.

Does this mean that I have somehow rejected high-mileage training as a pathway to running greatness? Not at all. We know that high-mileage works. But I think it's fair to ask if it works for everyone all of the time and also to ask if the long-term damage incurred by high-mileage training is worth the short-term performance benefits.

And in asking those questions, I would encourage all runners and triathletes—whether novices or veterans—to consider the concepts and principles that MacKenzie discusses in this book. Adopting some or all of them just may lead to improved performance, and I'm convinced that they will lead to better health and greater longevity as an athlete.

T.J. Murphy

Editorial Director

Competitor

Triathlete

Velo

Inside Triathlon

PREFACE

In ten plus years as an athlete and coach, I have seen every type of training fad known to the endurance-sports world, implemented many of these fads in my own training, and experimented with them on the athletes I've coached. Through much trial and error, I have found most of them, while seemingly rooted in good science, to be missing a crucial "something." But when I met Dr. Nicholas Romanov and "Coach" Greg Glassman, everything fell into place. And that's how *Power, Speed, Endurance* came about. Throughout this book, you will see why the Pose Method, devised by Romanov, and how CrossFit, founded by Greg Glassman, so profoundly influenced my own training methods and how the synergy of these coaches, my experience, and many other professional athletes and trainers went into the creation of CrossFit Endurance, which is explained herein.

While founded on hard data compiled over years of keen observation and scientific process, this book is meant to be a manual to make you a better athlete or trainer, not turn you into a science nerd. But don't underestimate the power of your own observations and intuition. Don't take my methods as gospel. Try them on and measure the advantages. I'm sure that you will experience fewer injuries and fewer endurance-training frustrations and reach new performance highs—because why else would I have bothered to write this book?

INTRODUCTION

A Paradigm Shift

When I first started coaching endurance athletes and competing in endurance events back in 2001, my training and coaching protocol was fairly straightforward. I followed a typical long, slow distance (LSD) endurance periodization program—increasing time and distance by 10 percent a week for three weeks, decreasing by 15 percent for the last week, and then repeating. It was all about volume, volume, and more volume. How many miles could I (and my clients) rack up in a day, week, month, year? The program seemed to make perfect sense: If you wanted to be fast over a long distance, you had to perform long workouts to simulate that goal. It had worked for a lot of endurance athletes in the past, but I started to notice certain holes in the method and began to wonder: Is this the most efficient way to train for endurance sports?

The vast majority of athletes measure their fitness according to three factors: how they feel, how they look, and, most important, how they perform. When I started competing, I felt good, experienced a steady increase in my aerobic capacity, and although I lost some weight from poor eating habits and the lack of strength training, I looked reasonably healthy and in shape. The same could be said about the endurance athletes I was coaching. We were all experiencing some positive results in that we continued to build our stamina, but it ultimately came at a cost.

This went on for a few years, as I competed in ultra marathons, triathlons, ironmans, and the like. I performed well, but the training volume started to wreak havoc on my body. While I was training for Ironman Canada in 2004, I developed plantar fasciitis as well as a plethora of other injuries. Put simply, my body went on strike. I was overtrained, losing muscle mass, constantly in pain, chronically fatigued, and worse still, I was bored to death with the time-consuming training.

As I started to reevaluate my situation, I was forced to ask some very important questions: What was my purpose in training/coaching? And why was I adhering to the LSD program?

The answer to the first question was quite simple: I wanted to continue to enjoy the sport that I loved and provide clients with the most efficient training program in existence so that they could continue to make performance gains while living a long and healthy life without injury. To answer the second question, I first have to break down the LSD training protocol, which looks like this:

- ☐ **Volume** relates to the distance or the amount of work that you're putting into a given training session or routine. For the majority of endurance athletes following the traditional model, this makes up 80 percent of their training.

- ☐ **Intensity** refers to the amount of force or power you have to exert in order to achieve a desired goal—how much work do you have to do? Because an endurance athlete has to be fast over long distances (or any set distance for that matter), intensity is almost always defined as an effort above 70 to 80 percent. Training above 80 percent, in the form of intervals or tempos, accounts for roughly 20 percent of the traditional LSD program.

☐ **Skill (Technique)** addresses efficiency of movement. This aspect of training is rarely if ever addressed in the traditional LSD model. Rather than breaking down the actual mechanics of the movement and learning to be more efficient through drills, repetition becomes your body's teacher, regardless of what that repetition is teaching you!

So the general M.O. of LSD training is to log as many miles as possible, throw in a sprint interval and a strength-and-conditioning or "core" session every so often (or in phases), and acquire skill through ad nauseam repetition. Although long training sessions at low intensity made sense to me from a sport-specific standpoint, avoiding high intensity and drills that focus on building technique didn't. After all, almost every other sport reverses the traditional endurance structure, putting technique at the top of the list, gradually increasing the intensity of the workouts to enable an adaptive response, and once that skill is performed at high intensity without fault, volume is added in the form of distance or repetition.

So why were endurance athletes going against the grain? Were we all so caught up in running, riding, and swimming long that we forgot about being efficient?

Although I already knew how important running technique was, I realized that I was on to something, so I replaced the long, slow distance efforts with lower volume training in the form of interval and tempo workouts. I tested new diets and started implementing power lifts such as squats and dead lifts—which had been introduced to me by my father at a young age—as well as functional movements such as kettlebell exercises and some basic gymnastics, with great results. This new approach opened my eyes to just how far my body had regressed.

When I trained with my father in the 1990s, I could squat more than 300 pounds and had perfect range of motion. Now, as an endurance athlete, I couldn't squat half that weight or drop my hips below my knee crease without compromising form. I thought, *Here I am in the prime of my life and I can barely squat my own body weight—what the hell have I done to myself?*

Everything I did, prior to stepping outside the traditional endurance box, was solely aerobic in nature. I had, like a lot of endurance athletes, assumed that anaerobic training (speed work, sprint intervals) and functional lifts didn't matter. But based on the results I was getting, I knew that there was more to what I was doing. I refined my purpose: my goal was to find a system that worked with the realities of life; that could be accomplished without compromising a marriage or time spent with family; something that wouldn't leave you broken and fatigued to the point of depression; a training method that allowed for continual growth as opposed to gradual decline. Not only for myself, but also (and more importantly) for the athletes I was coaching.

I continued to experiment with new training methods, but I struggled to find a perfect balance between developing strength without putting on too much muscle mass and still maintaining stamina and reducing breakdown. Then I was reintroduced to a coach that would help refine my approach to endurance training: Dr. Nicholas Romanov. A world-renowned Olympic coach, author (*Pose Method of Running, Pose Method of Triathlon Techniques*), educator, and sports scientist, Dr. Romanov developed and successfully implemented the Pose Method, which seeks to correct technique and improve movement efficiency.

This was not my first exposure to Dr. Romanov. In 2001 a friend took me to one of his Pose Method of Running seminars. At the time, I didn't realize the potential of his entire system, but I did begin to see running through a new lens. While I did embrace his Pose Method and saw the benefit of implementing and coaching athletes in proper running form, I didn't pay too much attention to his programming methodology or other training practices.

The second time I met Romanov, I asked him to mentor me. In addition to shedding more light on the Pose Method for running, cycling, and swimming, Romanov taught me how to identify weaknesses in an athlete's profile and develop a program to correct such weaknesses, and he taught me methods to determine what an athlete is capable of on any given day; how to program for specific goals; and the importance of recovery protocol before, during, and after training (or a race). It didn't take long before my training overhaul started to reap dramatic results. In only a few months, I became stronger, recovered faster, and had more stamina than ever. Not only that, but with all the four-hour, steady-paced runs and long bike rides hacked from my training schedule, I had more time than I knew what to do with. I started using the same strategy with the athletes I was coaching, and they got similar results. While I knew in my heart that this was a more efficient path, I was nevertheless astonished at how quickly everything improved. I couldn't help asking myself, *Why isn't everybody doing this?* As I would later find out, this program is not for everyone.

I studied with Romanov for several years—eventually earning my Level 5 Pose certification—learning the Pose Method for swim, bike, and run and the art of programming for endurance sports. During this time, I experienced a complete paradigm shift in the way I thought about endurance sports. As it turned out, my original intuition, which questioned the traditional model, was spot on. The keys to implementing an effective endurance program were: First, master the skill of the movement to improve movement efficiency; second, slowly add higher intensity workouts to build strength and test the limitations of your technique; then, once you can maintain technique with intensity, add volume.

Enter CrossFit

Although my work with Romanov was enlightening, I still hadn't found that perfect blend of functional strength and conditioning and anaerobic/aerobic sport-specific training I was searching for. I knew there was something I needed to add to the program, but I couldn't quite put my finger on it. CrossFit, as it would turn out, was the missing link.

Created by Greg Glassman, CrossFit is a highly effective strength-and-conditioning system that utilizes functional movements such as power lifts, Olympic lifts, and gymnastics, and then blends them into a constantly varied format. It is defined as "constantly varied functional movement executed at high intensity," and the goal is to improve fitness by "increasing work capacity across broad time and modal domains."

CrossFit defied the conventional strength and conditioning paradigm, which was based on isolated movements (bicep curls, triceps extensions, and leg presses) and structured periodization programs. CrossFit was designed to build an all-around athlete who didn't break down, yet still had the stamina to be competitive at a high level. A fit athlete, as Glassman put it, is competent in all general physical skills, meaning that he or she not only has stamina, but is also strong, fast, agile, coordinated, and flexible. With this base, you can add in sport-specific training for anything from running a marathon to fighting in the cage.

CrossFit was close to Romanov's approach in that its goal was to create a more efficient and well-rounded athlete. But CrossFit incorporated strength-and-conditioning workouts and a training methodology that was suitable for people of all ages and ability levels. After delving into CrossFit, I became convinced that it was the best model for tackling the strength-and-conditioning component of training, which was where most endurance athletes were deficient. It trained athletes in all metabolic pathways. If there was a weakness in the athlete's profile, CrossFit exposed it. If you replaced the slow/medium efforts with short and long intervals and CrossFit, I thought, you would create a bulletproof athlete. I put the theory to the test by competing in an ultra marathon with only 10 hours a week of training. In addition to finishing the race uninjured, I bested my previous ultra time. Having laid a foundation for a new way of training, I began to implement the system with my clients, and had similar results.

Putting what I learned from Romanov and Glassman together with my personal experience and knowledge of endurance athletics, I developed a system that maximized time and optimized performance gains without sacrificing stamina. The focus was on skill acquisition, smart programming, constant variance, functional movements, and sport-specific training executed at high intensity. CrossFit Endurance was born.

CrossFit Endurance: Understanding the Model

The goal of the CrossFit Endurance (CFE) program is twofold: 1) to allow you to have a life by cutting down the hours you spend training—quality versus quantity; and 2) to accelerate your performance gains in endurance sports without the long, steady-state workouts that can beat your body into submission. In other words, we want you to spend more time on technique, reduce your aerobic workouts, and develop all 10 general physical skills through constantly varied programming. When the CFE program is followed correctly, you not only reduce your susceptibility to injury, move more efficiently, and recover quicker, but you also look, feel, and perform better.

To better understand the CFE system and programming methodology let's revisit the definition of CrossFit: Constantly varied functional movement executed at high intensity.

- In CFE, however, functional movement is replaced with a sport-specific activity, such as a run, bike, swim, or row.

- Thus, CFE is defined as: Constantly varied *sport-specific movement* executed at high intensity.

- Just as CrossFit seeks to find a balance among metabolic conditioning, gymnastics, and weightlifting, CFE is a delicate dance between CrossFit and running, cycling, and swimming (or whatever endurance sport you are focusing on). Let's backtrack a little bit and compare LSD training and CFE.

LSD	CFE
1. Volume	1. Skills and Drills (Technique)
2. Intensity	2. Intensity
3. Skill	3. Stamina (Volume)

Skills and Drills

As I've already mentioned, learning correct technique—whether you're lifting, running, cycling, or swimming—is critical to not only preventing injury, but also maximizing performance. If you don't spend time drilling the various layers of the technique, you will never obtain mastery of the movement. For example, if you learn how to position yourself correctly on a road bike, but fail to develop proper pedaling technique, the integrity of your position will be compromised by your dysfunctional movement pattern. It doesn't matter if you're following the traditional LSD program or the CFE program, your body will fall apart and you will get injured.

CrossFit's General Physical Skills

In October 2002, Glassman wrote an article in CrossFit Journal titled "What Is Fitness?" which helped define the logic as well as lay the foundation for CrossFit's approach. Glassman included CrossFit's 10 general physical skills—compiled by Jim Cawley, the inventor of the Dynamax medicine ball—which are essential to maximize training and performance.

1. **Cardiovascular/respiratory endurance**—The ability of body systems to gather, process, and deliver oxygen.

2. **Stamina**—The ability of body systems to process, deliver, store, and utilize energy.

3. **Strength**—The ability of a muscular unit, or combination of muscular units, to apply force.

4. **Flexibility**—The ability to maximize the range of motion in a given joint.

5. **Power**—The ability of a muscular unit, or combination of muscular units, to apply maximum force in minimum time.

6. **Speed**—The ability to minimize the time cycle of a repeated movement.

7. **Coordination**—The ability to combine several distinct movement patterns into a singular distinct movement.

8. **Agility**—The ability to minimize transition time from one movement pattern to another.

9. **Balance**—The ability to control the placement of the body's center of gravity in relation to its support base.

10. **Accuracy**—The ability to control movement in a given direction or at a given intensity.

Source: http://library.crossfit.com/free/pdf/CFJ-trial.pdf

Intensity

Intensity comprises sport-specific interval training, which is based on a work-to-rest ratio; tempo training, which is a steady-state effort; as well as CrossFit strength-and-conditioning workouts of the day (WODs). This builds metabolic conditioning, improving endurance across an open plane, meaning not only in your sport of choice, but for all other activities—whether it's playing basketball with friends or snowboarding.

It's important to point out that the moment your skill is compromised by the intensity of your effort, that is an indication that you need to dial it back. For example, if you're unable to run 400-meter sprint intervals without crumbling to pieces afterward, you need to either reduce your distance or the amount of your intervals. Conversely, if you can perform a specific workout effortlessly or run an interval without your lungs burning, that might mean that you need to increase the intensity of your effort. It could also mean that you need to increase the distance of your interval or the number of intervals you perform over a given distance.

Volume

Stamina replaces long, slow distance. Volume is the amount of work you do in a given training schedule. For instance, the goal of the CFE program is to implement three to four CFE workouts a week (ideally, but not necessarily for everyone), either in the form of a CrossFit WOD or CFE strength-bias WOD, coupled with three to four sport-specific training sessions, either intervals or tempos. Unlike the conventional paradigm that prescribes running at low intensity, the majority of our stamina work is done at 80 percent effort or above. So instead of running 20 miles on a Sunday, most athletes will run a 10-mile time trial or a series of eight 100-meter intervals. The interval workout accomplishes everything you would by jogging 20 miles but doesn't put the same level of stress and damage on the body.

Volume also entails long-distance efforts, which is another way to build stamina. This is where the CFE program is often misunderstood. Although I've made a strong case against LSD efforts, I've never said, nor will I ever say, that you should *never* run, ride, or swim long. If you're training for endurance you do need some kind of stamina work or intervals that last more than 70 seconds to dial in technique, adjust rhythm, and formulate pace strategy. But in order to accelerate performance gains, you need to keep this kind of training to a minimum and prioritize skill work and intensity over long, slow distance efforts.

Remember, volume, like everything, is individualized. For example, a long-distance effort could be, although it is extremely rare, as long as 20 miles. Regardless of how smart you train or organize your life, your genetic potential will allow you to put in only a specific amount of work before your training is negatively impacted. To ensure continual improvement, long-distance efforts have to be incorporated into your program in a way that doesn't compromise your technique, instill dysfunctional movement patterns, or leave you unable to recover for your next training session. This is the art of knowing your body and understanding what you can and can't handle under this training paradigm.

Lydiard's Model

For years, the long, slow distance approach to endurance has dominated the minds and training practices of athletes and coaches worldwide. Originally made popular by New Zealander Arthur Lydiard—a self-trained endurance runner who meticulously experimented on himself and fellow endurance athletes back in the 1940s—LSD, which is based on high-volume periodized training, has proved to be an incredibly effective training model for competitive and recreational endurance athletes alike. In fact, Lydiard used his periodization program, which is based on successive phases of specified training aimed at peaking an athlete for a race or series of races, to train a number of world-class endurance athletes, including Peter Snell, three-time Olympic gold medalist in track. The phases of training are generally defined for a runner as follows:

- ☐ **The Base Phase:** The focus is on building an endurance base in the form of long, slow, easy runs. The goal is no less than 100 miles per week.

- ☐ **The Strength Phase:** Anaerobic interval base training in the form of hill runs and sprints.

- ☐ **The Speed/Race Phase:** Anaerobic work and volume are tapered so that you can peak for a race or series of races.

Although Lydiard stressed and advocated the implementation of anaerobic work, much of this is lost on the typical endurance athlete. Instead, the notion of accumulating 100 miles or more each week, which is a requirement during the base phase, infects the minds of most endurance runners. This dogma has created a deep connection between success and high-mileage, low-intensity training in the endurance community.

What Is Endurance?

Endurance is defined as the ability to exert energy over a prolonged period of time or distance. Most of us have been led to believe that to improve endurance all you have to do is perform a specific task until you achieve your goal. For example, say you want to improve endurance as well as overall fitness. Some people who subscribe to the LSD (aerobic) training philosophy would say that all you need to do is run: it doesn't matter if you run at low intensity; as long as you run often and for a long time, you'll experience improvement across your entire athletic profile.

If you're sedentary, going out and simply running slow and long will definitely elicit an adaptive response, which is necessary to improve fitness, specifically endurance. However, at some point you are going to adapt to the stress of long, slow distance efforts and ultimately plateau performance-wise.

If you're a competitive endurance athlete who trains often, you may not see any improvements at all. In such a situation, you have to increase the intensity of your efforts and adopt a training program that involves shorter high-intensity intervals, such as sprints, to challenge your body's natural adaptation response. In other words, if you don't cause a disruption of oxygen homeostasis (get winded and feel your muscles burn), you're never going to get stronger, faster, or build stamina beyond your aerobic base, which adds credibility to Lydiard's second phase.

Let's use a simple example to help make this easier to understand and shed more light on the flaws of steady-state training. Take an inactive individual who struggles to run a mile without stopping. If you told him to run one mile consistently, he would (over time) undoubtedly get positive results as it relates to his fitness base. But how long do you think it would take until running that same mile at a slow pace is no longer a challenge? Although it depends on the individual, it probably wouldn't take very long. In such a case, the conventional theory would advise keeping intensity low and increasing distance to keep improving fitness rather than running that same mile at a faster pace: you would increase the distance to two miles, and then three, and then four, and so on, until you reach your target distance or until a foundation in endurance is built.

The important question is, *At what point does the scale get tipped from improving endurance and aerobic capacity to compromising recovery and even inviting injury?*

Again, it depends on the individual, but for the majority, running longer than 10K is not going to yield the benefits that sport-specific interval training and a well-rounded strength-and-conditioning program can provide. Running long is just not the most efficient way to improve endurance and become a better athlete. At a certain point, running more, riding more, or swimming more is not going to do anything but put unnecessary stress on your body. What are you doing it for? To get faster? Build lean muscle? Lose weight? Build cardiovascular fitness?

The LSD model is fundamentally flawed in this regard because it doesn't cater to a wide range of goals. Not only that, if you continue to train slow, you're going to race slow. As a result, the protocol doesn't develop speed, power, coordination, strength, agility, and mobility in athletes. Moreover, athletes whose training bible is LSD tend to have less lean muscle mass, acquire poor motor patterns, suffer from fatigue throughout the day, be more prone to injury, and have short life spans in their sport. In other words, it's a high-risk, low-reward model.

We are not one-dimensional creatures. While we're capable of sustaining efforts for long periods of time, we're also designed to lift, climb, sprint, carry, and jump. In order to express our true nature and maximize endurance gains, we must also develop all of these other attributes. As I already stated, I'm not saying there's no place for long, slow distance training. For some of you, going out for long runs or rides is an escape from the daily grind; it's your form of meditation and is required to maintain sanity. Moreover, if you're training for a marathon or your goal is to sustain a pace for a prolonged period of time (two or more hours), incorporating long, slow distance runs into your training program periodically is not a bad idea. In fact, it's something that is built into the CrossFit Endurance program. But you have to understand that it comes at a cost. The repeated volume is inevitably going to break your body down. To realize your potential and avoid injury, you have to look at how your body adapts to your training.

ANAEROBIC AND AEROBIC ENERGY SYSTEMS

Anaerobic Energy Systems: The rapid and immediate breakdown of nutrients to form ATP for energy without the use of oxygen. Examples: lifting weight, a 100-meter sprint.

Phosphagen System (ATP-CP): To replenish ATP levels quickly, muscle cells contain a high-energy phosphate compound called creatine phosphate (CP). The phosphate group is removed from creatine phosphate by an enzyme called creatine kinase and is transferred to andenosine diphosphate (ADP) to form ATP. The cell turns ATP into ADP, and the phosphagen rapidly turns the ADP back into ATP. As the muscle continues to work, creatine phosphate levels begin to decrease. The phosphagen system supplies the energy needs of working muscle at a high rate, but only for up to 10 seconds. For any exertion longer, the body must tap into the glycolytic, lactate, or aerobic system to generate ATP for energy.

Glycolytic System: Glycolysis is the process by which carbohydrate (sugar or glucose) is broken down to form ATP without the use of oxygen, which is then converted to energy.

Lactate Shuttle: As creatine phosphate runs out, the body uses stored glucose and glycogen for ATP. The process is still anaerobic because there isn't enough oxygen to break down pyruvate (the enzyme used to break down glucose), producing lactate. Lactate then enters muscle cells, and blood, and the lactate is either broken down into immediate fuel (ATP) or used in the creation of glycogen.

Aerobic System: The aerobic system can use carbohydrate and fat as fuel. Using carbohydrates produces 36ATP per molecule. Beta oxidation, or oxidation of fats, yields approximately three times this amount. Beta oxidation can be thought of as the overdrive of energy systems. It takes a long time to get there, and once there, the body settles in for a long trip. Examples: prolonged walk, run, bike, or swim.

In Summary: The phosphagen system uses CP to convert energy into ATP. The glycolytic system converts glucose into ATP. The lactate shuttle system breaks down lactate into ATP, and beta oxidation breaks down fat into ATP.

You could look at it this way:

☐ Fast glycolysis uses CHO and creates lactic acid as a byproduct.

☐ Slow glycolysis can use CHO or fat as fuel.

☐ It takes a longer duration (30 plus minutes just to start this system) and a lower intensity to burn fat as a primary energy source—one of the main detriments of the LSD paradigm.

The objective of any training program is to develop energy-production systems so you can meet the demands of your sport. The fundamental weakness with the LSD training model is that it targets only one energy-production system (aerobic). In order to perform well in endurance activities, you have to train across all energy systems, not just one. But before I explain why, it's important for you to understand how these pathways work.

The Energy Pathways

To perform any movement, your body must use nutrients from food—carbohydrate, fat, and protein—to create energy in the form Adenosine-triphosphate (ATP).

☐ **Carbohydrate** provides fuel for moderate- to high-intensity exercise (sprints, CrossFit WODs).

☐ **Fat** provides fuel for low-intensity exercise (walking, long runs).

☐ **Protein** can be used as fuel (protein is converted to glucose via gluconeogenesis), but functions primarily to repair, maintain, and help facilitate growth of the body's tissue.

Put in simple terms, ATP converts these vital nutrients (carbohydrate, fat, and protein) into usable energy. The body isn't great at storing ATP for more than a few seconds, so you have to continually create ATP in order to keep your muscles firing. However, you will pretty much do this as long as you focus on your sport of choice—by doing either high-intensity (anaerobic) efforts less than two minutes in duration (weightlifting, sprints), which promotes strength, speed, and power, and stamina, or low-intensity efforts (walking or jogging), which promote endurance. Depending on the intensity and duration of the exercise, you will tap into the anaerobic system, aerobic system, or both.

To keep improving in your sport, you want to develop energy systems that support, rather than impede, performance. Say you're a competitive Olympic weightlifter. Your only goal is to lift a heavy load from the ground to overhead (or to your shoulders if you're isolating a clean) in one explosive movement. Because each movement lasts less than a few seconds, you're favoring the phosphagen energy system.

So do you think that running 400-meter sprints would help increase your one rep max? Not likely! Remember, you're really training only within those narrow parameters, meaning that you need to be using only the phosphagen system for your energy needs. If you introduce workouts that use other systems, you compromise your ability to perform the sport-specific task of performing one explosive movement. The training principle of specificity states that your body adapts to the stress and stimulus you throw at it. So if you start throwing long-duration workouts into your training mix, when what you need is strength and power, you can say goodbye to winning the gold in Olympic lifting.

If your goal is to run, ride, and swim long, on the other hand, then it makes sense to run, ride, and swim for long distances every time you train. Assuming that you run, ride, or swim using correct technique, LSD or aerobic training effectively improves endurance. However, unlike Olympic weightlifting, which typically targets only one energy pathway (phosphagen), endurance activities utilize anaerobic and aerobic energy systems.

Endurance is not just about long, slow distance efforts; it's about the breakdown of tissue and the ability to maintain an efficient position for extended periods of time. By isolating the aerobic system, you ignore the development of other quintessential attributes, such as strength, speed, and power, which are critical in preventing the breakdown of tissue. All of us break down at a certain point (some faster than others), regardless of volume, intensity, or load. The key is to slow that process, maintain the ability to explode when necessary—whether you're trying to close a gap between you and another racer or sprint to the finish line—and, most important, not to lose form once fatigue sets in.

The only way to accomplish that is to: 1) master technique by putting skills and drills at the forefront of your training, 2) incorporate high-intensity workouts in the form of CrossFit or CFE to develop strength, speed, and power, and 3) continue to train your aerobic system in the form of long-distance workouts, but not to the point where it compromises your form or recovery.

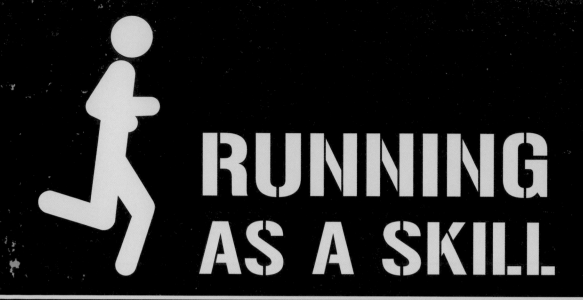

RUNNING AS A SKILL

"NOTHING WILL UNRAVEL AN ATHLETE FASTER THAN FATIGUE OR FEAR OF FATIGUE"

TONY BLAUER,

FOUNDER & CEO OF BLAUER TACTICAL SYSTEMS

S.P.E.A.R SYSTEM, & HIGH GEAR

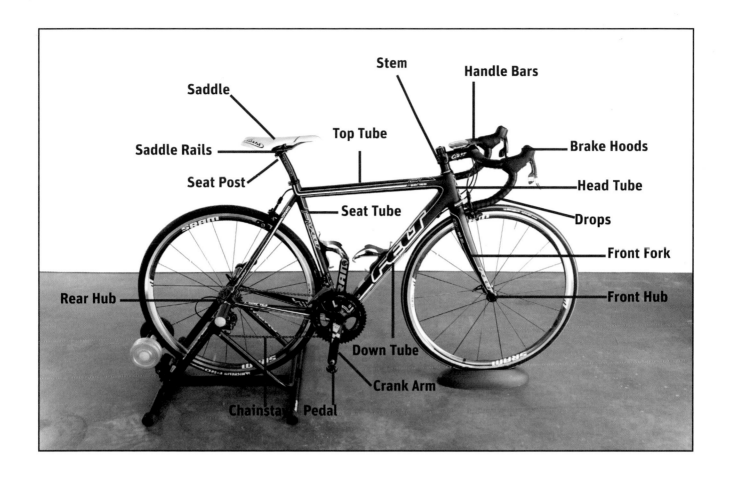

The bicycle is a wondrously complex yet elegant human-powered machine that serves a variety of functions. As a result, the bicycle means different things to different people. For some, it is merely a low-cost, efficient means of transportation. For others, the bicycle represents a tool used for recreational fitness. For a child, a bike might be a right of passage and a means to gain independence. For us, the bike is all of this and more. It represents freedom, transportation, and fitness, and above all, the bike is the link to the crucible of competition, where what we strive for as athletes is laid bare—determination, heart, the will to succeed.

When you think of cycling today, you probably picture lightweight, body-friendly, ergonomic bicycles made from space-age materials forged in wind tunnels. It wasn't always this way.

Early bicycles had vaguely insect like names (the velocipede) or slightly off-putting ones (the Boneshaker). Like the first automobiles, early bikes weighed a ton, were constructed of heavy-gauge steel, were difficult to pilot, and were dangerous. Although the fundamental geometry and appearance of the road bike has not been significantly altered since its inception in the 1800s, modern technology has produced a far superior machine. The bicycle has graduated from steel to titanium, and thence to aluminum to carbon fiber, and surely yet more ingenious composites will be discovered on alien worlds. The purpose of all this advancement isn't purely manufacturer's one-upmanship, but a quest to deliver the most efficient, most powerful, and fastest machine without entirely sacrificing comfort.

While advances in technology continue to improve the bicycle, its unique tradition keeps cycling a communally rich activity. In this age of sports science, the cycling culture has maintained an identity apart from cold science. Ever since Baron Karl von Drais introduced the first credible bicycle in 1818, there has been a strong connection between man and this machine.

To competitive and recreational riders alike, the bicycle can be viewed as an extension of the body—like a katana to a samurai. Consider the allure of the cycling culture—aerodynamic gear, professional tours on TV, Gran Fondos, regional races, local group rides that turn a workout into the social event of the week—and it is easy to see how cycling has become a way of life. Unlike with so many other sports, which can be watched from afar, but not engaged in by fans, cyclists can get on the road any time they want and pedal, just as their favorite racers do. It has created its own passionate subculture, appealing to all ages regardless of fitness.

Now while all that community and tradition stuff is great, I don't want you to think that getting on a bike and pedaling away into the sunset is just what the pros do, because it isn't. An intangible known as skill separates the elites from everyone else, and that's what we're going to address here. Don't make the mistake of thinking that you can learn how to ride by simply buying a bike and getting on it. That's like saying you can learn to run by buying a pair of shoes and hitting the track. You need to educate yourself on the proper mechanics by isolating movements and position.

Unless you're a professional cyclist or competitive endurance athlete, much of the technique—positioning, shifting, braking, climbing, descending, and steering—is self-taught. It's unlikely that proper skill development is taken into consideration by the do-it-yourself cyclist. Poor technique is then compounded by thousands of miles in the saddle, and it becomes necessary to unlearn before you can improve. Just like learning how to run or swim, learning how to ride is critical to both enjoyment and maximizing performance.

The goal of this chapter is to reclaim or strengthen that connection by teaching the principles that yield success on a bike, which include bike fit, proper positioning, pedaling mechanics, climbing, descending, and cornering (turning). Remember, cycling is a demanding sport. The margin for error is slim. Where you place in a race may be a matter of hundredths of a second. Sprint wins may come down to a bike throw. To ride well and ensure sustainable longevity in the sport—whether riding a road, time-trial, or mountain bike—you must remain focused on the science of skill.

In my 20 plus years of coaching and racing, I've come to understand the delicate balance among training, bike fit, mental preparation, and positioning. Cycling is a practical lesson in math, geometry, physics, aerodynamics, and human movement. Unlike running, you have two key factors that must work in concert to maximize or achieve a desired goal: the bike and the body. You can adjust the size and dimensions of the bike, but you can't change the length and size of your bones. For that reason, you must first understand how to fit the bike to your body so that you can achieve a position that will allow you to maximize your power, speed, efficiency, position, and control. Then you can focus on skill training, which is covered later in the chapter.

Bike Fit

Bike Fit Checklist

Proper bike fit is the first step to maximizing power, speed, efficiency, comfort, sustainability, recovery, and enjoyment of your bike. However, bike fit is not as simple as measuring your inseam (although measuring you inseam is an important step) and picking out a bike that corresponds to it. There are several things to consider: leg and torso length; skeletal structure; the individual's experience, mobility, and athleticism.

Another important fact to consider when shopping for a bike is the different makes and models. Not all bikes are created equal even though frame sizes may be the same. For example, a 54 cm Brand A may not fit the same way a 54 cm Brand B does. Just like when shopping for an automobile, you should test-drive as many makes and models to find the right match. There is a big difference in acceleration, responsiveness, and comfort from bike to bike. Style, color, and design are also important—after all, there is a lot of pageantry and fashion in this sport!

Don't be in a rush or pick out a bike because your favorite pro cyclist rides a particular model. Remember, everyone is different. Do a lot of research. What works for the pro, may not work for you. The pro is being paid to ride a particular bike, and the bike is usually custom-built for him. They also have the luxury of having their body position and angles analyzed in microscopic detail to maximize performance.

If possible, find a qualified coach or bike fit expert to guide you through the process, ideally someone with experience as both a cyclist and a fitter. Imagine that you're buying a custom-made suit. The tailor has to not only take your measurements, but also know why you're purchasing the suit: are you going to a wedding? A funeral? Will you wear it to business meetings? A bike fit is no different: the fitter needs to know whether you're going to be riding recreationally or racing, whether you've been riding for years or are just getting into the sport.

It's important to note that there are numerous approaches, opinions, theories, and systems that can be applied to the bike fit process. To avoid confusion, you may need to research and interview a qualified coach who understands how to address the points outlined in this chapter.

In the subsequent section, I outline three steps that you can take to determine the proper bike fit. Whether you're attempting a solo bike fit or trying to educate yourself on the process before seeing a bike fit doctor, it's imperative that you understand how and why each step is used. If you overlook this critical process, you not only compromise comfort, posture, efficiency, and control, but also increase your susceptibility to injury.

Tools

Before you start the do-it-yourself bike fit process you will need: a goniometer (it measures angles), a plumb line (a string with a bolt/weight attached), and a selection of allen wrenches. It's also useful to have a Sharpie pen on hand so that you can mark both the rider and components on the bike. Also, to ensure you can perform all the bike fit steps, you need a bike stand or trainer (something that holds the bike up) so that you can sit on the saddle and pedal without losing balance.

1. **Bike Fit Goniometer:** measures the angle of your knee. One can be purchased at bikefit.com.
2. **Allen Wrenches:** to adjust saddle, handlebars, seat post.
3. **Plumb Line:** to confirm proper knee alignment.

There are three main points of contact on the bike, which help determine positional strength and stability: your rear end on the saddle, your feet on the pedals, and your hands on the handlebars. These points of contact are the support structures that allow the bike to move, turn, climb, accelerate, and stop effectively. This is also where the three main measurements are taken for the bike fit. In order of importance, you want to measure the saddle height, the forward and backward positioning of the saddle, and the handlebar height and width. It's important to note that the bike fit system can be used for all three types of bikes (road, time trial, and mountain); any variations will be noted.

HOW TO DETERMINE THE RIGHT SIZE BIKE FRAME

Inseam	Frame Size Range (Road)	Frame Size Range (MTB)
Less than 28 cm	46cm or under	Less than 17 inch
28-32 cm	46-54	17-18
32-36 cm	54-60	18-20
36+ cm	60+	20+

NOTE: Mountain bikes are typically measured in inches, and road bikes are typically measured in centimeters.

The above chart is meant to be a general guideline to help you decide what size frame/bike to buy. Note: buying a bike based solely on your inseam measurement isn't necessarily going to get you the most accurate frame. Your arms and torso may be entirely different lengths than those of someone else who wears the exact same pants size. For that reason, it can be difficult to determine with tack sharp accuracy the exact frame size based solely on your inseam measurement. But it's a good place to start if you don't have a bike fit expert at your disposal.

Another important point is that just because Brand A's frame is 54 cm and so is Brand B's, it doesn't mean they will fit the same way! Seat tube, top tube, and head tube angles will vary and thus affect how you and the bike will fit together. Moreover, top tube lengths are generally designed for men, whose torsos are generally longer, so women need to shop around for either female-specific frames or brands that have slightly shorter top tubes.

To get the most accurate information, follow the guidelines outlined in the checklist, which are pretty simple and will get you pretty close to that bull's-eye of perfect fit.

1. Stand facing a wall with your feet directly under your hips. Ideally, your feet should be spaced the same distance apart as if you were on your bike. Place the spine of this book in your groin against your pubic bone and make a short line or dot where the top of the book meets the wall, keeping the book as level as possible. Now measure the distance from the ground to this mark. This is your inseam measurement. If you are fitting for a road bike, you generally want to take the measurement in centimeters, and if you are fitting for a mountain bike, you generally want to take the measurement in inches. Another crude method that can be used is to measure the inside of your leg with a tape measure. To do this, step your inner heel over the hook and draw it up the inside of your leg to your groin.

2. Multiply your inseam measurement by .65. This is for a center-to-center (C-to-C) sizing versus a center-to-top (C-to-T) sizing. Be careful when reading specifications for a frame. If the bike size is measured C to T, multiply your inseam measurement by .67. *Note: For mountain bikes, complete the same process for inseam measurement, but subtract 3.9 inches after you multiply your inseam by .65 (C to C).*

Here's an example:

> **Road Bike/Time-Trial Bike: Inseam measurement of 84 cm; 84 x .65 = 54.6 (C to C).**
> **Mountain Bike: Inseam measurement of 33 in; 33 x .65 = 21.45; 21.45 − 3.9 = 17.55 in.**

Another way to determine frame size, which is even more elementary, is to do a stand-over test. On a road bike, stand directly over the bike with the top tube between your legs: you should have at least two and a half inches clearance between your body and the top tube. On a mountain bike, you should have at least a four-inch clearance. If the bike has a sloping top tube, however, the stand-over test doesn't work.

Remember, these tests are just starting points. The guidelines in the checklist will offer more specific measurements so that you can get the most exact fit on your bike possible without going to a pro—which is always a possibility and which I do highly recommend.

BIKE FIT CHECKLIST

- ☑ **SADDLE HEIGHT**
- ☑ **SADDLE FORE-AFT**
- ☑ **HANDLEBAR HEIGHT AND WIDTH**
- ☑ **FINAL CHECK**

Saddle Height

Determining saddle height is the first and most important measurement. If this step is not carried out correctly, the subsequent measurements will be off and the rider will not be able to achieve the ideal position. It's important to note that there are two phases to this initial setup. The first phase is meant to warm the rider up and get him into a comfortable position on the saddle; the second phase is meant to find an ideal knee bend to ensure that the saddle is set at the correct height. To begin the first setup, stand next to the bike and set the saddle height a few inches below your belt line. Technically, you want it positioned on your greater trochanter, which is at the top of your femur.

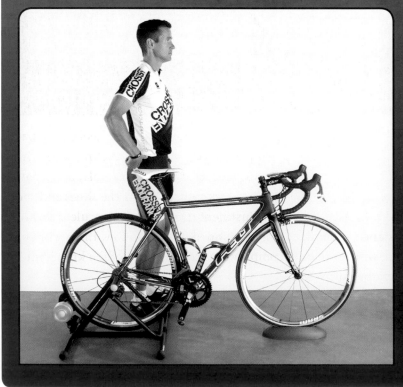

I'm standing next to the bike. My right hand is positioned on my greater trochanter. This is my saddle height. After you've set the saddle height, slide the saddle into a neutral fore and aft position, meaning that an equal amount of saddle rail is exposed front and back. Now get on the bike and ride for at least three minutes. This light warmup will loosen up your legs and allow you to find a sweet spot (comfortable position) on the saddle.

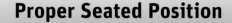

Proper Seated Position

Positioning on the bike starts with the saddle. If you glance at the photos, you'll notice that I sit my pubic bones on the saddle right where it starts to widen. That is your sweet spot.

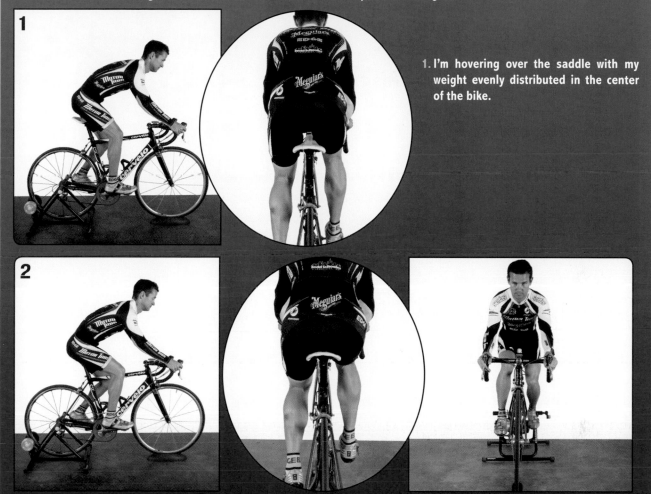

1. I'm hovering over the saddle with my weight evenly distributed in the center of the bike.

2. I place my pubic bones around the middle of the saddle, right where it starts to widen. This may vary slightly depending on the brand of saddle, so be sure get fitted on the saddle you will be riding on.

Once the first phase is complete, set the crank arm to the six o'clock position and place your heel on the pedal axle. Your leg should be fully extended (straight). If you're wearing a touring shoe or a cycling shoe with a raised heel, you have to measure the height of the shoe stack and adjust accordingly. For example, if you have a 2 mm heel lift, you should raise the saddle 2 mm. (Note: To avoid any discrepancies, wear the shoes and socks you'll be using on the bike you're being fitted for.) Although the adjustment may seem minuscule, a few millimeters can make a huge difference. For instance, if the saddle is positioned 3 mm too low, there will be an exaggerated bend in the knee when you pedal, which not only compromises the integrity of the knee joint but also sacrifices power, making for a less-efficient pedal stroke.

Another way to offset the shoe stack is to place the arch of the shoe on the center of the pedal axle. Regardless of your approach, the goal is to achieve a straight-leg position with your foot centered on the pedal axle as demonstrated in the photo on the next page. If you're unable to reach the pedal axle with your leg straight and your foot parallel to the ground, drop the saddle height until you can. Conversely, if there is any bend in the knee, raise the saddle until your leg is completely straight. Any deviation from this ideal position will compromise the accuracy of the bike fit.

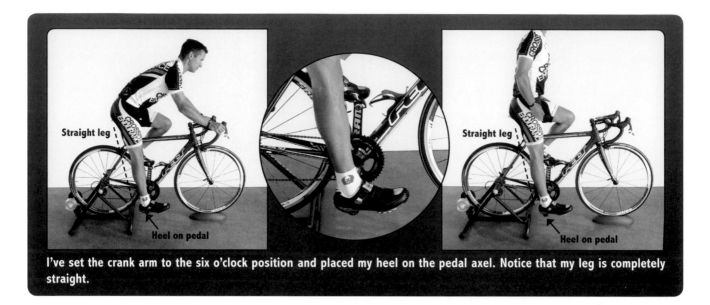

I've set the crank arm to the six o'clock position and placed my heel on the pedal axel. Notice that my leg is completely straight.

Once you've set the saddle to a height that allows for a straight leg at the bottom of the pedal stroke, the next step is to remove your heel from the pedal and clip in. If the previous steps were carried out correctly, there should be a 25- to 35-degree bend in the knee. In addition to maximizing the efficiency of pedaling mechanics and reducing your susceptibility to injury, this bend allows you to pedal using the full musculature of your leg—quads, hamstrings, and glutes.

It's important to note that your ability to feel muscle activation during the fit process does not indicate proper bike fit. Many factors affect which muscles are required to pedal at any given time. For

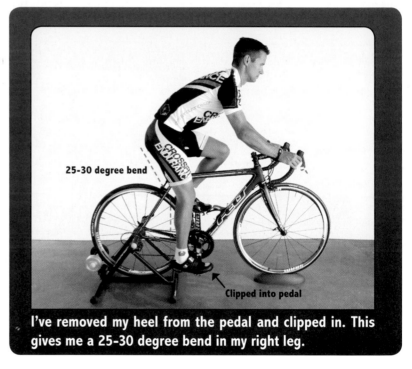

I've removed my heel from the pedal and clipped in. This gives me a 25-30 degree bend in my right leg.

example, the type of saddle you're riding, the angle of the nose, your understanding of proper positioning, and whether you're wearing a regular shoe or a cleat, can dictate which muscles are fired as you engage the pedal system. It also depends on your mobility and flexibility, as well as your hip angle when you sit.

At this stage, it's helpful to take a Sharpie and mark a spot on the outside of your leg parallel to the knee's flexion point, which is at the center of the patella. This not only marks the placement of the goniometer, but also helps with the subsequent stage of the bike fit, which is to determine the fore and aft position of the saddle.

After you've made the mark, place the center of the goniometer over it to ensure that you've achieved a 25- to 35-degree bend in the knee. Note that the lower part of the goniometer should be in line with the lateral malleolus (ankle bone), and the top part should be in line with the femur bone.

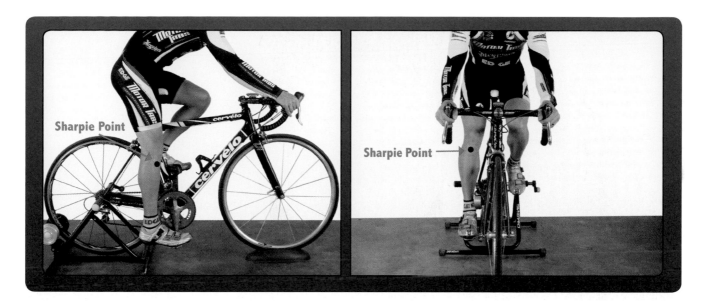

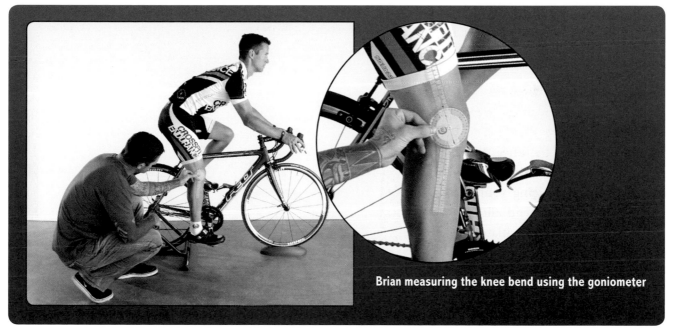

Brian measuring the knee bend using the goniometer

Adjusting the Fit: If the knee angle is 40 degrees, move the saddle up. Conversely, if knee angle is 20 degrees, move the saddle down.

Key Points:

☐ Measure the saddle height based on the positioning of your greater trochanter.

☐ Find the sweet spot on the saddle and pedal for a few minutes to warm up—see correct seated position and pedaling mechanics.

☐ Set the crank arm to six o'clock and achieve a straight-leg position.

☐ Engage into the pedal system.

☐ Use the goniometer to make sure you have a 25- to 35-degree bend in the knee.

☐ If the angle is greater than that, raise the seat. If the angle is less than that, move the saddle down.

With a mountain bike, you're usually seated a little bit lower than on a road or time-trial bike because you move up and down and get out of the saddle more often because of the constantly varied terrain. For that reason, you may want to lower the saddle a few millimeters after you've completed the first step in the bike fit checklist. This allows for a more comfortable and safe position because you can slide and shift your weight around the saddle as you navigate obstacles and undulating terrain without compromising stability or pedal efficiency.

It's important to note that the extent in which you lower the saddle is highly individualized and should be based on the type of terrain you're going to ride, your skill set, and your level of comfort. It's also important to note that if you're touring or riding on a fire road that is mostly flat you probably don't need to lower your saddle. In such a situation, set the saddle to a height that allows for the 25-35 degree bend just as you would on a road bike. There are also adjustable seat posts that allow you to raise or lower your saddle with a push of the button. Although this is an expensive option, it is great if you're riding on trails that transition from single track to fire roads.

The crank-arm length is also worth mentioning. On most mountain bikes, the crank arm is a little shorter than on a road or time-trial bike. For example, if your road bike crank arm is 175 mm and the crank arm on your mountain bike is 170 mm, you can make up for the discrepancy by lowering your saddle 5 mm.

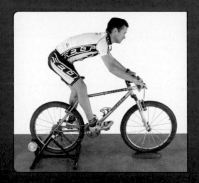 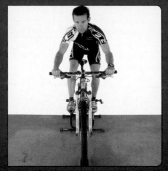

The seat is slightly lower, giving me more maneuverability with the bike.

SADDLE ANGLE

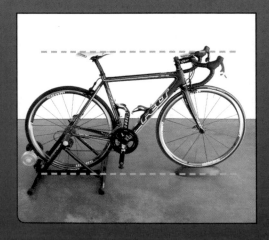

As a general rule, the saddle should be essentially level with the ground. Unless the cyclist has a physical abnormality, there is no documented performance advantage to tilting the saddle nose up or down. An improper tilt can compromise stability on the bike and may affect the reach of the leg in relationship to the pedal system. Another factor worth noting is saddle wear and tear: most pro cyclists or amateur racers change out their saddles several times a year. To check the integrity of your saddle, place a straight edge on the center of the saddle and look for more than a quarter-inch drop or sag in the middle. If it's more than a quarter inch, it's time for a new saddle.

Saddle Fore-Aft

After you've determined the correct saddle height, the next step is to position your leg in the proper power position, which is accomplished by sliding the saddle either forward or backward (fore or aft). The goal is to position the saddle so that the previously marked center flexion point of the knee is directly over the pedal axle. To begin this process, place the crank arm at three o'clock, and then using the plumb-line drop, have a friend pin the string to the center of your patella (knee cap), allowing the line to hang. The string should align perfectly with the front of the crank arm or bisect the center of the pedal axle. If the string hangs behind the front of the crank arm, slide the saddle forward. If the string hangs in front of the pedal, slide the saddle backward. To ensure an accurate measurement, your foot must be completely parallel to the ground.

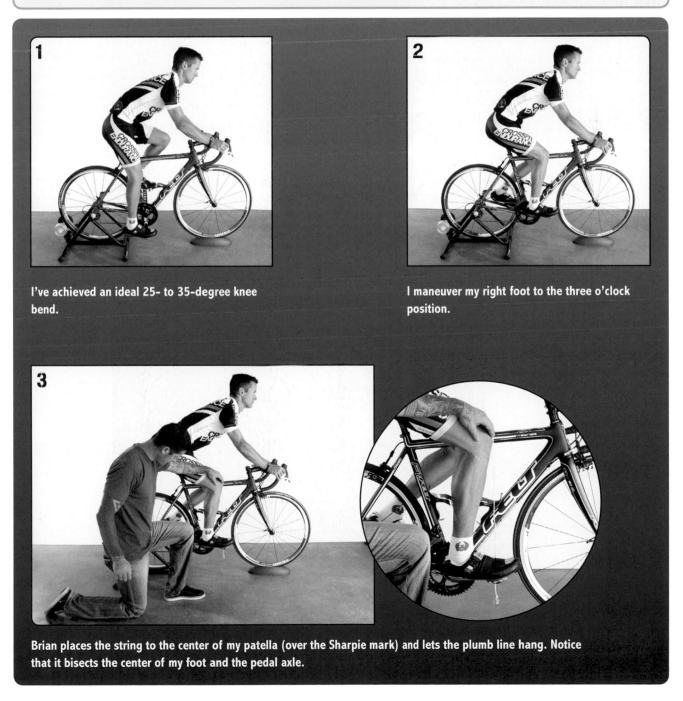

1 I've achieved an ideal 25- to 35-degree knee bend.

2 I maneuver my right foot to the three o'clock position.

3 Brian places the string to the center of my patella (over the Sharpie mark) and lets the plumb line hang. Notice that it bisects the center of my foot and the pedal axle.

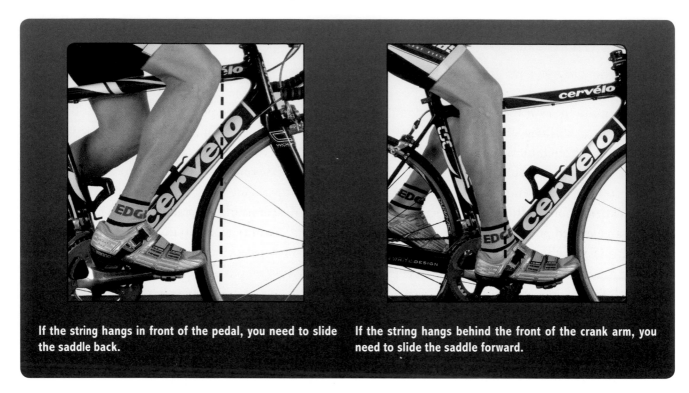

If the string hangs in front of the pedal, you need to slide the saddle back.

If the string hangs behind the front of the crank arm, you need to slide the saddle forward.

Another important step, which is often neglected at this stage, is to measure both legs to make sure there isn't a discrepancy in their lengths. If one leg happens to be slightly shorter than the other, address your position to ensure you're seated correctly on the bike. In some cases, this is a musculoskeletal issue and should be addressed using the mobility techniques in the Mobility as a Skill chapter. If there is an actual difference in leg lengths, I suggest you seek your doctor's advice so you can make accurate cleat adjustments.

Once the fore and aft is set, it's important to recheck the saddle height and measure the knee bend. Sometimes fine-tuning the fore and aft can affect saddle height, so you may have to redo the previous step so you can adjust accordingly. Once everything is set, it's important for you to pedal again for several minutes to confirm your position.

Key Points:

☐ Make sure the saddle is level with the ground and the saddle height was assessed properly before you adjust the fore-aft.

☐ Position the crank arm at three o'clock.

☐ Have a friend place the plumb line to the front of your patella (knee cap).

☐ Adjust the saddle fore-aft so that the string hangs in front of the crank arm, bisecting the pedal axle.

☐ Check the saddle height and measure the knee bend to ensure an accurate fit.

☐ Pedal for a few minutes to confirm the position.

Handlebar Height & Width

For the majority of riders, the height of the handlebars should be roughly the same as the height of the saddle (in the beginning). However, if you're not used to being in the cycling position, your erectors/quadratus lumborum and low back may not be conditioned to this loaded position and you may not have the mobility to achieve the proper position—this takes time and progression. You may have to add some spacers to the stem to raise the handlebars. Using the setup for the dead lift as a test should shed light on your positional deficiencies/requirements for adaptation. For example, if you can't set up for a dead lift correctly—see Strength-and-Conditioning as a Skill—you probably won't be able to achieve the correct bike position. In that case, you should spend some time dead lifting (or starting in the hang clean) from an elevated position until you develop the strength and mobility to set up from the ground. In the meantime, you should raise the handlebars to compensate for the deficiency in strength and flexibility, making proper positioning on a bike easier to maintain. With strength-and-conditioning training and enough time on the bike with proper form, you'll be able to lower the handlebars into a more aggressive and aerodynamic position.

Handlebars come in standard widths of 38 cm, 40 cm, 42 cm, and 44 cm, with the majority of riders using 40 cm or 42 cm. To maximize control, comfort, and stability, the width of your handlebars should be roughly the width of your shoulders. A lot of riders think that such a narrow position restricts the ability to breath, rendering it ineffective. If you're breathing correctly, meaning that you are inhaling and exhaling with your diaphragm, a handlebar as wide as your shoulders is just fine. In fact, anything wider will reduce your control over the bike, and it could increase the possibility of banging bars with another racer during a sprint, which could result in a crash. It's important to note that a lot of this boils down to personal feel.

Time-Trial Variation

For time-trial bikes, the handlebars are generally as low as possible to create minimal frontal surface area for a highly aerodynamic position. Again, this is also a function of midline integrity, strength, and experience. Handlebar fore-aft on the time-trial bike is equally important. Your arm bend (measured at the elbow) should be close to 90 to 100 degrees to place your body in a falling position to support the pedaling drive.

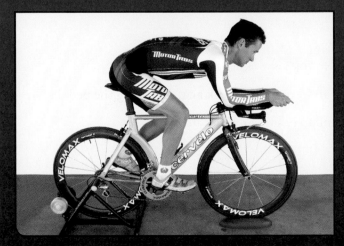

I've established the proper time-trial position. Notice that my arms are angled at roughly 90 to 100 degrees.

Mountain Bike Variation

For most riders, setting the handlebar height about level with the saddle is usually a comfortable start. From there, you can experiment to find the optimal fit. The goal is to set the handlebars in a position that allows for maximum leverage while riding on the varying terrain that is indicative of mountain biking. When making the final adjustment, be wary of raising the handlebars too high, as this will affect your ability to control the bike while climbing up a steep hill.

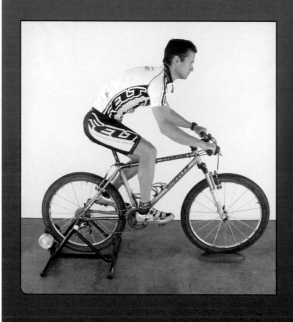

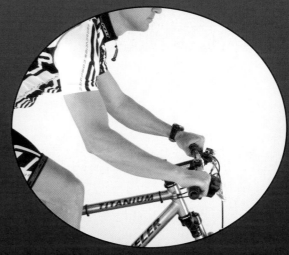

I've established the proper position on the mountain bike.

Final Check

An often-overlooked element to bike fit is the *mechanical motion of mass and body weight:* meaning, once you start pedaling, your mechanics may shift. The final check to confirm your bike fit is to go out for a ride. The position should be comfortable and efficient. If you're shifting in the saddle, your pedal stroke feels choppy, or you can't effectively steer the bike, you may have to reassess the fit, or address proper position and mechanics, which I cover in the following pages.

ADHERE TO THE BIKE FIT CHECKLIST

To repeat, if your bike is not fitted correctly, everything from your position to your mechanics is compromised. In addition to not being as efficient as possible, you dramatically increase your susceptibility to injury.

USE THE FOLLOWING STRATEGIES TO PRESERVE YOUR BIKE AND EQUIPMENT:

- To save the sidewalls on your tires, deflate 20 to 30 pounds of tire pressure after each ride.

- Wipe down your bike after each ride, and use Pledge to preserve the finish. The three most important cleaning areas are the chain, chainrings, and pulleys.

- Lube and clean your cleats at least every 500 miles to help extend the life of the springs (i.e., speedplay).

- Put a little baby powder on your spare tube so when it comes time to fix a flat, the tube/tire will slide on easier.

THE SHORTER THE EFFORT THE LONGER THE WARM-UP

A lot of riders get injured because they don't warm up properly before short sprints or time trials. Before any ride or race, I recommend doing at least five roll-ups, 10- to 15-second accelerations in the saddle. In addition to warming up your body, this helps prevent the shock of the first hard hit of intensity on a ride.

THINK ABOUT THE MOVEMENT, NOT THE MUSCLES BEING USED

A lot of riders make the mistake of thinking about the muscles they need to fire while pedaling. More often than not, this will cause you to forget about your position, resulting in a breakdown of mechanics. Instead, focus on maintaining an ideal position and using proper mechanics. Your muscles will follow suit.

ADJUST YOUR BIKE FOR THE COURSE

For example, if you're going to be doing a long, extended climb, experiment with tilting your brake hoods up slightly. It can make for a more comfortable position when you stand, which is common on long climbs.

PACK-SURF WHEN POSSIBLE

A good skill to get comfortable with when you're pack riding/racing is to "pack-surf": changing your position in the peloton. Practice this by moving from the back third to the middle third, then to the front third of the pack on your local group ride.

ALWAYS IMPLEMENT MOBILITY EXERCISES BEFORE AND AFTER EACH RIDE

Riding hard can take a terrible toll on your body if you don't put the necessary time into recovery protocol, especially for your feet, ankles, legs, and hips. To avoid stiffness and injury, pinpoint your areas of weakness and implement the necessary mobility exercises before and after each ride.

BREATHE DEEPLY

To practice diaphragmatic breathing, lie flat on your back with a book on your bellybutton and focus on limiting the movement in your chest while you raise and lower the book.

WHEN IN DOUBT COVER YOUR KNEES AND ARMS

Being cold can seriously restrict your performance. Wearing arm and knee sleeves will help you stay warm in colder conditions. Remember: You never know when the weather will change, and you can always shed clothing if you're too warm.

DESCENDING TIPS

- To maintain control on fast, straight downhill descents, brace your knees/legs against the top tube and keep your chest down to prevent the bike from wobbling.

- On steep descents, feather your rear brakes prior to cornering and avoid hitting your front brakes.

- For stability, control, and easier access to your brakes, keep your hands in the drops instead of on the brake hoods.

- When coming into off-camber* corners, shift your weight back slightly in the saddle to allow for better body weighting on the bike.

CLIMBING TIPS

- Lightly resting your palms about 4 to 6 inches apart on the handlebars will help you relax and stay focused on establishing rhythm.

- To get a "head start" on the climb, accelerate to the base of the climb. This will allow inertia to carry you up the first part of the climb. Then, continue to keep your cadence at or above 80 RPM to carry you through the rest of the climb.

- On long, sustained climbs, you can unzip your jersey to stay cooler and stick your sunglasses on your helmet to avoid sweat from getting on them. This will also keep you dry as you enter the descent, at which point you better put your glasses back on or risk losing them.

- Usually people get to the top of a hill and shut it down, which is not what happens in a race. This is where you want to punch it. To increase your work capacity and simulate a realistic race scenario, accelerate for 200 meters or more when you get to the top of a climb.

- On climbs with multiple switchbacks, shift up one to two cogs (from, say, a 21 to a 19). As you hit the beginning of the switchback, stand and accelerate through the corner, and then sit back down and resume your original tempo and gearing. This skill helps to keep speed going through switchbacks, especially those that are off-camber.

- On climbs with occasional lulls or less-steep sections (going from, say, 7 percent to 2 percent), try using a bigger gear (your 15 rather than your 19) on the climb, instead of taking time to keep reshifting. Again, this saves time on the climb.

*Off-camber: Turns in which the ground slopes toward the outside, making it harder to keep traction as speed increases.

KEEP ONE THUMB HOOKED AROUND THE HANDLE-BARS AT ALL TIMES WHILE MOUNTAIN BIKING

A lot of mountain bikers become complacent while riding on fire roads and even on single-track. The most common mistake is to monkey grip the handlebars by hooking your thumb over the top, reducing your control over the bike. This modified grip puts you at serious risk: bumps and obstacles can come out of nowhere so you always have to be ready. By keeping your thumb hooked around the handlebars you can ensure optimal control and reduce your chances of crashing.

USE STOPLIGHTS OR STOP SIGNS TO PRACTICE TRACK-STANDING AND ACCELERATION

To practice track standing while stopped at a traffic light, remember to turn your front wheel at an angle while you weight and unweight each pedal. The moment the light turns green, or when the road is clear, accelerate instead of slowly rolling across the intersection.

SKILL TRAINING

Once you've completed the bike fit checklist, you can address the skill of cycling. In this section, I will break down proper positioning (of body to bike), pedaling mechanics, climbing, descending, cornering, as well as the common faults associated with each technique. To make navigating through this section easier to manage, I've broken up the section into three categories: road bike, time trial, and mountain bike. It's important to note that if you haven't been fitted correctly on the bike, achieving proper form will be difficult.

Road Bike

In many ways the road bike started it all. It was the horse and carriage that evolved into the car: other bicycle frames, such as the time trial and mountain bike, evolved from the road bike. Although technological advancements have wrought slight adjustments to the frame (i.e., shape and sizing of the tubing), the fundamental geometry has changed very little.

The reason the road bike is so popular, aside from its efficient design, is its versatility. Unlike time-trial bikes, mountain bikes, hybrid bicycles, utility bikes, and touring bikes, which are designed for specific purposes, the road bike is designed to do just about everything on the road. Whether you're going uphill, downhill, cornering, traveling on flat road, or sprinting, as long as you're riding on a paved road (or sometimes not so paved) the road bike can handle it.

The road bike's versatility extends beyond its practical application in that it can be used in a variety of cycling competitions and applications. For instance, it can be used for recreational touring or racing. It can be used in competitive criterium races (a closed short course of typically a mile or less). It can be used in circuit races (a series of generally two- to eight-mile laps).

The best-known implementation of the road bike is in stage racing—think Tour de France, but usually only three to seven days long. Because a stage race is a mix of everything (climbing, descending, sprinting, and time-trialing), it is the best overall measurement of fitness for a cyclist. Of course, the most practical application of riding a road bike is to commute or go from point A to point B.

To get the most out of each of these skills, which I am about to discuss in detail, it's important for you to spend time training each skill before packing up your car and heading to your first stage race. Whether you're a recreational rider or competitive cyclist or specialize on a different bike, learning the proper mechanics on the road bike translates well to other bikes because of the diverse nature and fixed geometry of the road bike. Remember, the key to successfully implementing the strategies outlined in this section is to isolate each technique and become familiar with its common faults. Although you want to absorb and practice only the correct techniques, it's helpful to be aware of the dysfunctional positions and movement patterns to avoid making those mistakes on the road.

Drafting reduces wind resistance and conserves energy. Riders ride one behind the other, the rider in front basically blocking the wind and pulling the rider behind him forward. To ride efficiently en masse, whether in a small group or a large pack, you need to learn drafting technique. Properly executed, drafting can save 15 to 30 percent of energy expenditure. In addition to saving energy and increasing your average speed, drafting teaches you balance and how to control the bike in a straight line. The closer you are to the person in front of you, meaning the closer your front wheel is to the rear wheel in front of you, the better the draft. Experienced riders can keep their wheels just an inch and a half away from the wheel ahead of them. If you are more than a bike length behind somebody, you're not getting a draft.

The art of drafting boils down to three things: being confident in your ability to control the bike and speed, knowing the rider in front of you, and the direction of the wind. For example, when I ride with training partners I'm comfortable with, I get so close that I may actually momentarily rub tires with them. While this can be extremely dangerous and is not recommended, the risk is decreased by the fact that we know one another's riding styles and we're experience riders. The point is: The more comfortable you are with the people you're riding with and the more experienced you are on the bike, the closer you will feel comfortable drafting.

It's important to note that your drafting position is dictated by the direction of the wind as well as your position in the pack. If you have a strong head wind, you want to draft directly behind the wheel in front of you. If you have a crosswind, you want to draft to the leeward side of the rear wheel in front of you in what's called an echelon. If you're in a very large group, riding two or more abreast, the best drafting position is in the front third or middle because you're protected all the way around, which is why in big bike races you're never going to see the great sprinters at the front. They're trying to conserve as much energy as possible and draft off everybody for as long as they can so that when it comes time to stick their nose into the wind, they have the energy to go all out.

Safety Tips

* Learn to draft behind one person before drafting in a group. Ideally, you want to draft behind an experienced rider going at a slow pace.

* When learning the art of drafting, the person in front of you should ride at a consistent pace in a straight line—there should not be a lot of stopping and starting or weaving back and forth.

* In the beginning, start out at about a bike length or half bike length away. As you get more comfortable, start inching closer and closer.

* When drafting, you never want to overlap your front wheel with the rear wheel in front of you. That is how crashes most commonly occur.

PROPER ROAD BIKE POSITION
(FLAT ROAD)

Cycling is no different than running, swimming, or lifting in that body position dictates power output and efficiency: if your body is not positioned correctly on the bike, power is going to leak out at the weakest point. For example, if you roll your hips from side to side as you drive through the pedal stroke, which is usually a result of poor midline stability (or incorrect bike fit), your lumbar spine will flex and bow out. Weighting and unweighting the bike will cause your body to drift subtly from side to side as a response to the pedaling motion (see Hip and Knee Alignment).

Just like running with bad form or lifting weights with poor mechanics, this positional compromise forces the larger muscle groups to work harder to make up for the lack of stability, which ultimately slows you down, speeds up the onset of fatigue, and increases your risk of injury. Not to mention that you will be working against gravity rather than allowing it to work for you.

The key to establishing an ideal position on a road bike is to keep your lower back (lumbar spine) as flat as possible, which allows for efficient hip movement, centers your body weight between the front and back tires, and keeps your hips, knees, and ankles in alignment. You also want to keep your upper body compact and fairly relaxed, with your knuckles, wrists, arms, and shoulders in line. Any break in this chain will result in an immediate loss of power and efficiency.

HIP AND KNEE ALIGNMENT

Any time your ankles, knees, hips, and shoulders are out of alignment, you sacrifice efficiency, power, and energy, as well as place additional torque on the body, which can lead to injury.

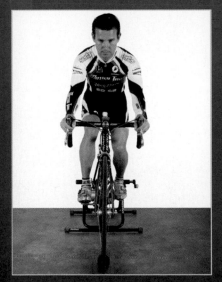

Correct Alignment
I'm in the ideal riding position, with my hips, knees, and ankles directly in line.

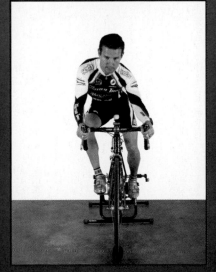

Tilted Out
My right knee is tilted out, the left side of my hips is being forced toward my left side, and I'm leveraging off the handlebars in an attempt to create power.

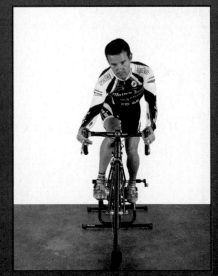

Tilted In
My right knee is tilted in, the left side of my hips is being forced toward my left side, and I'm leveraging off the handlebars in an attempt to create power.

It's important to note that your upper body stabilizes and balances you on the bike so that your lower body can generate power through the pedal stroke. Remember, cycling is about what happens below your waist. To generate the most amount of power, you need to minimize upper body movement without sacrificing control of the bike. That's why if you look at accomplished or professional cyclists, it's difficult to tell how hard they're working because their upper bodies barely move. They keep a relatively relaxed position with a flat lower back and only stray from the proper position when necessary to corner, climb, or descend. Even then, the deviation is slight and at times hardly noticeable. If your upper body moves excessively in any direction, it's a strong indication that your mechanics are faulty and that the bike is in control of you. Although it's the powerful muscles of the legs that do the majority of the work, you must have a strong upper body to maintain a stable position and push off the handlebars.

Proper Road Bike Position

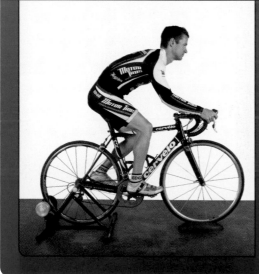 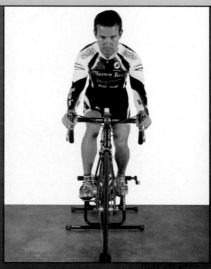

I'm in the proper road bike position. My lower back is flat, my midline is engaged, my head is straight, and my weight is centered between the front and back tires. My knuckles, wrists, arms, and shoulders are on the same vertical plane. To maintain a stable yet comfortable position, I bend my arms slightly and avoid crunching my trunk.

HAND POSITIONS

As I mentioned before, whether you're climbing, sprinting, riding on flat road, or descending, the biomechanical chain from your handlebars up to your neck should always be in line. Any deviation will result in an immediate loss of power. In the following sequences, I demonstrate all the fundamental hand positions that you can implement on the road bike.

Hoods Grip

Hands on the hoods is the most casual, fundamental, and comfortable grip on the road bike. If you're touring, on a training ride, cruising on a flat road, and not racing hard, keep your hands on the brake hoods as demonstrated below.

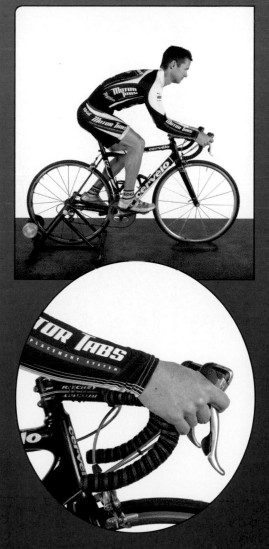

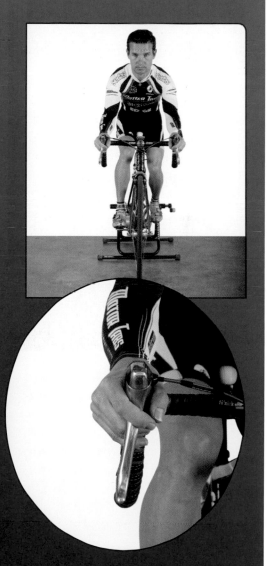

My hands are comfortably wrapped around my brake hoods. Notice that my index finger is wrapped around the front of my brakes and that my wrist, arm, and shoulder are in alignment.

Drops Grip

Riding in the drops is a slightly more aggressive position than the hoods grip in that it is primarily utilized when you're racing hard and trying to maintain high speeds. With your upper body low, you have more stability to corner, and you can leverage off the handlebars to generate a bit more power for sprinting or accelerating. To maximize efficiency, position your hands high on the drops as illustrated below. In addition to giving you more control, it puts your hands close to the brakes and shifters should you need to get to them quickly.

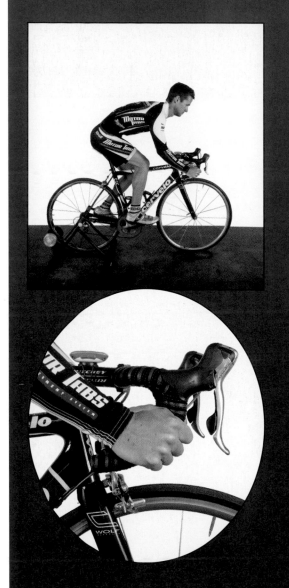

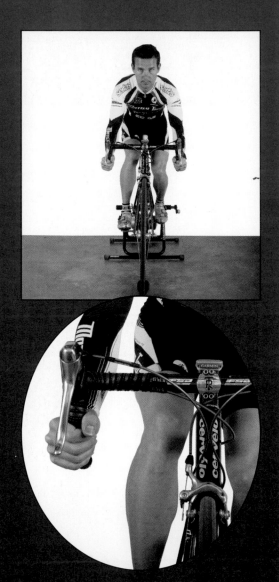

I've lowered myself slightly to achieve a more powerful position and repositioned my hands in the drops. Just as in the previous grip, my knuckles, wrists, and shoulders are straight. It's also important to notice that there is no break in my wrist. Remember, the body needs to be one unified instrument with no loss of energy or strength.

Casual or Recovery Ride and Seated-Climb Grip

The handlebar grip is most commonly used when climbing. With your hands on top of the handlebars, you can get into a comfortable position and focus on using the strength of your legs, rhythmic breathing, and gearing to conquer the hill. You can also incorporate this grip when you're warming up, cooling down, or trying to recover after a hard sprint interval. However, it's important to mention that if you're doing interval training or any type of race simulation, you should be riding on the brake hoods or in the drops. I see far too many inexperienced riders place their hands on the handlebars during interval training, which is a complete waste of time. If you glance at the photo below, you'll notice that the position forces you into an upright seated position, which limits your ability to drive the pedals (when on flat ground), reduces leverage and control of the handlebars, and increases wind resistance. In a nutshell, it's not a very powerful and efficient position unless you're climbing.

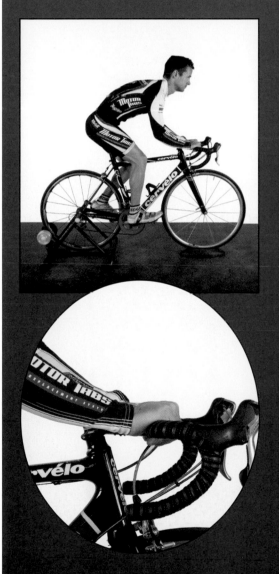

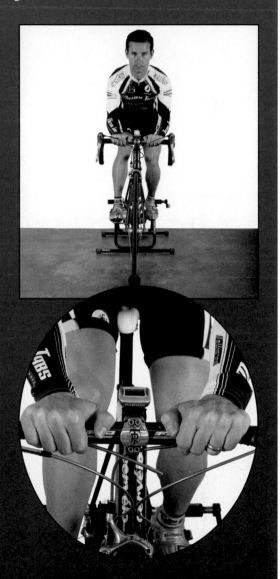

I've positioned my hands on the handlebars. Notice that my thumb is hooked over the bar and that my knuckles, wrists, and arms are still in line. Because this grip is for powering up a hill, you don't need to be as concerned with control or steering. Generally you're going straight up. For that reason, you want to keep your hands relaxed and keep everything in alignment so that you can pedal with maximal efficiency.

POSITIONAL FAULTS

The majority of the positional faults detailed below (assuming correct bike fit) are a direct result of a rider who lacks the skill or strength and capacity to maintain the proper position. A weak, inexperienced rider will try to get more comfortable by shifting into another position, which offers temporary relief but will ultimately result in a rapid loss of power, speed, and stamina, as well as increase the risk of injury. The bottom line is endurance sports such as cycling entail some suffering and muscular fatigue, but mitigating suffering can be accomplished only through proper attention to technique, smart strength-and-conditioning training, and sport-specific training.

Common Fault: Seated Too Far Back

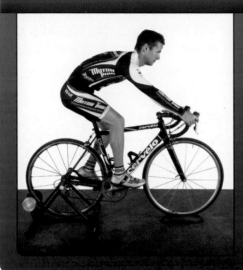

Sliding too far back in the saddle causes your arms to straighten, which reduces your ability to control the bike and forces your lower back into forward flexion. In addition to causing lower-back issues, being too far back in the saddle forces you to reach for the pedals with your legs, causing a rapid loss of power.

I'm seated too far back on the saddle. My arms are extended, the integrity of my lower back is compromised, and my knee is no longer bisecting the middle of the pedal axle, which indicates that I can't properly pedal.

Common Fault: Seated Too Far Forward

If you're too far forward on the saddle, your arms have to stabilize the majority of your body weight by putting more pressure on the handlebars, which not only increases fatigue and reduces your ability to control the bike, but can also cause impingement syndrome of the shoulders and elbows. This forward shift in body mass also places additional pressure on your knee, compromising the integrity of the joint.

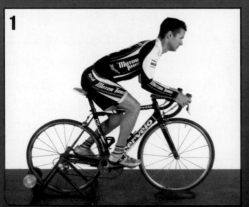

It may appear that stronger riders are falling forward on the bike when attacking, bridging a gap, or attempting a solo breakaway. This is a technique that may create greater speed but has somewhat limited sustainability depending on skill level.

1. I'm positioned too far forward on the saddle. Notice that my arms are supporting the majority of my body weight and that my knee is in front of my foot. The former increases fatigue, while the latter puts stress on the knee joint every time I engage the pedal system.

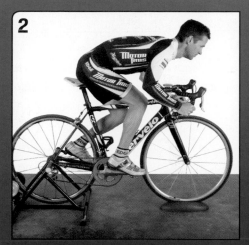

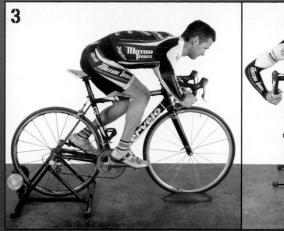

2. With my arms supporting the majority of my body weight, I begin to collapse forward.

3. Unable to support the pressure of my body weight, my arms externally rotate out of alignment, placing stress on my wrists and shoulders.

Common Fault: External Rotation

Everybody responds differently to fatigue. Some slide back on the saddle, while others slide forward. The same is true with alignment faults. As fatigue sets in and the back starts to round, additional weight is placed on your arms. Unable to support the weight of your upper body, your arms will eventually roll out, from the elbow, wrists, or both. By strengthening and conditioning the muscles as well as practicing correct form you can eliminate and slow down the effects of fatigue.

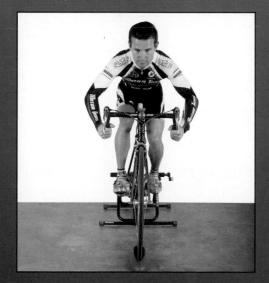

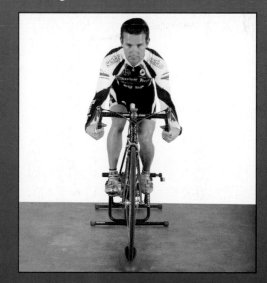

Broken at the Elbows
I'm rounded slightly forward as a result of fatigue, and unable to support the pressure of my body weight with my arms, I externally rotate at the elbows, which puts additional stress on both of my shoulders. This also often causes a midline break and an elevated chin, which may lead to neck/shoulder pain.

Broken at the Wrists
Here I'm illustrating the same fault, only now I'm broken at the wrists. My gripping power has failed, and all the weight of my upper body is driving into my externally rotated wrists. If your hands slip from this position, which does happen, you risk a nasty fall.

Common Fault: Internal Rotation

Internal rotation of the arms is not as common as the external rotation, but this does happen with inexperienced riders without upper body strength. Just as the previous fault, this one causes you to lose power through your arms, making it difficult to drive powerfully into the pedals and control the bike.

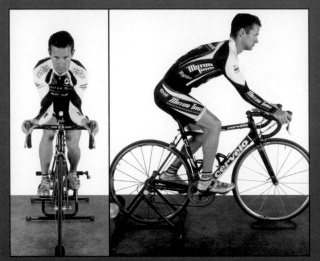

Broken at the Wrists
Here I'm illustrating the same fault, only now I'm in the drops, with my wrists internally rotated. It's the same break in position, in that my wrists, elbows, and shoulders are out of alignment and my ability to control the bike is reduced to a dangerous point.

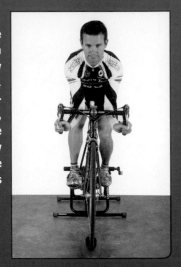

Broken at the Elbows
I'm in the ideal seated position, but I'm broken at the elbows. Over time this can lead to impingement of the shoulders and pain in the elbows and wrists.

Common Fault: Straight Arms

As riders get tired, it's common to see them straighten their arms, shrug their shoulders, round their back, and drop their head. If you're in a race and see a biker with this posture, it's a good time to attack and pass. These movements are primarily a result of fatigue and not having the strength to maintain the proper position on the bike. It's almost as if they're pushing themselves away from the hub of the front wheel. In addition to limiting your control, you take away your shock-absorbing system, which is your arms, thereby increasing your chances of crashing or flying over the top of the handlebars should you hit a bump or obstacle.

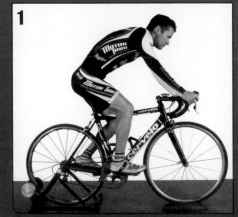

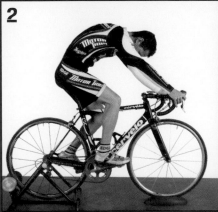

1. As my upper body starts to fatigue and break down, I straighten my arms and begin to push my upper body away from the hub of the front wheel.

2. Unable to maintain the integrity of my posture with straight arms, my upper back rounds forward into flexion and my head drops.

Common Fault: Low-Drops Grip

Another fault common among novice riders is to take a low grip in the drops. As your palms get clammy with sweat, the risk of your hand slipping off the drops dramatically increases. Not only that, it's difficult to reach your brakes and shifters and effectively steer the bike from such a low position.

1

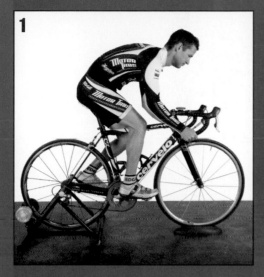

My hands are positioned too low in the drops and I'm unable to effectively reach my brakes or shifters. Controlling the bike as I pedal or steer around corners is also difficult.

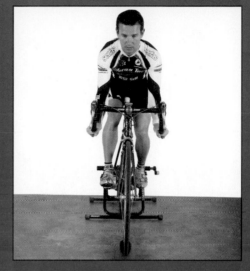

2

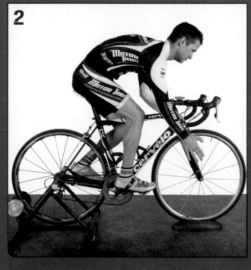

Unable to maintain a solid grip on the drops, my hand slips off (either from sweat or a bump in the road), which will most likely result in a horrible crash.

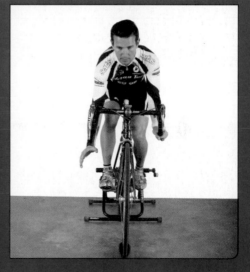

Common Fault: Top-Hoods Grip

Gripping the top of the hoods is another fault that restricts your ability to reach the brakes and shifters or steer the bike. If you hit something, you're going to Superman over the top of the handlebars; if your palms get slippery with sweat, your hand can slip off the handlebars and cause you to crash.

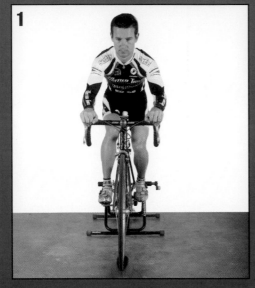

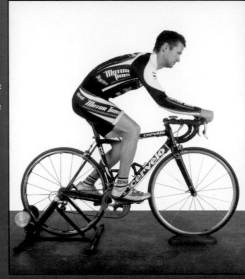

I'm gripping the top of the brake hoods to give my forearms a rest.

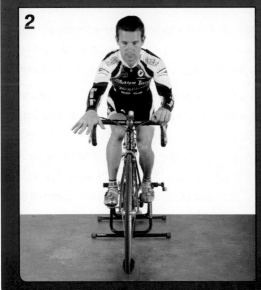

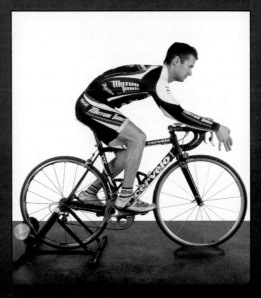

The moment I hit a bump in the road, my hand slips off the top of the brake hoods, causing me to crash.

PEDAL STROKE

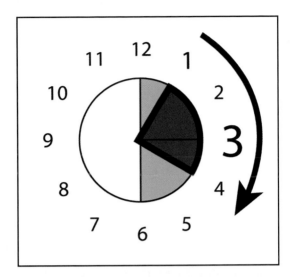

When you watch an experienced cyclist pedal, it's almost as if he's floating in space. You really can't tell how hard he is working or how much power is being generated. The legs fire like pistons and the stroke is perfectly circular, fluid, and rhythmic. Watch an inexperienced rider, on the other hand, and it looks as if he's drawing squares with his feet—the pedal stroke his choppy and unrhythmical. In order to maximize efficiency and power, you have to minimize movement, develop a circular rhythm, and engage the pedal system with proper technique. You need to work with nature and use physics to support your movement.

To help you understand the proper pedaling mechanics, think of the pedal stroke as a clock. To generate the most power and torque out of the lever, which is your leg and crank arm, you want to strike into the pedal system at the power phase, which is at three or four o'clock. Contrary to popular belief, there is no such thing as pushing and pulling in the pedal stroke. A lot of people make the mistake of thinking that you should push down on one side while pulling up on the opposite side. There is always one side working (power phase) and one side resting (relaxation phase). Using the clock analogy, you preload at about one o'clock, start engaging at about two, and then exert the most drive through three and four. Still driving down as you pass through the power phase, you begin to ease off through five and six and then completely disengage at about seven o'clock. At this stage, the opposite leg is entering the preload phase, and the cycle is repeated on the other side.

It's important to mention that when you're entering the power phase you must push the middle of your foot down on the center of the pedal. If you place more pressure toward the inside (knees flaring in) or outside (knees flaring out), you instantly sacrifice power. To create the most power and torque, your legs should move straight up and down in perfect alignment with minimal horizontal movement. It's like a hammer driving down into a nail. If you hit the nail straight on, it will sink directly into the wood without restriction. But if you hit the nail at an angle, it still goes in the wood, but you lose power and compromise the integrity of the nail and hammer. Come down with enough force and your tools can break. The same is true with the pedal stroke. If your hips, knees, and ankles are out of alignment as you strike, you risk a break in the system. In a nutshell, the moment you break the alignment of your hip, knee, and ankle, you lose power and risk injury.

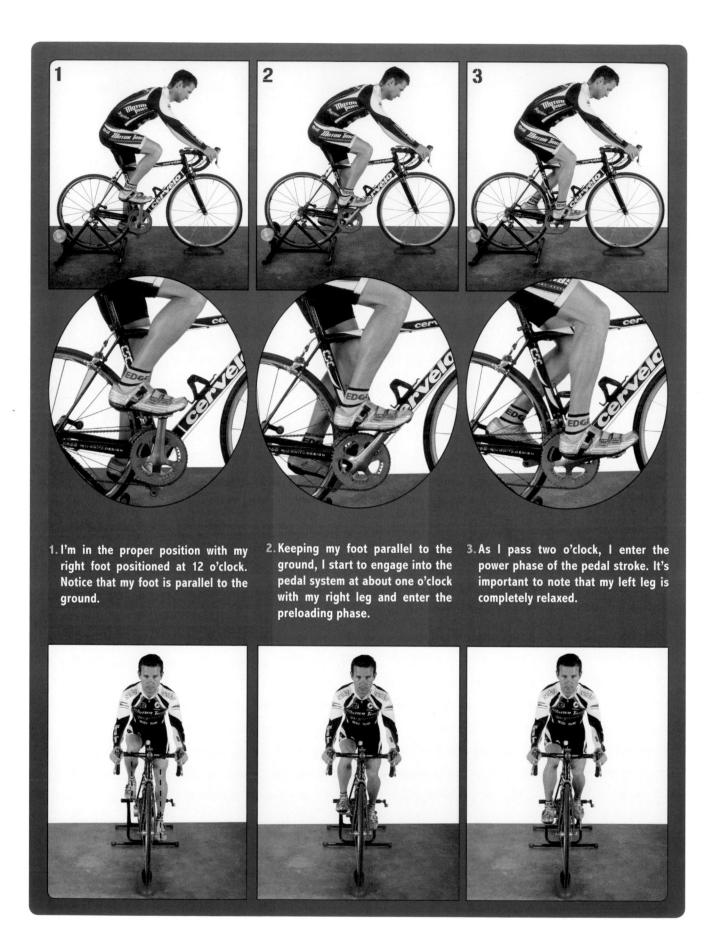

1. I'm in the proper position with my right foot positioned at 12 o'clock. Notice that my foot is parallel to the ground.

2. Keeping my foot parallel to the ground, I start to engage into the pedal system at about one o'clock with my right leg and enter the preloading phase.

3. As I pass two o'clock, I enter the power phase of the pedal stroke. It's important to note that my left leg is completely relaxed.

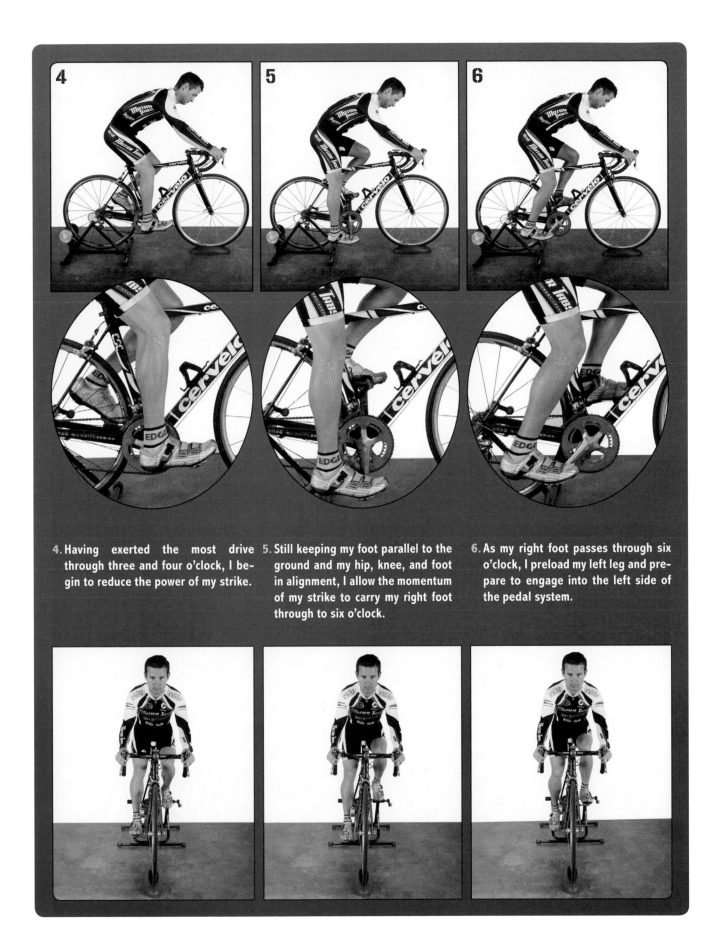

4. Having exerted the most drive through three and four o'clock, I begin to reduce the power of my strike.

5. Still keeping my foot parallel to the ground and my hip, knee, and foot in alignment, I allow the momentum of my strike to carry my right foot through to six o'clock.

6. As my right foot passes through six o'clock, I preload my left leg and prepare to engage into the left side of the pedal system.

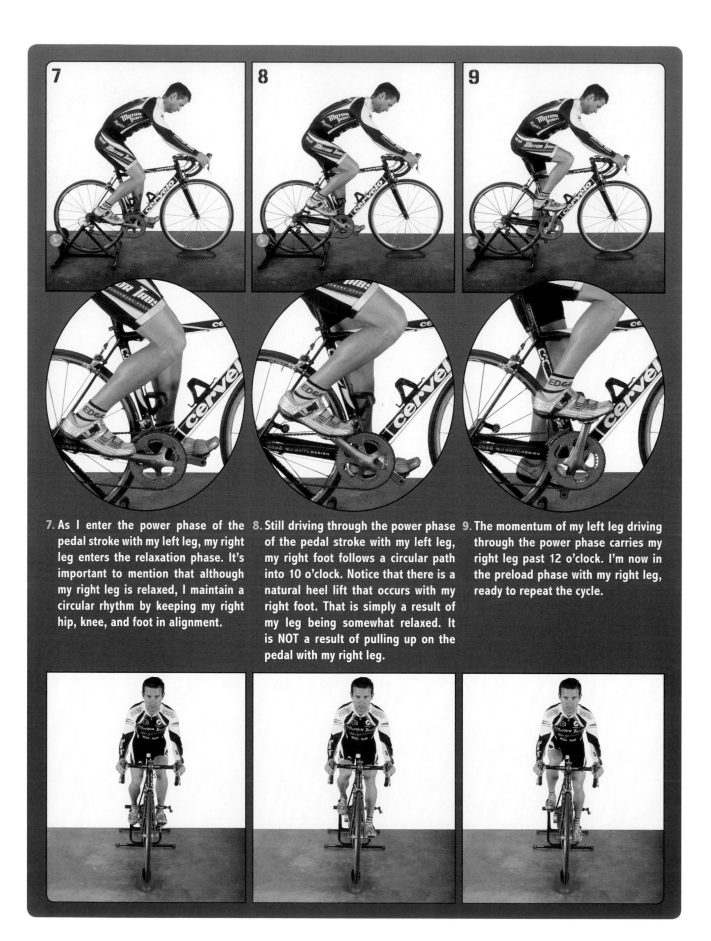

7. As I enter the power phase of the pedal stroke with my left leg, my right leg enters the relaxation phase. It's important to mention that although my right leg is relaxed, I maintain a circular rhythm by keeping my right hip, knee, and foot in alignment.

8. Still driving through the power phase of the pedal stroke with my left leg, my right foot follows a circular path into 10 o'clock. Notice that there is a natural heel lift that occurs with my right foot. That is simply a result of my leg being somewhat relaxed. It is NOT a result of pulling up on the pedal with my right leg.

9. The momentum of my left leg driving through the power phase carries my right leg past 12 o'clock. I'm now in the preload phase with my right leg, ready to repeat the cycle.

Common Fault: Heel Down

As illustrated in the previous sequence, your foot should be essentially parallel to the ground at all times. Aside from the natural heel lift that occurs at the top of the relaxation phase, you want to avoid driving into the pedal system with the heel of your foot. In addition to losing power, you open the door to a plethora of discomforts and injuries. If you notice that you're driving down with your heel, it could be that your saddle is too low or that you're midline is not engaged, causing you to rock your hips back and forth.

The former is a bike fit fault, and the latter is a mechanics fault, which can lead to hip and lower-back problems. The only time a slight heel drop is warranted when engaging the pedal system is if you're climbing a steep hill.

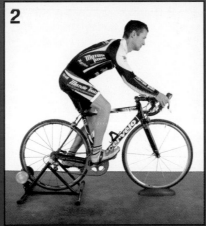

My right foot is positioned at 12 o'clock.

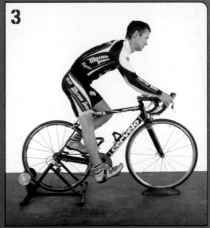

As I engage the pedal system, I make the mistake of pressing my heel down. Note that in addition to losing power, I compromise the integrity of my knee and ankle.

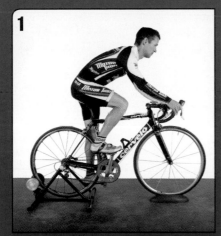

My leg straightens as I reach the bottom of the pedal stroke. This exaggerated stretch not only makes it difficult to maintain a fluid, circular rhythm, but also increases my chance of injury.

Common Fault: Elevated Heel

Just as with the previous fault, driving into the pedal system with your toes can be a result of poor mechanics or bike fit. If your saddle is too high, chances are you will reach for the pedals, which can cause you to elevate your heel. This is also a common fault among riders who haven't spent time developing their erectors, glutes, and hamstrings. If you're not strong in the areas of the body that you can't see in the mirror, you'll have the tendency to pick up the heel so that you can shift the load to your quadriceps. This not only restricts your ability to effectively drive through the power phase of the pedal stroke, but also compromises the integrity of your knee joint. (In the experienced racer/rider mentioned earlier who slides forward on the saddle for short-term speed, the heel may have a slightly more pronounced lift.)

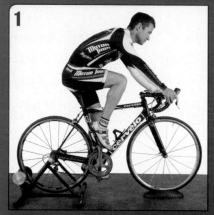 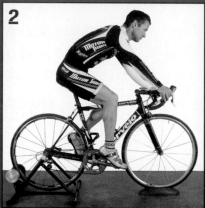 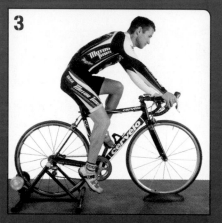

1 My right foot is positioned at 12 o'clock.	**2** I engage into the pedal system using the ball of my right foot. In addition to placing unnecessary stress on the ankle, this mechanics fault shuts off my hamstrings and glutes, causing me to lose power.	**3** I pedal through the power phase with my toes down, which not only puts the knee into a compensated position, but also disrupts the rhythm of the pedal stroke.

Common Fault: Knees In

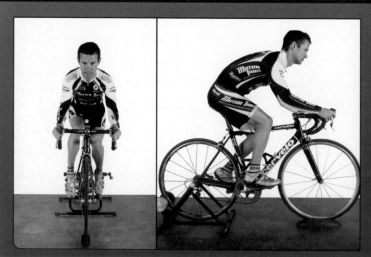

In an attempt to be more aerodynamic, some riders will tilt their knees in and strike into the pedal using the inside of their foot. This shuts off the lateral quadriceps (vastus lateralis) and glutes, reducing power, and shifts the majority of the demand to the medial quadriceps vastus medialis (VMO), which can invite injury.

My knees are internally rotated, causing my ankles, knees, and hips to fall out of alignment.

Common Fault: Knees Out

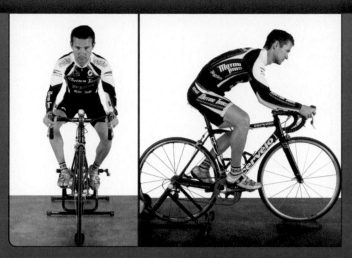

My knees are externally rotated, causing my ankles, knees, and hips to fall out of alignment.

As I mentioned before, when riders start to break down and fatigue they start to shift their position in an effort to save energy, but it usually has the exact opposite effect. The moment you deviate from proper riding position, you sacrifice power and efficiency. For example, if your knees are bowed out and you engage the pedal system with the outside of your foot, you're not only going to lose power by shutting off your VMOs, but you're also putting additional shear stress on the hip, knee, and ankle. It's like driving a nail down at an angle. You put down enough angular force and you're going to bend that nail.

Common Faults in Hip and Knee Alignment

Sometimes a rider will try to wrestle the bike to generate more power from the pedal system. This can also occur when you're in the wrong gear or you're putting too much effort into the pedal stroke. As you should already know, anytime your ankles, knees, hips, and shoulders track out of alignment, you sacrifice efficiency, power, and energy, as well as place additional torque on the body, which can lead to injury.

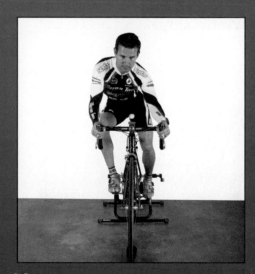

Tilted Out
My right knee is tilted out, the left side of my hips is being forced toward my left side, and I'm leveraging off the handlebars in an attempt to create power.

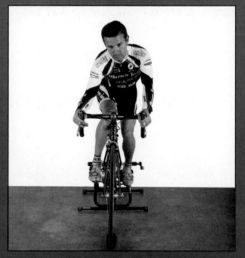

Tilted In
My right knee is tilted in, the left side of my hips is being forced toward my left side, and I'm leveraging off the handlebars in an attempt to create power.

SEATED CLIMB

As a rule of thumb, you need a reason to get out of the saddle, otherwise stay seated. If the hill is steep, you may have to stand to power over the top. But if you can stay in the saddle throughout the entire climb, that is the most efficient and effective strategy. To execute a seated climb, you need to slide back in the saddle slightly and reposition your hands on the handlebars. This gives you more stability on the bike, increases your ability to generate power through the pedal stroke, and is ergonomic.

If you make the mistake of leaving your hands on the brake hoods as you slide back, you end up reaching for the handlebars, effectively limiting the amount of power you can generate with your larger muscle groups. Another common mistake regarding grip is for your arms to be too wide on the handlebars. This is like doing a push press with your arms too wide, in that you lose power and place additional stress on the wrist, shoulder, and elbow joints.

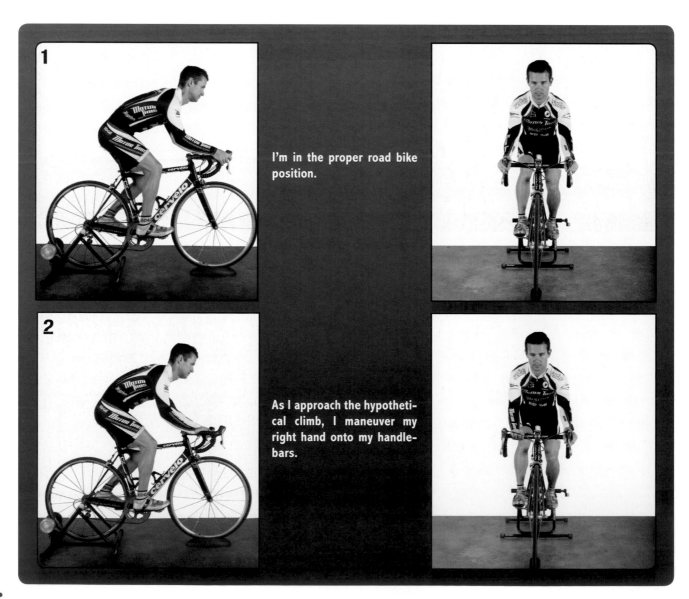

1 I'm in the proper road bike position.

2 As I approach the hypothetical climb, I maneuver my right hand onto my handlebars.

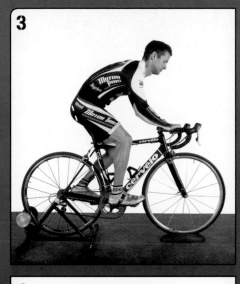

3

I place my left hand on the handlebars and assume the seated-climb position. It's important to notice that my knuckles, wrists, and shoulders are in line.

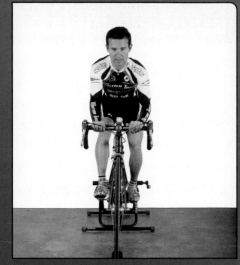

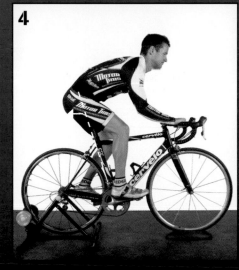

4

To compensate for gravity and the grade of the climb, I slide back slightly in the saddle.

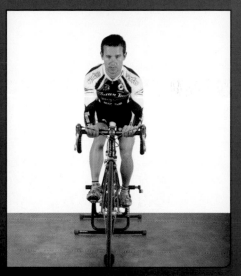

Common Fault: External Rotation

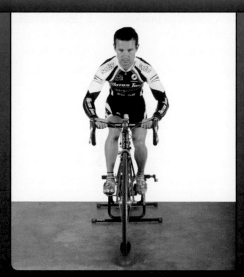

A lot of cyclists will position their hands too wide on the handlebars, which makes it difficult to keep their knuckles, wrists, and shoulders in line. Just as with all the positional faults illustrated in this chapter, this causes you to fatigue at a faster rate and limits your ability to control the bike.

I've formed my grip on the handlebars next to the brake hoods. Unable to keep my wrists and arms in line because of my wide grip, my triceps give way and my elbows bow out.

SLIGHT HEEL DROP

Executing a slight heel drop as you pedal can be a good technique when climbing from the seated position. It not only maximizes power output by engaging the powerful muscles of your posterior chain, but also helps to work with gravity. But make sure you've still got that 25- 35-degree bend in your knee. To avoid a loss of power, be careful not to exaggerate the heel drop to the point that your leg straightens.

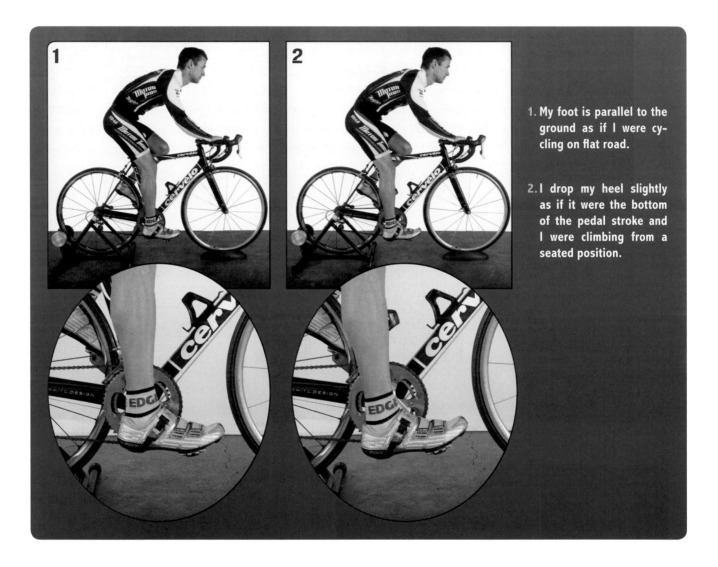

1. My foot is parallel to the ground as if I were cycling on flat road.

2. I drop my heel slightly as if it were the bottom of the pedal stroke and I were climbing from a seated position.

STANDING CLIMB

As I have mentioned, climbing should be done mostly in the saddle, which is the most sustainable and energy-efficient position. The moment you stand up, you have to use your upper body to stabilize the bike (maintain GCM) and you exert more energy to power through the pedal stroke. That said, if you're climbing an extremely steep hill and you can't maintain momentum while seated, you might have no other option than to stand. In such a situation, you should stand up, power over the top of the hill, and then return to the seated position as fast as possible. Timing is critical. To avoid losing momentum or sacrificing a break in cadence, you have to time your position change with the pedal stroke. As your crank arm passes 12 o'clock and you enter the power phase of the pedal stroke, stand up and use your weight to drive through the power phase of the pedal stroke. If you stand up before your crank arm passes 12 o'clock, you may actually fall backward, which will cause you to lose power and momentum. A bike computer that measures your RPMs and cadence can also be used to indicate when to stand. For example, on most climbs your RPMs should be between 60 and 80. If you're going up a steep hill and your cadence drops below 60, it's either time to stand, or you need to drop into a more efficient gear.

Another situation, which may warrant getting out of the saddle, is on long climbs: say it's a 10-mile climb at an 8 percent grade. Although staying the saddle is more efficient, standing for 10 to 20 pedal strokes and then sitting back down will help you reestablish rhythm and flush out (open up) your legs.

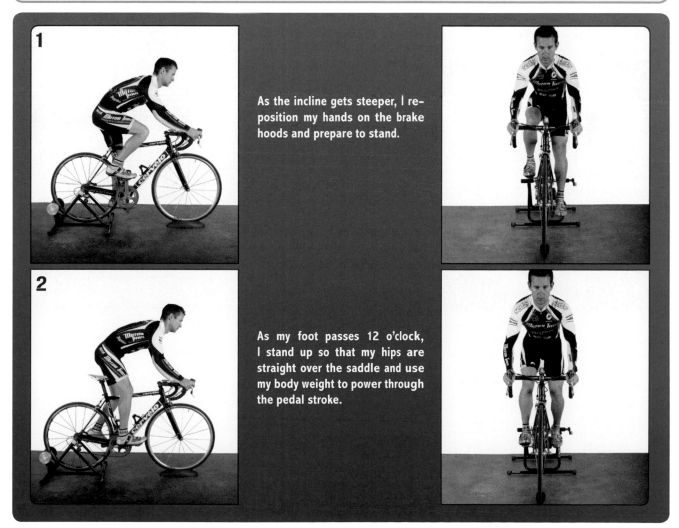

1

As the incline gets steeper, I re-position my hands on the brake hoods and prepare to stand.

2

As my foot passes 12 o'clock, I stand up so that my hips are straight over the saddle and use my body weight to power through the pedal stroke.

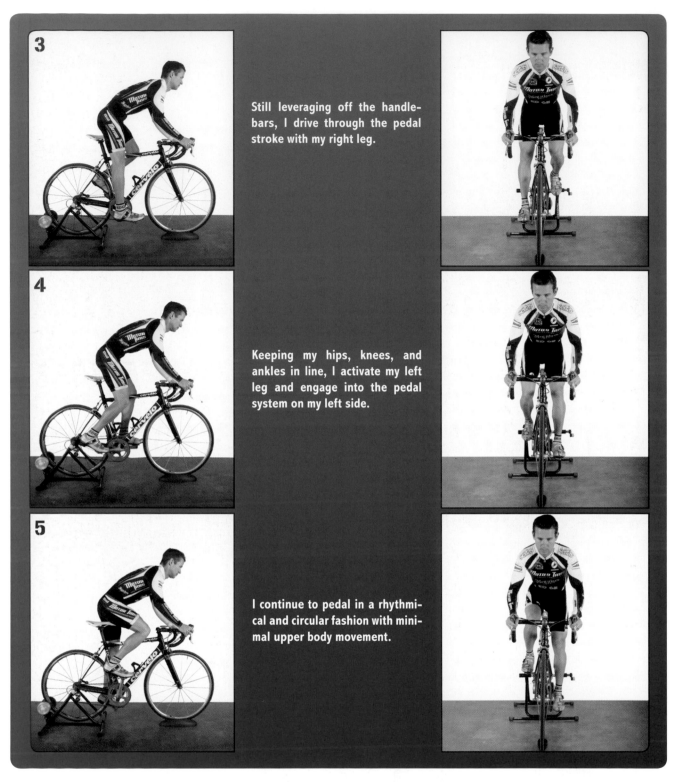

3 Still leveraging off the handlebars, I drive through the pedal stroke with my right leg.

4 Keeping my hips, knees, and ankles in line, I activate my left leg and engage into the pedal system on my left side.

5 I continue to pedal in a rhythmical and circular fashion with minimal upper body movement.

Technical Note: Although it's difficult to illustrate in photos, there should be as little upper-body movement as possible. Remember, your body moves the bike, not the other way around. For example, if you're riding a road bike up a hill, you can leverage off the handlebars using the power of your upper body (shifting body weight from hand to hand). As a result, the bike moves from side to side, but your upper body moves very little. This not only allows you to pedal more efficiently, but also maximizes power and energy output. If you're on an indoor trainer, on the other hand, your upper body may move a little more because of the limited mobility of the bike.

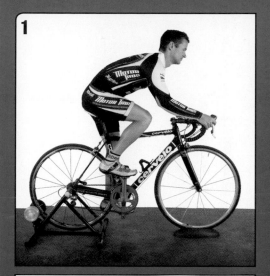

When you get out of the saddle your body should be centered over the bike and you should maintain good posture. A common fault is for riders to lean over the handlebars. By shifting your body weight over the front tire, you reduce traction from your back tire, limit your ability to control the bike, and decrease the power you can generate through the pedal stroke. In short, you slow down, risk crashing, and expend twice as much energy.

As the incline gets steeper, I reposition my hands on the brake hoods and prepare to stand.

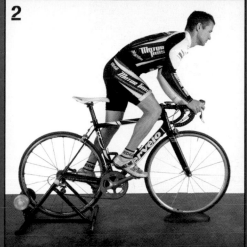

I make the mistake of leaning forward as I get out of the saddle. Notice that my head is over the front hub. With my arms supporting the full pressure of my upper body, it's difficult to steer the bike.

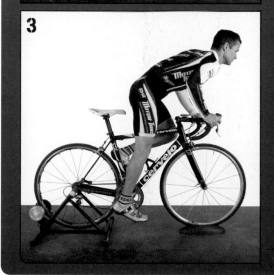

As a result of my forward lean, my pedaling mechanics break down into short, choppy strokes, causing me to lose power, and I lose the ability to steer the bike.

SHORT-RANGE ACCELERATION

There are moments in a race when you need to bridge a gap, pass a rider who is losing it, or prevent someone from overtaking your position in the field. In these situations, you don't want to expend too much energy by transitioning to the drops and standing for a full-on sprint. Save that for the finish. Instead, you should transition into a slightly more aerodynamic and powerful position so that you can put the hammer down and accelerate for a short distance—200 meters or a gap of more than 30 seconds.

If you glance at the photos, you'll notice that I've assumed a modified time-trial position by sliding forward in the saddle and establishing a modified grip on my brake hoods. The former puts a little more bend in the knee, which places a lot more demand on the quadriceps and VMO, while the latter is a more aerodynamic position and allows you to leverage off the handlebars to generate more power. It's important to mention that shutting off the posterior chain in this manner is usually a strategy to avoid, but for a short-range acceleration it's acceptable. Your quads will burn like crazy as you hammer down, so having your hamstrings and glutes fresh when you settle back into the saddle will work to your advantage.

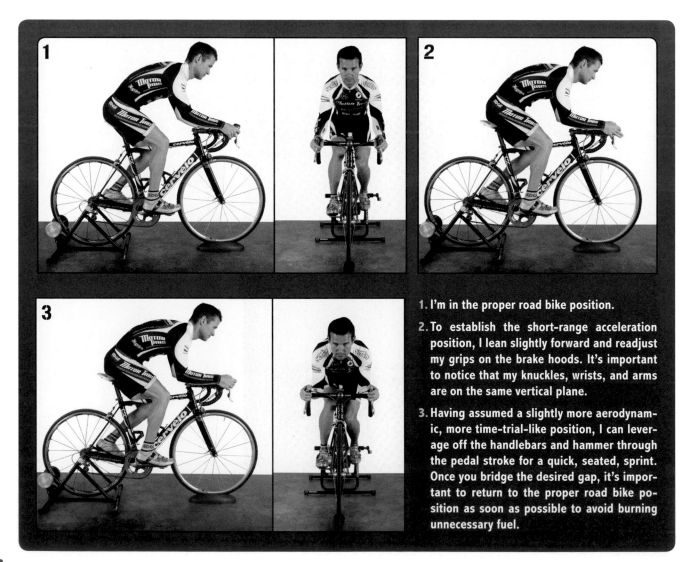

1. I'm in the proper road bike position.

2. To establish the short-range acceleration position, I lean slightly forward and readjust my grips on the brake hoods. It's important to notice that my knuckles, wrists, and arms are on the same vertical plane.

3. Having assumed a slightly more aerodynamic, more time-trial-like position, I can leverage off the handlebars and hammer through the pedal stroke for a quick, seated, sprint. Once you bridge the desired gap, it's important to return to the proper road bike position as soon as possible to avoid burning unnecessary fuel.

STANDING FINISH

There is much to be said about taking an emotionally calm yet strong mind into the final leg of a race. When it comes down to the wire (or the city sign in your local group ride) all hell breaks loose. With the finish line in sight, the lead group goes all out for the final sprint. Riders are leaning and bumping into each other to jockey for position.

It is during this last leg, in which fatigue, adrenaline, and a reckless sense of abandon take hold, when critical mistakes are made. The most common mistake is standing up too early for the final sprint, causing riders to blow up, slow down, and ultimately lose position. Remember, you pay the cost for standing in the form of energy. The longer you stand, the more energy you have to dole out. To prevent blowing up before the finish line, stay seated, click into a higher gear as you approach the 1,000-meter mark, and hammer down. As a rule, you should pop out of the saddle only in the last 30 seconds to get some leverage off your handlebars so you can go hard, harder, hardest, throwing caution to the winds and completely emptying your tank in one spectacular sprint.

Sequence A: Standing Sprint

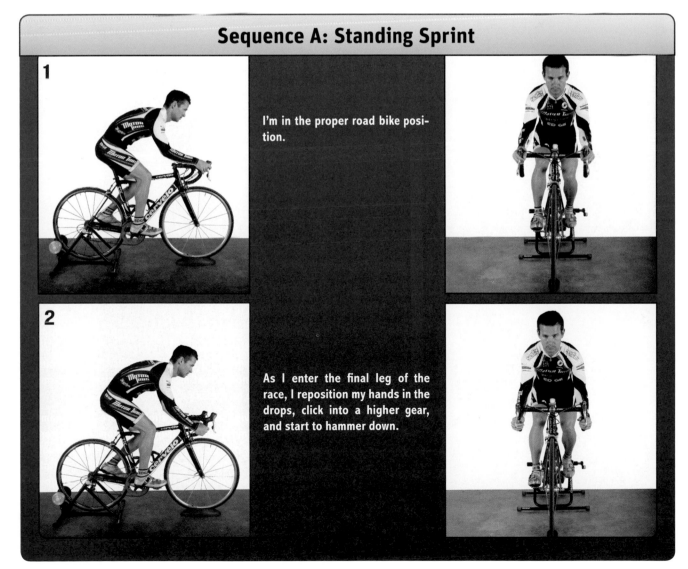

1 I'm in the proper road bike position.

2 As I enter the final leg of the race, I reposition my hands in the drops, click into a higher gear, and start to hammer down.

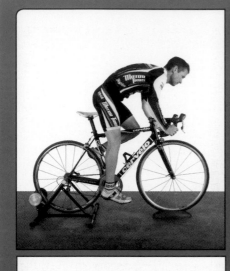

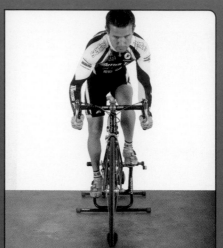

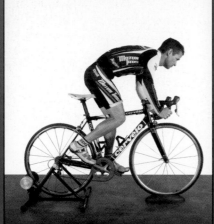

3

As I approach the finish line, I get out of the saddle, lean forward slightly, and use my body weight to help power through the pedal stroke. It's important to note that although I'm leveraging off the handlebars, I'm not moving my body excessively to one side or the other; rather I stay almost vertical (see Sequence B). It's also important to note that just as in the standing climb you shouldn't get out of the saddle until your dominant leg passes 12 o'clock. This allows you to strike down using your body weight, which generates more power.

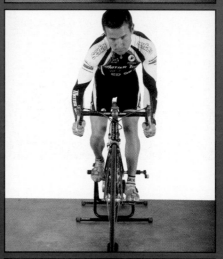

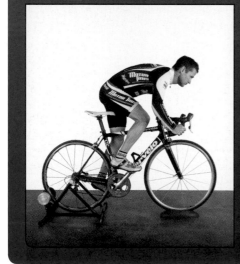

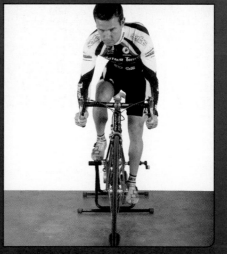

Sequence B: Bike-to-Body Lean

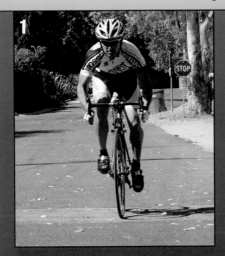

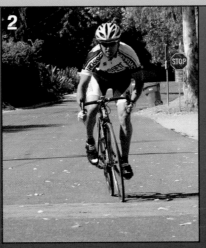

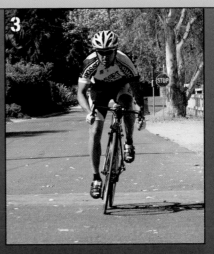

I get out of the saddle and lean slightly forward just as my right foot passes 12 o'clock.

As I stand up and drive my right leg through the power phase of the pedal stroke, I leverage off the handlebars and tilt the bike toward my right side. It's imperative to notice that my upper body remains perpendicular to the bike.

Keeping my upper body vertical, I continue to pedal and leverage off the handlebars, tilting the bike toward my left side.

Common Fault: Excessive Bike Whip

It's important to mention that a little bit of bike whip is fine when you get out of the saddle and really start pedaling hard. However, you want to avoid excessive bike whip, meaning that your body and bike lean in opposite directions. To generate the most power possible, upper-body movement should be kept to a minimum. In other words, your bike will move as a result of you leveraging off the handlebars, but your upper body should remain in roughly the same position.

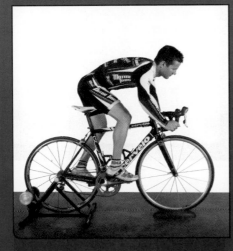

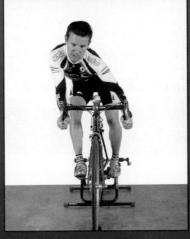

Although it's difficult to illustrate on a stationary bike, excessive bike whip occurs when you're leaning too far to one side. Here I illustrate this by leaning too far to my right side as I leverage off the handlebars. In reality, my bike would be tilted toward my left. However, here, I'm still out of position. In order to keep pedaling, I wrestle the bike to my opposite side while trying to maintain a fluid cadence.

Common Fault: Leaning Too Far Forward

Another common fault riders make when standing for the final sprint is leaning too far over their handlebars. Just as on a standing climb, you should limit the distance between your butt and the saddle. The moment your hips track over the nose of seat, you lose control of the front of the bike, pedaling mechanics devolve into choppy, inefficient strokes, and your legs can no longer generate maximum power. Compounded with the fact that it's the end of the race and you're already suffering from exhaustion and you're asking for trouble.

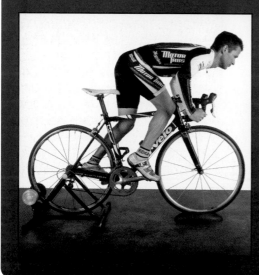

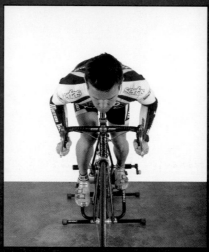

Here I'm illustrating a forward lean in the sprint. Just as I demonstrated in the standing climb, this positional fault causes a mechanical breakdown of the pedal stroke, causing you to lose power, and reduces your ability to control and steer the bike.

DESCENDING

Descending is an undervalued art form. It's part technique and part madness. Just as in running, to be efficient you must understand the importance of body control, using a slight lean to dictate direction, and using gravity and momentum to your advantage. A lot of riders, whether out of fear or neglect, overlook this aspect of racing in their training and focus solely on building power and stamina on the climb.

While it's imperative that you train for the climb, you must also spend considerable time working on your descending skills. You go downhill every time you get to the top of a mountain, so take the time to master the skill—you could be the first to the top but the last one to the finish line (unless, of course, it's a mountaintop finish). In other words, don't mindlessly cruise downhill after a hard climb as if you're taking a Sunday stroll. Adjust your grip, get into an aerodynamic position by leaning forward, pinch your thighs against the top tube for control, and attack the descent with as much determination as you did the ascent. I've seen a lot of riders who are not strong climbers close the gap to the lead group because they are masters at descending. There are, of course, different strategies for bombing down a mountain. Choosing which technique to implement is based on the course and your skill set. And don't forget to enjoy the ride: for me, descending is an opportunity to experience freedom and appreciate the feel of the road beneath me.

Descending: Drops

If you're going down a hill with a lot of curves, it's better to be in the drops so as not to compromise your ability to corner. This is also a great position for novice and intermediate racers because it gives you a lot of control over the bike and allows you to easily reach the brakes should you hit speeds outside your comfort zone.

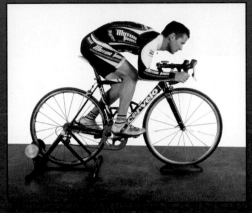

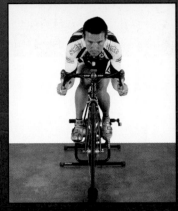

1. To assume the proper position, I place my hands in the drops for optimal control, bring my upper body as close to the bike as possible to reduce wind resistance, and pinch my knees against the top tub to stabilize against speed wobbles. It's important to note that your weight should be evenly distributed between the front and back tire and that you think of your body and the bike becoming one machine as you lower your upper body into position.

Descending: Handlebars

If you're an experienced rider bombing down a straight hill, you can place your hands on the handlebars next to the stem, drop down into an aerodynamic position, and aggressively attack the hill. Note that you will lose the ability to corner sharp curves, so you really have to know the course.

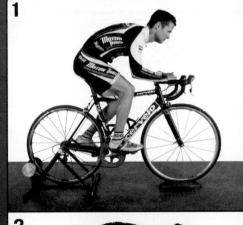

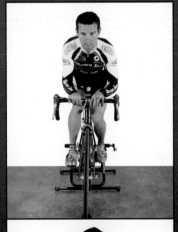

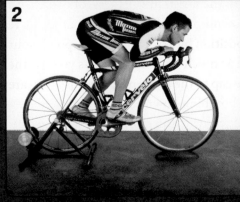

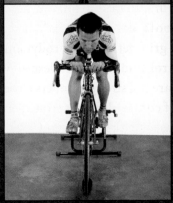

1. I'm in the seated-climb position. It's important to notice that I hook my thumbs around the handlebars for control as I position myself for the descent. Although this is not as important, but still advisable, when climbing, it is absolutely imperative when descending a steep hill.

2. To assume the proper position, I lower my upper body and become as one with the bike as possible by tucking my head between my hands and bringing my chest as close as possible to the top tube.

Descending: Behind the Saddle

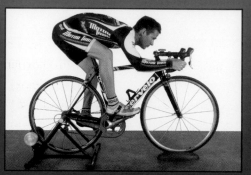

To assume the behind-the-saddle position, I place my hands in the drops, maneuver my hips behind the seat, and then rest my abdomen on the saddle.

Dropping behind the saddle is a highly advanced technique that not a whole lot of riders utilize, and for good reason. It can be extremely dangerous if you don't know what you're doing. Just like the former option, you have to really know the course because your ability to corner is limited. If you glance at the photo, you'll notice that I'm actually resting my abdomen on the saddle. From here, I can control the bike lean with my chest and use the pedals as rudders to help steer the bike. Although I would not recommend this strategy to most riders, it's an excellent way to pick up additional speed and give your legs a rest on long downhills.

CORNERING

Cornering is similar to going downhill in that it is an undervalued skill and often exposes the rider's confidence in his ability to properly weight and unweight the bike. Like other skills, cornering takes time to develop. You have to attack the corner in an aggressive fashion, which takes self-assurance, guts, and at times a touch of recklessness. I've broken down cornering into three distinct, yet simple, categories: the approach, in the corner, and the exit.

The Approach:

As a rule, you should always ride the straightest line possible through a corner to avoid losing speed and expending excess energy. To ensure the best entry and exit, you have to set up your position during the approach, which is the brief window of time you have before you enter the corner. It's the time to measure the angle of the turn to determine your best line of attack.

For example, if you're approaching a sharp corner, you have to set up for the turn by taking the outside lane and then cut the corner as tightly as possible: think of a NASCAR racer approaching a sharp turn. Taking the straightest line in and out of the corner maximizes speed, distance, and energy expenditure.

If you're approaching a wider and longer corner, on the other hand, you can cut your approach closer, meaning that you don't have to float to the outside as you enter the turn, while still maintaining a straight line through the turn. As you calculate your approach, it's important that you set your gearing so that you can accelerate out of the corner, as well as factor in the next turn, your position in the pack, and your desired velocity. All of these factors affect how you should attack and safely exit the corner.

Regardless of the angle, the goal is to maintain speed going into the corner and to minimize braking. When riders are apprehensive, they often tap their brakes or take the wrong line, causing them to lose a lot of speed. As a result, they not only compromise their position in the corner, which increases their chances of a crash, but also have to exert additional energy in the exit.

To approach the corner correctly, transition into the drops—the safest and most stable position—and continue pedaling as you approach the corner. It's important to mention that if you need to brake while cornering you should do it prior to initiating any significant lean to avoid compromising your position and velocity. As you enter the corner, stop pedaling to avoid scraping or catching the inside of the pedal on the road, lift your inside leg to the twelve o'clock position, and "point" that knee and your head (eyes) in the direction you want to "exit" the turn. As you stop pedaling, start leaning toward the inside of the corner by shifting your body weight to the inside. To maintain speed and proper balance, be sure to keep pressure on both front and back wheels by keeping your body centered on the bike (front to back).

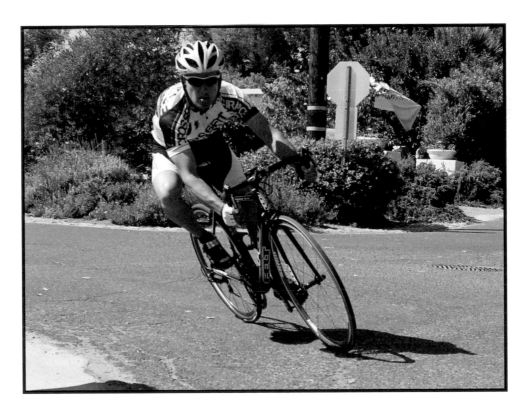

In the Corner:

While in the corner, most riders will either have a rush of adrenaline or a rush of fear! Regardless of your response, you want to stay seated and maintain a solid, rigid, and confident body position. This is your time to surf through the corner and allow your speed to carry you through as if you were riding a wave. Note that you should brake and pedal only if the corner is wide and long. The key is to trust your approach, commit to the corner, and allow your bike to react to your lean as gravity and inertia take you through it.

It's important to note that the more aggressive your lean, the faster you will get through the corner. But be extremely careful not to lean too far. If you miscalculate by loading too much weight on the inside or outside of the bike, chances are you will crash. To prevent this, keep your rear end firmly rooted in the saddle and your inside knee and eyes pointed toward the exit.

The Exit:

As you emerge from the corner, you should already be in a favorable gear, which you set during the approach, so that you can accelerate out of the corner as you transition back into a vertical position.

The two most common faults in cornering are changing gears several times while accelerating and hesitating out of the corner. The former can compromise the rhythm of the pedal stroke and distract the rider's focus, causing him to slow down, while the latter is usually a brain fart. Sometimes riders become complacent after successfully attacking the corner and then forget to accelerate as they exit. To prevent a delay, imagine that a pack of ravenous dogs are chasing you—that should do the trick! Another important point is your grip. To ensure a fluid and rapid exit, your hands should be in the drops and you should maintain a powerful body position (engaged core). That way, if you need to change gears or momentarily get out of the saddle to generate additional speed, you can do so without wasting time or compromising the efficiency of your position.

Technical Note: Cornering on wet or sandy surfaces requires practice and an attention to safety. In most cases, you should slow down, adjust your center of gravity on the bike, and reduce the degree of your lean.

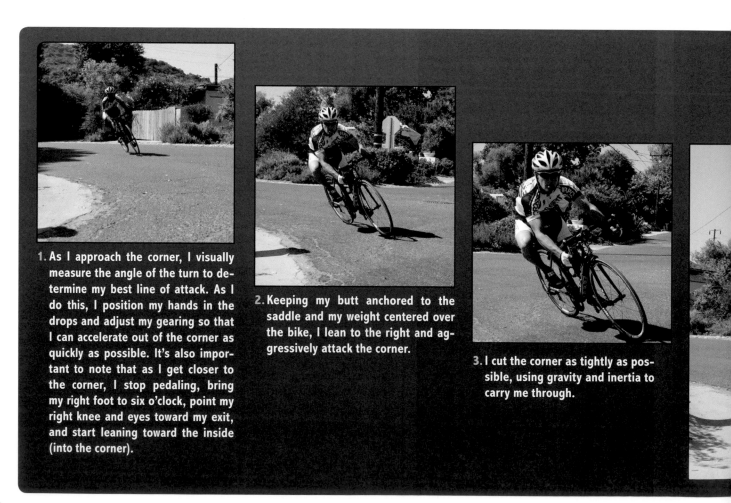

1. As I approach the corner, I visually measure the angle of the turn to determine my best line of attack. As I do this, I position my hands in the drops and adjust my gearing so that I can accelerate out of the corner as quickly as possible. It's also important to note that as I get closer to the corner, I stop pedaling, bring my right foot to six o'clock, point my right knee and eyes toward my exit, and start leaning toward the inside (into the corner).

2. Keeping my butt anchored to the saddle and my weight centered over the bike, I lean to the right and aggressively attack the corner.

3. I cut the corner as tightly as possible, using gravity and inertia to carry me through.

Cornering Faults

Although capturing the bike-to-body lean is impossible to illustrate on a stationary bike, I've detailed a few common faults that are important to note when learning proper cornering mechanics.

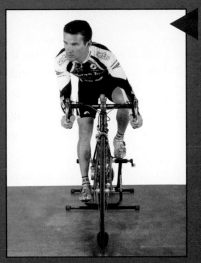

Common Fault: Pedal Down
If you fail to pull your inside leg up coming into a turn, you risk clipping your pedal or foot on the ground as you lean into the corner. To prevent this from happening, be sure to pull your inside leg up to the twelve o'clock position as you approach the corner.

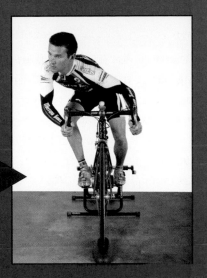

Common Fault: Too Much Lean
Sometimes cyclists will lean too far off the bike and slide off the saddle as they enter the corner. With your tires unweighted, you will lose traction and wash out. To prevent this from happening, keep your butt glued to the saddle and be cautious when you lean.

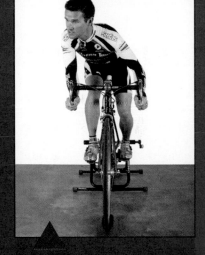

4. As I exit the corner, I start pedaling, transition to a vertical riding position, and work on accelerating as fast as possible without sacrificing rhythm.

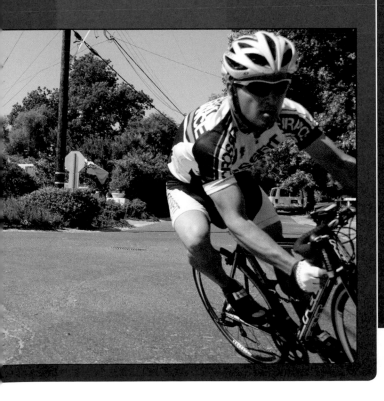

Common Fault: Upper-Body Lean
A lot of inexperienced riders lean their upper body into the corner but make the mistake of failing to point with their knee. As a result, the rider's ability to steer the bike is compromised, which increases the likelihood of a crash. To avoid this, point your knee and eyes in the direction of your exit and then shift your upper body over that leg while keeping your butt in the saddle. This allows you to control the bike lean and hug the corner without compromising speed or control.

Time-Trial Bike

Unlike the road bike, which has a lot of versatility, time-trial bikes are built for one thing: speed. Think of the time-trial bike as a dragster and the road bike like a fine Audi or Porsche. The former does really well on straight, flat roads, while the latter can handle pretty much anything you throw at it. For that reason, the time-trial bike—just like the dragster—is primarily used in events or courses that are short, flat, straight, and fast.

By definition a time trial is a race against the clock. No hiding, no drafting, no pack-surfing—just raw power. Time-trial races can be anywhere from 8 to 40 kilometers. They are usually the prologue in a stage race, with each rider going off separately. The time trial is also popular among triathletes.

With the majority of races taking place on straight, flat roads, the TT bike is engineered to be way faster than a road bike. Not only that, the bike's geometry places the rider in a position that demands more from the quadriceps, which leaves the hamstrings fresh for the run that follows in a triathlon. It's important to mention that although some courses have undulating terrain, the TT bike is not designed for efficient turning, climbing, or descending. If you're racing in a time-trial event that has a lot of hills and turns, you may want to consider using your road bike.

Another point worth mentioning is the positional stress and strength requirements of the time-trial bike. In addition to putting you in a lower, more physically demanding and aggressive position, the majority of TT bikes have only one huge chainring—with 54 or 55 teeth—which makes turning over a heavy gear more difficult.

If you haven't done proper strength-and-conditioning training or spent enough time on the TT bike, you're going to fatigue faster than you would on a road bike. To be a good time-trialist you have to spend time on your TT bike, regardless of how experienced a road rider you are. While there are some parallels that can be drawn between the road bike and the TT bike, it's a completely different animal. You have to give your body an opportunity to adapt to the new position and mechanics, which can be accomplished only through sport-specific training. In this section, I will break down the ideal TT position, discuss essential strategies, and shed light on some common faults.

PROPER TIME-TRIAL POSITION

The TT cyclist is a lot like a ballet dancer in that there is a lot of power and body control involved but it's not obvious. For example, when a ballerina spins on her toes, it looks effortless, but in fact it takes a lot of strength, power, and stability to perform the movement. The same is true with the TT position. An experienced rider will look relaxed, fluid, and rhythmic as he powers through the pedal stroke with minimal upper-body movement. Although he's working very hard—pedaling mechanics, shifting of the gears, drinking, and breathing—everything is working in concert, making the rider look as though he's not exerting that much energy.

To create the least wind resistance, the proper TT position puts you in the most aerodynamic and efficient position possible so you can ride as fast as you can. With your upper body blending in with the bike, you want to slide slightly forward so that you can generate maximum power with your legs without compromising efficiency and energy. If you glance at the photos, you'll notice that the back of the saddle is visible. This variation in position shifts slightly more demand onto the powerful muscles of your quadriceps, which allows you to generate a little bit more power.

It's important to note that unlike on a road bike, a good TT rider will rarely change his hand positions. The command center is in front of the bike. Your weight is distributed over your forearms, which are responsible for steering, while your hands control the gears. The only time you should deviate from this position is if you hit a steep climb or a sharp curve. Aside from those situations, you want to remain locked and loaded in the proper position for the duration of the race or training interval.

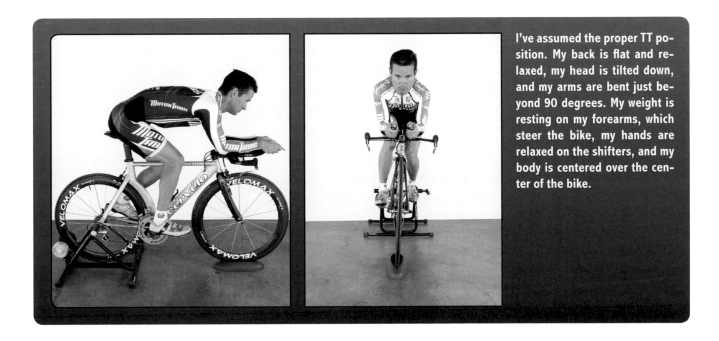

I've assumed the proper TT position. My back is flat and relaxed, my head is tilted down, and my arms are bent just beyond 90 degrees. My weight is resting on my forearms, which steer the bike, my hands are relaxed on the shifters, and my body is centered over the center of the bike.

Common Fault: Rounded Back

Remember, if the bike fit wasn't carried out correctly it can be difficult to achieve the proper position on the bike. For example, if the top tube is too short or if the aero bars or saddle is positioned too far forward, you'll end up with a rounded back. If you had a good bike fit, a rounded back is a result of fatigue or a lack of strength to maintain the proper TT position. So if your low back is weak, you don't have good midline stability, and you haven't spent time strengthening your posterior chain, you're probably going to round forward the moment you start to get tired. Think of it like sitting in a chair. The longer you sit in that chair without consciously being engaged in a correct ergonomic position, the more you shift into a sloppier and less efficient position.

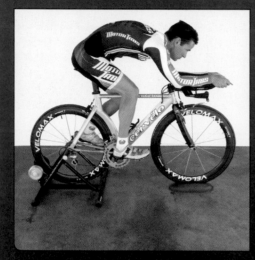 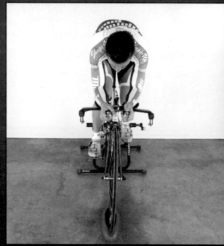

I've compromised the integrity of my position by rounding my back.

Common Fault: Head Lift

A lot of riders make the mistake of lifting their head up to see. In addition to compromising the integrity of the neck, you reduce the aerodynamics of your position. To keep your spine in the proper alignment, keep your head tilted slightly down with your eyes gazing forward.

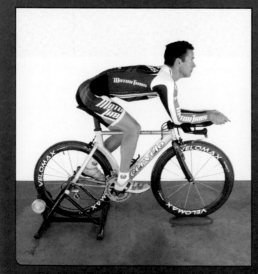 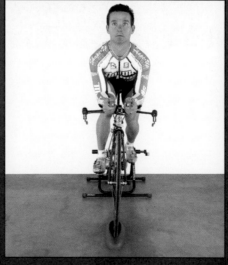

I've made the mistake of lifting my head up to see. This not only weakens my position, but also increases wind resistance.

Common Fault: (Saddle Position) Too Far Forward

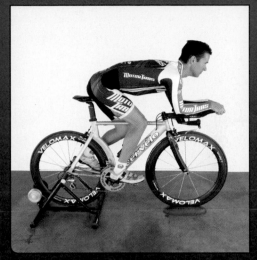

It's important to note that there is a difference between sliding forward in the saddle and being too far forward in the saddle. For example, sliding forward from the proper TT position is warranted when you're climbing up a short incline. However, if you're too far forward in the saddle during the duration of your ride, you're going to put too much pressure on your upper body, which causes an uneven distribution of weight on the bike. With the rear wheel un-weighted, you compromise your speed as well as your ability to control the bike.

I'm too far forward in the saddle. With my arms supporting the weight of my upper body and my hips positioned over the nose of the saddle, I'm unable to effectively steer the bike or generate power through the pedal stroke.

Common Fault: (Saddle Position) Too Far Back

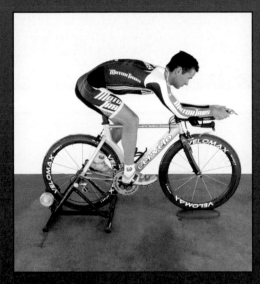

A lot of people make the mistake of sliding too far back in the saddle. If you glance at the photo you'll notice that my hips are positioned over the rear hub of the wheel and my arms are extended. This causes a loss of power and efficiency in your pedal stroke, places additional stress on your low back, which makes it more difficult to stabilize on the bike, and impedes your ability to steer.

I'm positioned too far back in the saddle. This not only compromises the mechanics of my pedal stroke, but also forces me to reach for the aero bars, giving me less control over the bike.

Common Fault: Hands Too Far Back

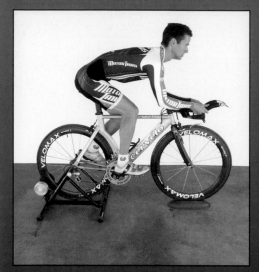

I've positioned my hands too far back on the aero bars. This not only reduces the aerodynamics of the position, but also limits my ability to control the bike.

Positioning your hands too far back on the aero bars is common with riders who haven't spent enough time in the proper TT position. Just as with sitting too far back in the saddle, this position reduces power and efficiency, increases the onset of fatigue, and reduces your ability to control the bike. Again, maintaining the proper TT position is not easy. In fact, a lot of riders find it difficult to maintain the proper TT position longer than five minutes.

The only way to get comfortable with the proper TT position is to spend time skill-training the position. By that I mean, sit on your trainer at home and practice maintaining that position for prolonged periods of time. As a rule, you should spend one out of every three rides at home on the trainer practicing just the position when first starting out. As your body adjusts, adapts, and strengthens, you can devote more time to actual training rides.

Common Fault: Shoulders Up

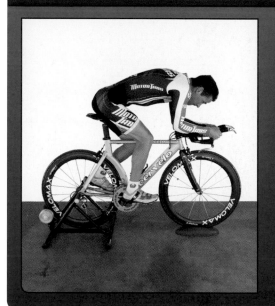

Shrugging your shoulders and dropping your head is another clear indication that fatigue has set in. As I mentioned before, in order to maintain the proper TT position you must have a strong upper body. If your upper body is weak, the pressure of your weight will eventually cause your shoulders to collapse into a shrugged position. This almost always leads to a head drop, which places additional stress on your cervical spine and makes it difficult to see.

Unable to maintain the proper position, my shoulders shrug and my head drops.

Common Fault: Mechanics Breakdown

As I mentioned before, everyone responds differently to fatigue. Some riders exhibit the faults previously illustrated, while others sit up and revert to a road bike position. Again, if you haven't trained to maintain the proper TT position, as you get tired you're going to shift into less aerodynamic positions that compromise your ability to generate power and steer the bike.

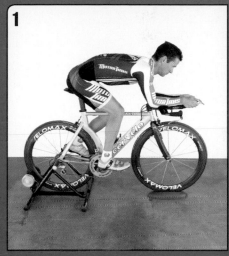

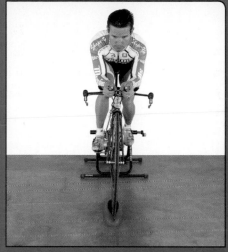

I'm in the proper TT position.

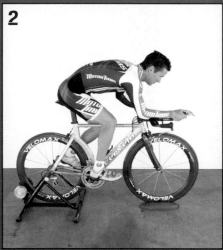

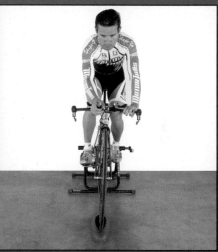

As fatigue sets in, I'm unable to maintain the proper position, and I start to default into a road bike posture in an attempt to relieve the suffering.

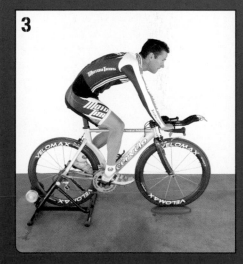

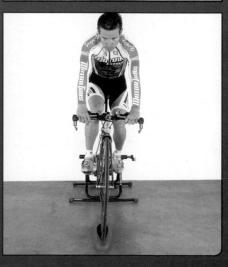

I assume a road bike position. All is lost at this point.

PEDAL STROKE

Aside from your position, the pedal stroke on the TT bike is the same as on the road bike in that you want to keep your heel parallel to the ground and your hips, knees, and ankles in line. The common faults are also the same. You want to avoid tracking your knees in or out, pointing your toes, and striking down with your heel. For a more elaborate explanation of the mechanics of the pedal stroke, flip back to the section devoted to the road bike.

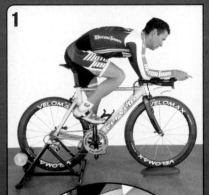

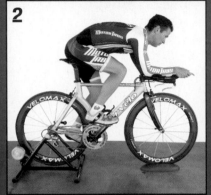

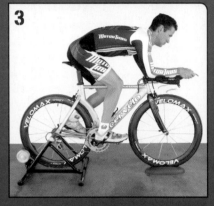

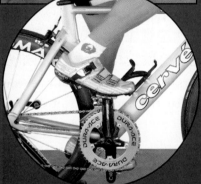

1. I'm in the proper position with my right foot positioned at 12 o'clock. Notice that my foot is parallel to the ground.

2. Keeping my foot parallel to the ground, I start pedaling at about one o'clock with my right leg and enter the preloading phase.

3. As I pass two o'clock, I enter the power phase of the pedal stroke. It's important to note that my left leg is completely relaxed.

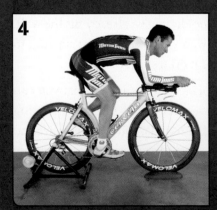

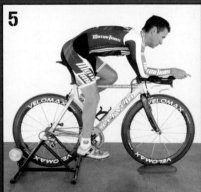

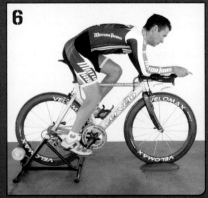

4. Having exerted the most drive through three and four o'clock, I begin to reduce the power of my strike.

5. Still keeping my foot parallel to the ground and my hip, knee, and foot in alignment, I allow the momentum of my strike to carry my right foot through to six o'clock.

6. As my right foot passes through six o'clock, I preload my left leg and prepare to engage into the left side of the pedal system.

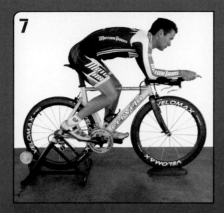

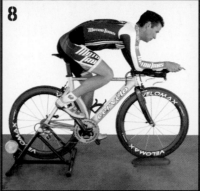

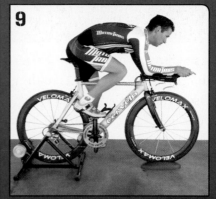

7. As I enter the power phase of the pedal stroke with my left leg, my right leg enters the relaxation phase. It's important to mention that although my right leg is relaxed, I maintain a circular rhythm by keeping my right hip, knee, and foot in alignment.

8. Still driving through the power phase of the pedal stroke with my left leg, my right foot follows a circular path into 10 o'clock. Notice that a natural heel lift occurs with my right foot. That is simply a result of my leg being somewhat relaxed. It is NOT a result of me pulling up on the pedal with my right leg.

9. The momentum of my left leg driving through the power phase carries my right leg to 12 o'clock. I'm now in the preload phase with my right leg, ready to repeat the cycle.

COUNTDOWN START

If you're racing in a short-time trial event—anything less than 20 kilometers—the race can literally be won or lost out of the blocks. Although the majority of time-trial athletes realize the importance of starting strong, not too many riders have a strategy for the start.

Here's what often happens: As the countdown begins, you place your hands on the handlebars. With 10 seconds to go, you clench the grips and tense up in anticipation. The moment the whistle blows, you take off, hammer down on the pedals, and accelerate up to speed. There is a massive adrenaline dump; your heart rate is through the roof, your lungs are on fire, and your muscles are burning. And you're not even through the first third of the course. By the time you reach the halfway point, you've already hit the wall. Your rhythm is off, you're no longer able to maintain an ideal position, and your muscles are starting to shut down. Finishing strong is no longer feasible. You lost the race before it even started.

To avoid making this all too common mistake, you want to stay as relaxed as possible so that you can maximize your acceleration from the start and reserve energy. As the countdown begins, remain sitting up with your midline stabilized. Take a couple of deep breaths. At about 10 seconds, spin your legs around and position your feet in the power position (assuming you have a holder). At five seconds, start to slowly lower your body and position your hands on the handlebars. The moment you hear the gun or whistle, blast off in a standing sprint and accelerate up to speed. After about 10 or 12 pedal strokes (or 10 or 12 seconds), find a comfortable gear, settle down into the saddle, and get into a rhythm. Your heart rate should be steady, and you should have plenty of energy reserves to carry you through the entire race. Assuming that you've trained properly, finishing strong and leaving everything you have on the course shouldn't be an issue.

1

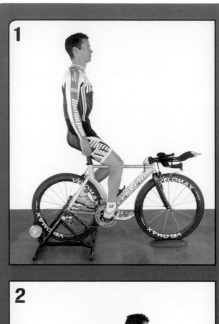

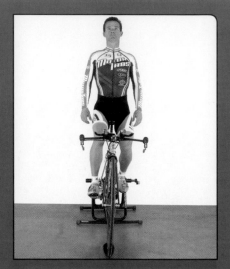

I'm sitting comfortably on the saddle with my midline stabilized. I'm breathing deep and staying as relaxed as possible.

2

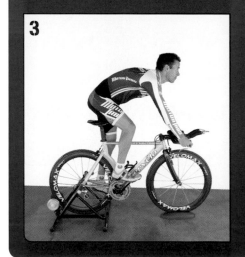

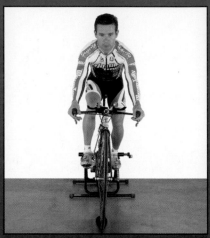

As the clock counts down to five seconds to go, I slowly lower my torso and assume my grip on the handlebars.

3

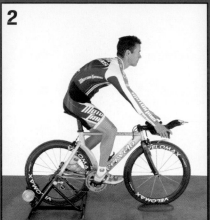

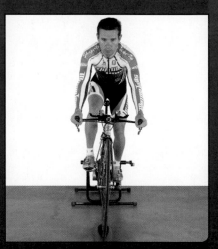

Still counting down from five, I maneuver my dominant leg (right) to two o'clock.

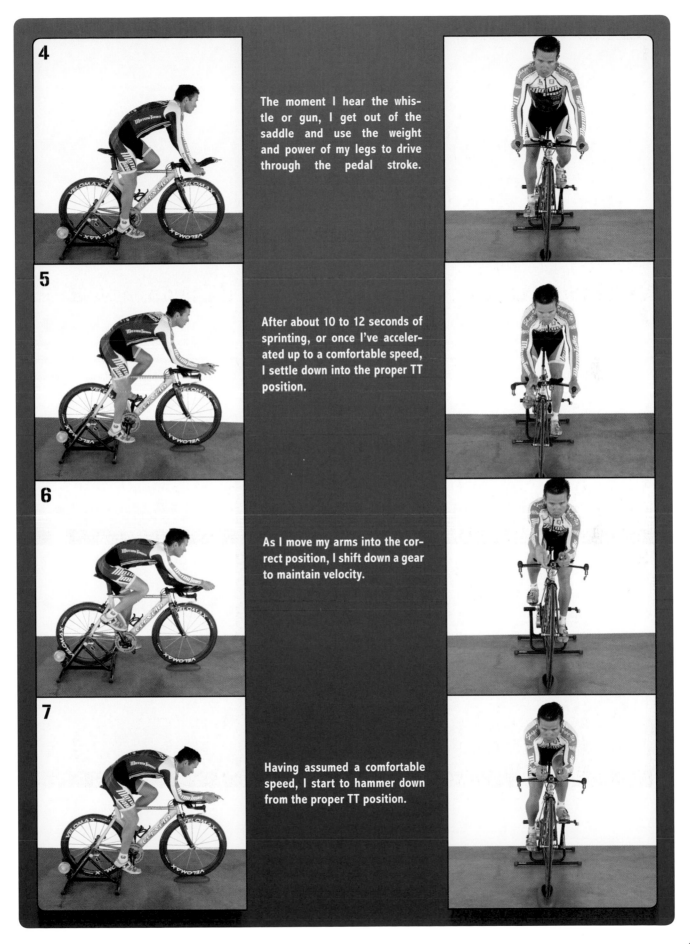

4

The moment I hear the whistle or gun, I get out of the saddle and use the weight and power of my legs to drive through the pedal stroke.

5

After about 10 to 12 seconds of sprinting, or once I've accelerated up to a comfortable speed, I settle down into the proper TT position.

6

As I move my arms into the correct position, I shift down a gear to maintain velocity.

7

Having assumed a comfortable speed, I start to hammer down from the proper TT position.

IDEAL SEATED-CLIMB POSITION

The key to climbing on a TT bike is to maintain an aerodynamic position and use the power of your legs and gearing to get you over the hill. Be careful about standing up or adjusting your grip. If the climb is short (two minutes or less) or the incline is slight (1 to 3 percent grade), you should be able to maintain the proper TT position and spin your way over the hill. If the hill is steep or it's an extended climb, you may have to simulate a road bike position by repositioning your hands on the handlebars or standing up. However, it's important to note that this situation should be a rare occurrence.

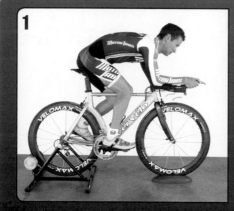

1. I'm in the proper TT position.

2. To offset gravity and keep my weight distributed over the center of the bike, I slide forward in the saddle slightly. From here, I will use the power of my legs and gearing to conquer the hill. It's important to notice that although I slide forward, I maintain the integrity of my posture and stay low to remain aerodynamic.

SEATED-CLIMBING POSITION

If you're going up a steep hill (4 to 6 percent grade) or an extended climb (anything over two minutes), you may need to put your hands on the handlebars and slide back in the saddle slightly. As you can see from the photos below, it's very similar to a road bike position in that my hands are narrow, my hips are positioned over the hub of the rear wheel, and I'm in a nice aerodynamic position.

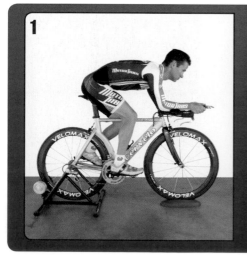

I'm in the proper TT position.

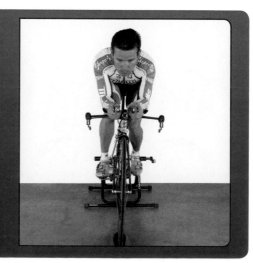

2

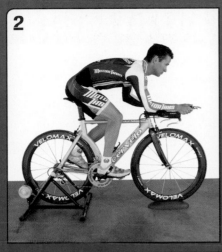

As the hill gets steeper, I place my left hand on the aero bar pad next to the stem.

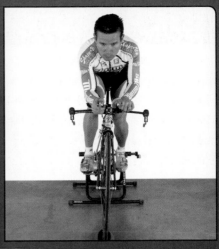

3

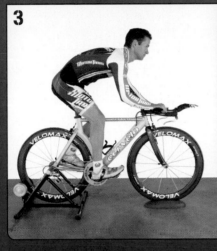

I assume a narrow grip on the handlebars and slide back in the saddle slightly.

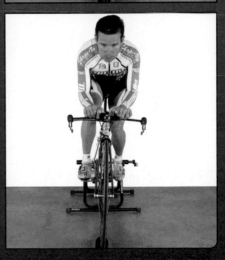

Common Fault: Gripping the Handlebars

When you transition into the road bike seated-climb position, avoid placing your hands on the outside of the handlebars. You will not only lose power, speed, and efficiency, but also sacrifice your aerodynamic position.

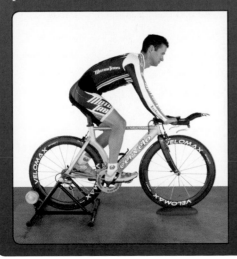

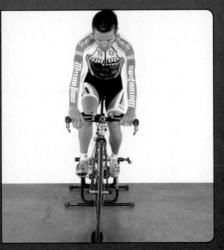

By placing my hands too wide on the handlebars, I inadvertently lift my upper body, compromising my aerodynamic position.

STANDING CLIMB

If the climb gets really steep and you're unable to maintain speed from the seated position, then you can stand up and power over the hill as a last resort. You can also use the standing climb if you're riding through a section that has a lot of undulating terrain. In such a situation, you may have to get out of the saddle to power over the lower climbs.

To avoid slowing down or reducing your cadence, make sure to shift into a higher gear and use the leverage of your body weight to power into the pedal system as you stand. It's important to remember that the moment you stand, whether you're powering over a steep hill or trying to maintain momentum over a lower climb, there is diminishing return in energy spent, meaning that the longer you stand the more energy you expend. For that reason, you want to use this technique sparingly and always sit back down in the saddle as fast as possible.

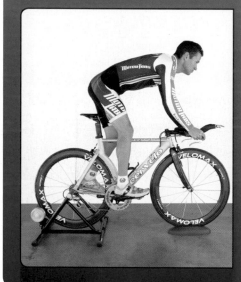
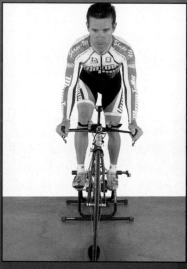

To assume the standing-climb position, I reposition my hands on the handlebars and stand straight up from the saddle. Note that my weight is still distributed directly between the front and back tires. Although I don't illustrate this in the photo, it's worth noting the timing with the pedal stroke. When you make the transition from seated to standing, you should stand as your dominant foot travels past 12 o'clock. (To see this technique performed as a step-by-step sequence, see page 111.)

TIME TRIAL TIPS

- In any race against the clock, don't worry about chasing those ahead of you on the course. This can make you lose focus and rhythm. Instead, focus on staying consistent and keeping the highest cadence possible in the largest gear possible. Remember, you need to be just below your redline to achieve your fastest time.

- Split your time trial into thirds. Take the first third to establish a balance between legs and lungs. (Going 100 percent out of the gate is a common mistake.) The middle third is the time to establish a high but manageable speed and consistent cadence. The final third is the time to lay your cards on the table. The goal is to give an all-out effort in the final kilometer, meaning that there should be nothing left in your tank when you cross the finish line.

- Warming up for a time trial may take as long as 45 minutes. Be sure to do a sufficient number of threshold/time-trial efforts of at least three minutes before rolling to the start line. As a rule, you should go to the start line with a sweat, but cooled down enough to be ready to hit the first third at a fast pace.

- The harder you ride, the calmer you should be. As you begin to work/breathe hard, focus on being calmly strong. Work to eliminate excessive body movement and concentrate on becoming one with your bike.

- Start fast and finish faster. Inexperienced time trialists will reduce cadence over the course of the race. Work on maintaining or increasing cadence as the time trial wears on.

- Write down three key phrases and tape them to your handlebars to maintain focus (i.e., "Breathe," "Solid Body," "Cadence").

DO DIAGNOSTIC TESTING (MINI TIME-TRIAL)

If you are an inexperienced racer, you need to get an idea of how you perform. For road cyclists and time trialists, pick a 10K course and test yourself on it once a month. For MTB/cyclocross riders, pick a 5-mile course with a mixture of hills, corners, and descents. Be sure to record your time after each effort. That will give you some baseline data so you can determine whether your training program is working for you. For example, every 4 to 6 weeks, I ride the same course on my cyclocross bike and time it just as I would time a CrossFit workout. If I improve my time from the previous month, I know my training is working. If I get slower, I know something is wrong. I also recommend that you keep a training diary and record the following key factors: time in the saddle, terrain (flat, hills, rolling), watt/power/speed average, distance covered, how you felt (strong, fatigued, etc.), outside factors (cold, wind, etc.), and dynamic of ride (solo, group, race, etc.).

Mountain Bike

Riding a mountain bike is like being a kid again. You get to play in the dirt, jump over stuff, get in the water, and be outside in nature. It's pure fun. Like the road bike, it's a very versatile piece of equipment in that you can climb, descend, and corner efficiently as well as use it on all different types of terrain. Whether you're riding on mud, dirt, rock, or road or going uphill, downhill, or around turns, the mountain bike can handle it. For recreational riders not used to being in the low position characteristic of road and time-trial bikes, the mountain bike allows for a more comfortable upright position, which lets you focus on bike-handling skills and pedaling mechanics.

The mountain bike is also one of the best cross-training tools for a cyclist. In the same way that CrossFit Endurance augments CrossFit with sport-specific training, mountain-biking is a great way to cross train for a road bike or time-trial event. For example, if you're a triathlete it's going to ask you to use muscles that you're not used to using and help you develop bike-handling skills. If you're a road cyclist, you can use the mountain bike in your off-season to teach you to climb with a slightly higher cadence while still maintaining an efficient pedal stroke. In a nutshell, the steep inclines, razor-sharp turns, and sketchy descents that are characteristic of mountain bike courses require you to shift your weight and adjust your body to constantly varied terrain, skills that will serve you well on the road and time-trial bike.

If you're competing in cycling events, generally you'll see the mountain bike used in XTERRA courses, which take place on dirt roads and single-track trails. The decision you have to make for such events is whether to use a hard tail or double-suspension frame. Although it primarily boils down to personal preference, I generally recommend double-suspension bikes for downhill courses that have a lot of ruts, holes, dips, and jumps. If you're riding on a fire road that is somewhat flat and open, full suspension may not be necessary. Hard tail bikes are more economical and versatile in that you can use them on aggressive single-track trails as well as straight, flat dirt roads. Just like when choosing a road bike over a time trial, it's part strategy and part personal preference.

PROPER MOUNTAIN BIKE POSITION

If you're truly mountain-biking, you're going to change positions a lot to adapt to variations in terrain. However, in order to shift into those positions, you must first understand how to properly situate yourself on the bike. Because of the difference in geometry, your basic setup on a mountain bike is very different than the road bike or time-trial position.

The top tube is shorter, and the wheels are closer together on a mountain bike, which forces a more dramatic bend in the upper back. The road bike and TT position your upper body closer to the top tube to reduce wind resistance so that you can maximize speed and power on hard-surfaced roads. The mountain bike, on the other hand, forces you into an upright position, which allows you to shift your weight on a moment's notice as you navigate around obstacles and sharp turns.

The key to positioning yourself correctly on a mountain bike, aside from getting a proper bike fit, is to establish a position that allows you to effortlessly transfer your weight, shift gears, and hit the brakes so that you can control the bike and react quickly to obstacles in your path. To accomplish this, you want to center your weight between the front and back tires and position your hands in the center of your grips with a slight bend in your elbows. The former allows you to shift your weight in any direction in the blink of an eye, while the latter gives you easy access to your brakes and shifters.

Although you're going to be shifting your position with the terrain, you should keep your shoulders, hips, and knees in line. If you look at the front-view photo, you'll notice that my shoulders, hips, and knees fall within a rectangle. As a rule, you should maintain the integrity of that rectangle—keep your arms and legs bent slightly—as you force the bike and adapt your body to ever-changing situations.

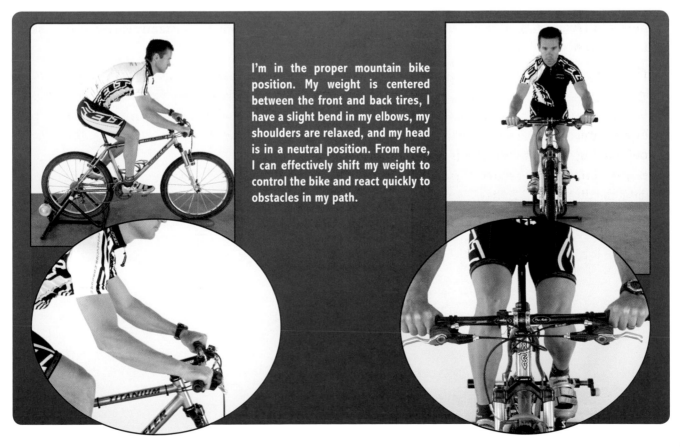

I'm in the proper mountain bike position. My weight is centered between the front and back tires, I have a slight bend in my elbows, my shoulders are relaxed, and my head is in a neutral position. From here, I can effectively shift my weight to control the bike and react quickly to obstacles in my path.

Common Fault: Thumbs Over

To avoid flying over your handlebars if you hit a rock, root, or other obstacle in your path, you should always loop your thumb around the handlebars and keep the grip positioned in the center of your palm.

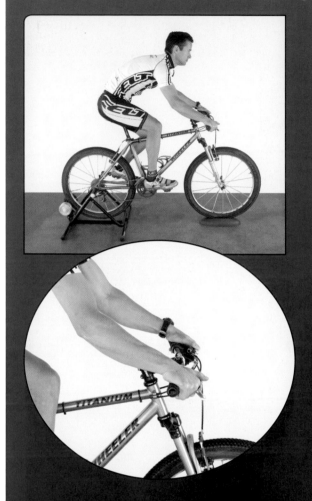

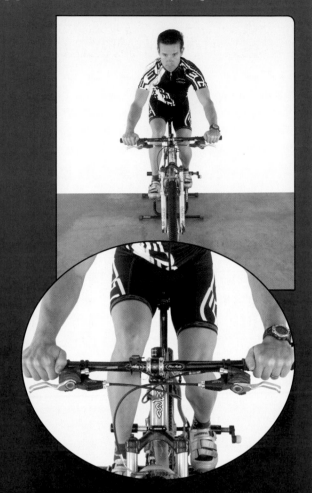

I've made the mistake of looping my thumbs over the handlebars. If I hit an obstacle, I risk losing my grip on the handlebars and crashing.

Common Fault: Grip Too Wide

The grip is simple on a mountain bike because unlike a road bike, which has several gripping options, your grip on a mountain bike never really changes. Your hands should always be in the center of your grips so you can get to your brakes and shifters without restriction. If your grip is too wide or too narrow, it restricts your ability to shift gears or brake on a dime, dramatically increasing your chances of crashing.

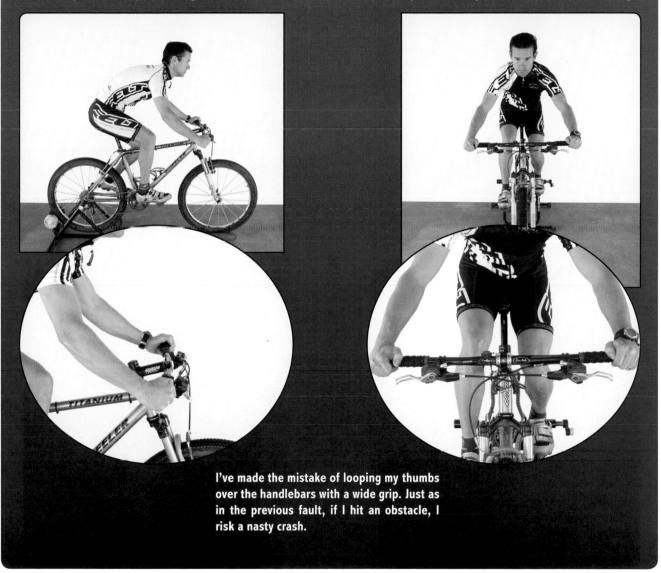

I've made the mistake of looping my thumbs over the handlebars with a wide grip. Just as in the previous fault, if I hit an obstacle, I risk a nasty crash.

Common Fault: Straight Arms

Remember that your arms are an extension of your front shocks. If you keep your arms straight, you not only reduce your ability to react to bumps in the road, but also place additional stress on your joints, which can wear you out and increase your chances of injury. To keep your response time razor sharp, you should always keep a slight bend in your elbows so that you can absorb the shock of seen and unseen obstacles.

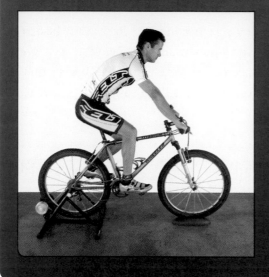

I've straightened my arms to relieve the pressure of my body weight. Unable to absorb the shock of obstacles in my path, I reduce my ability to control the bike and increase my chances of wrecking.

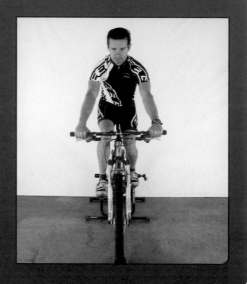

Common Fault: Rounded Back

Although the mountain bike forces a more dramatic bend in the upper back, you want to be careful not to exaggerate the position. A lot of riders will mistakenly tilt their head down, round their back, and straighten their arms as fatigue sets in. Mountain-biking is like skiing in that the majority of injuries occur later in the day when you're tired and your reaction time has slowed. If you notice that your mechanics are starting to fall apart, either take a break or slow down to avoid crashing.

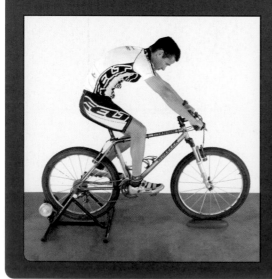

Unable to maintain midline stabilization and proper posture because of fatigue, I round forward, shrug my shoulders, and straighten my arms.

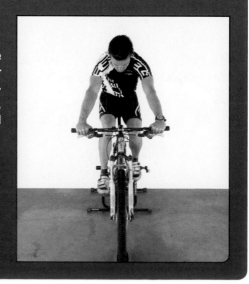

PEDAL STROKE

Assuming a proper bike fit, the mechanics of the pedal stroke on a mountain bike are no different than on a road bike. There is, however, a difference in cadence. For example, if you're going uphill your cadence is higher on a mountain bike than it would be on a road bike. Mountain bikers who transition to road bikes do really well because they are used to pedaling at a higher cadence and exerting more power into the pedal stroke.

Terrain also plays a role. As you navigate through an ever-changing environment, you have to be able to seamlessly shift into the appropriate gears to maintain speed and momentum. Not being in the right gear stops your momentum and forces you to reaccelerate up to speed every time you shift. This is a mistake that a lot of mountain bikers make and is responsible for more lost races than any other positional or mechanical fault. To see the proper pedaling mechanics, refer back to the road bike section of this chapter.

SEATED CLIMB: MODERATE CLIMB

If you're climbing up a hard-packed easy- to moderate-grade incline, you can slide back in your saddle and use gearing and the power of your legs to accelerate over the hill, just as you would on a road bike. If you glance at the photos below, you'll notice that I actually lower myself as I scoot my hips back. This places additional pressure on my handlebars so that I can keep my front tire grounded in the dirt, which is key for maintaining control of the bike. If you sit upright as you slide your hips back in the saddle, your front wheel will lose traction with the ground, causing you to lose control of the bike.

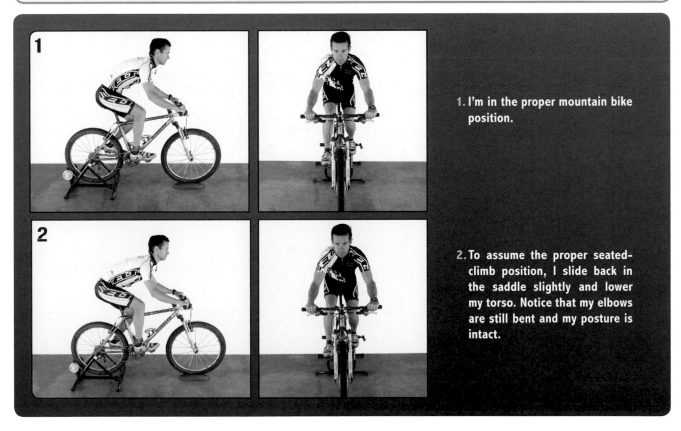

1. I'm in the proper mountain bike position.

2. To assume the proper seated-climb position, I slide back in the saddle slightly and lower my torso. Notice that my elbows are still bent and my posture is intact.

SEATED CLIMB: STEEP INCLINE

If you're attempting to conquer a steep incline, you have to keep your front tire grounded in the dirt to maintain traction and control of the bike by sliding forward in the saddle and lowering your center of gravity. A lot of mountain bikers fail on steep climbs not because they lack strength, but because they don't know how to properly weight the bike. Always remember that climbing on a mountain bike is all about keeping both tires grounded in the dirt. Unlike climbing on a road bike, you can't get out of the saddle and sacrifice traction on that back tire when charging up a steep hill. You have to keep at least an 80-to-20 percent weight distribution between the front and rear wheels. If one of your tires doesn't grab as you power up the mountain, you're going to lose balance, and to avoid falling over you will have to plant one of your feet on the ground. In addition to risking injury, this action stops your momentum, which in some situations may be impossible to reclaim. With gravity and grade working against you, getting settled in the proper climbing position, clipping your feet in to the pedals, and accelerating back up the mountain can be a huge challenge.

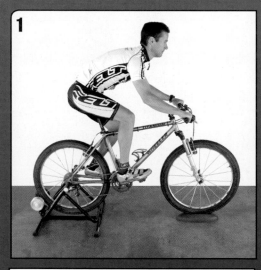

I'm in the proper mountain bike position.

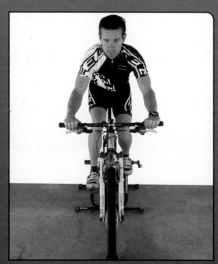

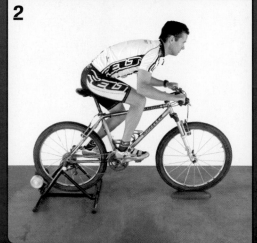

To establish the seated-climbing position for a steep incline, I slide forward in the saddle and lower my center of gravity to place additional pressure on the handlebars. This positional shift not only helps me offset gravity, but also keeps both tires firmly grounded in the dirt.

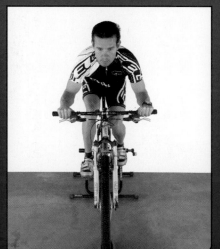

Common Fault: Standing Climb

It's common to see inexperienced mountain bikers stand up and lean over their handlebars in an attempt to power over a hill. In addition to shortening the pedal stroke, which creates choppy, inefficient pedaling, your back tire loses traction with the ground, causing you to spin out.

Your ability to control the front of the bike also changes. With the majority of your weight being distributed over your handlebars, you force your front shock to contract and recoil, creating a negative force on the incline. Unable to grip the ground thanks to no weight on the back tire or effectively navigate around bumps and objects, you lose momentum and you're forced to bail off the bike to avoid crashing.

Remember, standing up on a mountain bike is not efficient. There is a reason that mountain bikes have lower gears than road or TT bikes: so you can climb steep hills using the power of your gears without sacrificing your position.

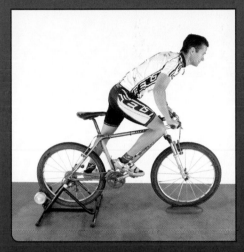 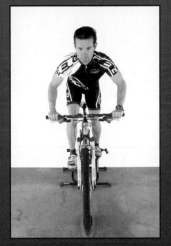

I'm standing with my weight distributed over the handlebars. With the majority of my weight centered over the front tire, my back tire loses traction with the road and I'm unable to steer the bike.

Common Fault: Seated Climb for Steep Inclines

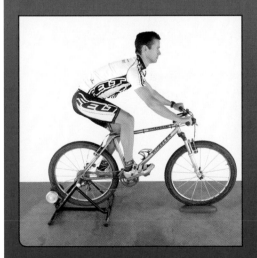 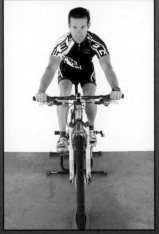

Although remaining in the saddle while traversing moderate grades is considered effective, mechanics change when you engage a steep hill. If you keep your weight back as you power up the incline, your front wheel will start wobbling all over the place, causing you to lose control of the bike. Remember, the steeper the hill, the more you have to slide forward in the saddle, the lower your torso must be, and the more pressure you have to put on the handlebars.

PROPER DOWNHILL POSITION

There are several things to keep in mind when going downhill on a mountain bike. The first is weight distribution and leg position. In order to navigate around objects and coast over shale or sandy, rocky, or gravelly terrain, you have to unweight the front tire, by sliding back in the saddle, and squeeze your thighs around the nose of your saddle. The former allows you to react quickly and manipulate the bike around and over objects protruding from the ground, while the latter allows you to steer and control the rear of the bike. If you lean too far forward, putting too much weight over the front wheel, or flare your knees out, you make it difficult to react to obstacles in your path, compromise your speed, and increase your chances of crashing.

Maintaining momentum is another critical component of riding downhill. To be effective, you have to find a comfortable speed that allows you to seamlessly coast over uneven terrain. Downhill tempo is like that of a skier bombing down a mountain: you need to make quick, fluid transitions while rolling effortlessly over bumps in your path, which is only possible if you're going somewhat fast. If you're going too slow, your rhythm and tempo will be affected by the obstacles, in which case it will take more energy for you to manipulate the bike up, over, and around objects and your chances of wrecking increase.

Knowing which brake to use and how to use it is another key factor when riding downhill. A lot of inexperienced riders will either brake with the front wheel or squeeze the rear brake for an extended period of time, both of which give you less control of the bike and can cause you to crash. The key is to grip the handlebar with your left hand to avoid defaulting to your front brake, and wrap your right hand (or index and middle finger) around the rear brake. As you coast down the trail, tap or feather the brake handle to slow down and skid around objects.

The last thing to keep in mind when you're bombing down a hill is perspective. Downhill tracks are filled with rocks, sharp curves, and drop-offs. To avoid crashing or slowing your momentum, you have to plot a path that allows you to navigate around objects without compromising your speed. This can be accomplished by focusing your gaze on the trail ahead. If you make the mistake of looking only at what's right in front of you, instead of what's ahead of you, you'll pass an obstacle before you can assess the situation and react accordingly. For example, if you're sliding down a shale surface heading into a sharp corner and you're staring down at your front tire, by the time you get to the sharp corner, it will be too late. Your brain won't have the necessary time to digest the situation and form a game plan. If, however, you're looking ahead, feeding your brain with data about what's to come, you can effortlessly respond to objects as you slide down the slippery surface while forming a strategy as to how you're going to enter and exit the corner without compromising your speed or safety.

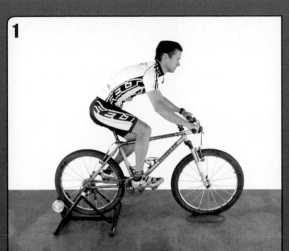

1. I'm in the proper mountain bike position.

2. To assume the proper downhill position, I stand slightly out of the saddle, drive my hips back, and pinch my thighs around the nose of the seat. It's important to notice that I maintain the integrity of my posture by keeping my back straight and my eyes locked ahead. From this position, I can see ahead of me and shift my weight to adjust to any obstacles that may cross my path.

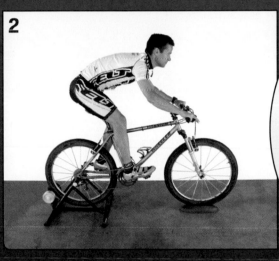

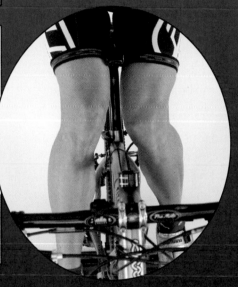

CORNERING

When you're cornering on a mountain bike, you need to lean your body just as you would on a road bike, but you have to be careful not to exaggerate the movement, especially if you're on dirt. If you lean too far, you're much more likely to wash out than if you were on a road bike. There are other parallels between cornering on a road bike and on a mountain bike, like keeping your inside pedal at 12 o'clock, looking in the direction of your exit, and not breaking in the corner.

Most of the cornering on a mountain bike is done downhill, though, which does change the dynamics. The degree of your lean is largely a function of how steep the grade and the angle of your turn. If you're approaching a really technical corner, meaning that there are a lot of obstacles such as rocks or roots, you can actually stand out of the saddle so that you can lift up on the bike and maneuver through/around the objects.

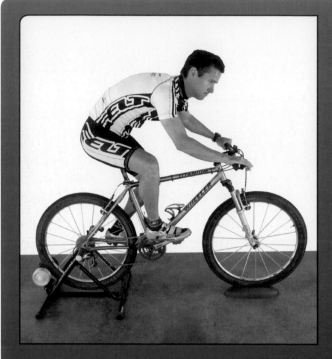 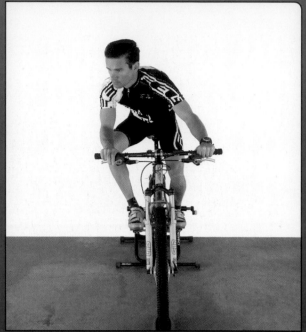

Although it's difficult to illustrate proper cornering technique on a stationary mountain bike, you can see that my right leg is at 12 o'clock to avoid catching my pedal on the ground and obstacles. I'm in a slightly lower position, and I'm pointing my eyes and knee toward my exit. The key is to not place too much weight over your back wheel as you slide back slightly in the saddle. Doing so will most likely cause you to wipe out.

For more technical corners, you can stand out of the saddle and kind of whip your hips from side to side to help steer the bike around obstacles and maneuver yourself around the corner. As you can see, the same rules apply. My right foot is still at 12 o'clock, and I'm pointing my knee and eyes toward my exit.

GETTING OVER OBSTACLES

As a rule of thumb, it's always better to go over an obstacle (assuming it's small and within your skill set) than to go around it, because you save energy and can maintain your speed and momentum. When you approach an obstacle, you should stop your pedal stroke at about two o'clock, stand up on the pedals slightly, and then pull up on the front wheel just as you're about to come in contact with the object. As your front wheel clears the object, shift your weight forward and pull up on your back wheel using the power of your hamstrings. Ideally, you want your back wheel to clear or brush over the object to avoid slowing you down.

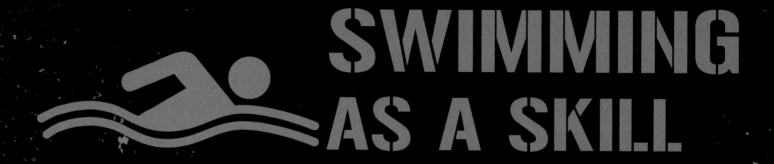

SWIMMING AS A SKILL

BY CHRIS MICHELMORE

"AS A COMBAT-ARMS MARINE OFFICER, I CAN ATTEST THAT THE CONCEPTS AND PRINCIPLES LAID OUT BY BRIAN MACKENZIE WILL NOT ONLY MAKE YOU A BETTER ATHLETE BUT WILL ALSO IMPROVE YOUR ABILITY TO DO YOUR JOB NO MATTER HOW AUSTERE THE CONDITIONS."

CAPT. P.J. NEWTON
USMC

While it can be convincingly argued that we as a species are designed to run, the same cannot be said about swimming. The moment you enter the water, you immerse yourself in an environment of constant resistance. Just keeping your head above the surface takes an incredible amount of energy. Try moving forward, and you expend even more energy. With every passing stroke and kick of your feet, the water's action of drag perpetually slows you down, making every movement an exaggerated effort. To avoid drowning, you must move each major body part, from your core to your extremities, in concert, as well as synchronize your breathing with the rhythm of your swimming stroke.

For the inexperienced swimmer, it can literally be a fight for life, but a trained, conditioned, calm swimmer can travel amazing distances in this seemingly hostile environment. However, because swimming doesn't come naturally to most people, it is certainly the most technical component of endurance athletics.

Knowing how to swim is a great skill to acquire. Whether or not you want to compete in endurance events like triathlons or survive the dreaded swim element in the CrossFit games, chances are you will certainly want to explore the coral atolls and Windex-blue waters of your next tropical vacation with confidence, and developing strong swimming skills is the only way to make yourself comfortable enough to do so. If you are an athlete, remember that everyone started in the same place with swimming and that many of your competitors will neglect swimming as a skill, assuming that their cycling or running times (or other WOD times in CrossFit) will make up for poor swim times. Ditch that mindset: if you are in a triathlon or other event, think of swimming as an opportunity to pull even further ahead.

Learning how to swim as a means of survival applies only if you've never learned this quintessential skill. Athletes who fall into this category need to get over their fear of drowning by taking it slow and working on fundamental drills. Put another way: They need to spend time in the water learning the basic mechanics. But convincing someone that doesn't know how to swim is not an issue. The problem is trying to teach recreational swimmers, who have already developed a basic knowledge or skill set, to swim as efficiently as possible. Here's why:

With drowning being one of the leading causes of accidental death, the majority of parents eagerly enroll their kids in swimming classes the moment they're of age. However, once the basics are mastered—meaning that you can put your head underwater with confidence, float on the surface without struggle, and move forward using a basic swimming stroke—developing technique to be more efficient is often overlooked or neglected altogether. For example, some (but not all!) endurance athletes who want to compete in a triathlon will start by swimming 10 laps; progress to 20, and then to 30, and so on until they meet their mark. While this method will undoubtedly improve an athlete's engine, it will do very little to improve swimming efficiency, which is far more important than fitness.

Swimming takes a lot more energy than any other activity because of the resistance of the medium (water), making technique extremely important. Water, in this particular case, is your worst enemy. The same is not true with running (or cycling, for that matter) because you don't have to overcome the water's drag or exert excessive energy to propel your body forward. You have a solid surface to drive off and nothing but air standing in your way. Water, on the other hand, is 800 to 1,000 times denser than air, making every movement an exaggerated effort. To compound the problem, you have nothing to grab to pull or push yourself forward. The only way to make moving through the element easier is to focus on body position and reduce drag with every passing stroke. In other words, you can't change water, but you can change how you move in it.

In this chapter, I will introduce a method that will make swimming much easier. Just as in the other chapters of this book, I'm not trying to reinvent the wheel or trademark any specific movement with new techniques. Instead, the CFE team of swimming coaches, which include myself, Brian Nebeta, and Sage Hopkins, have developed a sequence of drills and progressions that make learning how to swim simple and pleasant. The goal is to increase your learning curve by introducing important concepts and implementing drills in sequential order so that you can master the most technical component of endurance athletics, regardless of your skill set or background. Following the theme of breaking down movement into a series of defined positions based around midline stabilization and neutral spinal alignment, this chapter focuses on drills that will teach you how to swim faster and with less effort using the freestyle stroke, otherwise known as the front crawl.

The Freestyle Stroke:

The freestyle stroke is one of two long-axis strokes—the other being the backstroke—which allow you to cover the most distance humanly possible using the least amount of energy. With your body elongated in a stream-lined position, you spread your balance and buoyancy so that you can remain on the surface of the water, which in turn reduces the water's drag. In addition, with the continuous kicking of the legs and alternating action of the arms, you can propel yourself through the water without pause. For these reasons, the freestyle stroke is much more efficient than other common swimming strokes such as the breaststroke or butterfly stroke.

Here's a simple example to illustrate this concept. Imagine a sculling boat resting in the water with a team of accomplished rowers. Assuming that the boat is resting in calm waters and that the rowers are all paddling in rhythm, the boat should remain perfectly balanced over a single point in the water, meaning that it glides through the water over its balance point without bobbing up and down and maintains momentum with each passing stroke.

If we offset the balance point by having one person stand in the bow of the boat and another person stand in the stern, and together they teeter-totter it up and down as the boat progresses, would it still move forward without pause? Absolutely not. Such actions would cause the balance point to constantly shift from the front to the back, creating a start-and-stop motion that would slow if not stop the forward movement of the boat.

The boat teeter-tottering as it moves forward is similar to a swimmer doing the breaststroke or butterfly in that the constant up and down motion of your body changes your balance point in the water, compromises your hydrodynamics, and ultimately slows you down. In other words, you're not able to generate sufficient momentum to progress forward with every stroke. The freestyle stroke, on the other hand, is similar to a well-balanced sculling boat equipped with a team of Olympic rowers in that there is no up-and-down oscillation and you're able to move forward with every effort while keeping your balance point in the same position.

Although the freestyle stroke is the most efficient technique for endurance athletes to master, it is also one of the most difficult to learn. This is because of the different styles associated with the freestyle stroke and the process that most individuals got through in learning the skill. For example, if you were to watch the eight finalists in the Olympic freestyle event, you would see eight different styles of swimming, even though they are all using the same stroke. The problem with athletes who want to learn how to swim is that they try to emulate one of their favorite swimmers rather than hire a coach or learn proper swimming mechanics.

Although you may love the way Michael Phelps glides through the water, his swimming style may not be the most efficient for your body type and skill set. For example, say you're 5 foot 5 and 155 pounds and try to swim like Michael Phelps, who is 6 foot 4 and 205 pounds. Do you really think you can replicate his style even though you're shorter and have half his wingspan and a fraction of his experience? Although we should all work to swim as efficiently as Phelps, the timing of his stroke and beat of his kick may differ from yours, not to mention that you may need to make countless tweaks and adaptations to compensate for your unique frame. In other words, you have to understand and implement the fundamental laws that govern his movements before you can begin to mimic them. To aid your understanding of these universal guidelines, the CFE team of swimming coaches has created a checklist of categories that make synchronizing the complex motions of the freestyle stroke much easier to digest.

FREESTYLE SWIMMING CHECKLIST

It's important to note that the categories below represent a sequence of drills that work with the universal mechanics of swimming, meaning that they work for every individual regardless of body type. The drills are no different than in running, cycling, or lifting in that they start with midline stabilization and understanding how to position your body for movement. Once you know how to position your body in the water, everything else, from rotation to moving your arms and legs to breathing, becomes much easier to manage. It's also worth mentioning that although it's important to understand each category, there are techniques that are featured in the system that are not included in the checklist. The goal of this section is to break down the core principles (or guidelines) so that you can attach purpose and meaning to the sequential flow of drills in the skill-of-swimming section of this chapter.

FREESTYLE SWIMMING CHECKLIST

- ☑ **Balance and Buoyancy**
- ☑ **Body Position**
- ☑ **Rotation and Reinforcing Midline Stabilization**

Balance and Buoyancy

By the time you master the drills presented in this chapter, you'll be relaxed and confident in the water and be able to swim faster and longer than you ever thought possible. But to get to that point, you have to start by mastering the basics. For a swimmer, that means understanding how your body balances in the water. As I've already mentioned, the most difficult aspect of swimming is not the movement, but the water. In order to swim as efficiently as possible, you first must understand how your body naturally positions itself in this liquid medium.

To find your balance point, or natural position in the water, you need to perform a popular drill known as the dead man's float. Those of you who are experienced swimmers have probably performed this drill at some point in your learning process.

To execute this drill, take a big breath and let your body relax, allowing your arms and legs to dangle, with your head face down in the water. (For a more elaborate description of this technique flip to page 175.) What you'll realize is that your lungs act as floatation devices, which keep you balanced on the surface of the water. Another important takeaway is to realize that your spine naturally falls in line as you float on the surface of the water. For example, if you lift your head up, which is a common fault, your hips will sink. Conversely, if you tuck your chin to your chest, your hips will rise toward the surface. Although it's important to relax, the water will exaggerate any shift from a neutral spinal alignment, which can affect your position in the water.

It's important to note that there is no right or wrong with this drill. The point is to understand where your balance point is so that you can address what you'll need to work on as you advance through the sequence of drills. For example, if you have thick legs, your lower body will probably sink toward the bottom, which means you'll have to develop a powerful kick and rely on the strength of your legs to keep your body in a streamlined position. If you carry the majority of your weight in your upper body, your legs will probably rise toward the surface, which means you don't have to use your legs as much to maintain a level body position.

The point is that every individual is different. There are many variables to consider because everyone's body mass is proportioned differently, so don't get frustrated if you're not getting the same results as your swimming partner. The key is to find where your balance point is so that you can work on correcting your position in the water using the drills provided in this chapter.

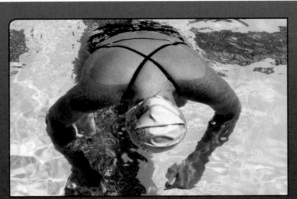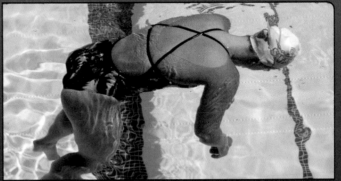

To assume the dead man's float position, Christina takes a big breath in using the full capacity of her lungs, completely relaxes her body, and falls forward. As you can see, she's floating on the surface of the water and her back is exposed directly over her lungs. This is her natural position in the water. To get the best results, it's imperative for you to stay totally relaxed and to avoid tensing your body or extending your neck to pull your head out of the water.

Body Position

In the running chapter, we shed light on Kelly Starrett's "position is power" mantra. As you should already know, position—the same thing as posture or stance—dictates your capacity for movement. For example, if you're setting up for a run, you first have to establish a strong neutral posture with your arms in the correct position before you initiate your fall. This is referred to as your running stance. If your stance is strong, falling forward and executing proper running mechanics is much easier to manage. If your stance is weak, you'll compensate with dysfunctional movement patterns, which increase your energy expenditure and open the door to injury.

To help illustrate my point, picture a boxer setting up a powerful punching combination. If that boxer is in a compromised stance, meaning that his feet are set in an awkward position or his balance is off, you can assume that the speed, power, and accuracy of his punches are going to be negatively affected. Not only that, but the more punches he throws, the harder it will be for him to reclaim a strong position because of the rotation and momentum of his body. If he starts his combination from a balanced stance, on the other hand, he can stabilize his position with each blow so that each one flows seamlessly into the next. Stance, in this case, dictates the boxer's ability to throw effective punches. Swimming is no different, in that assuming a strong stance dictates your ability to move your arms as efficiently and effectively as possible. However, because you have no platform on which to stand, a lot of athletes make the mistake of thinking that there is no swimming stance. Instead of trying to establish a strong position before initiating the swimming stroke, they jump in the water and start swinging their arms and thrashing their legs in a random and hectic sequence of motions. Although such a strategy will carry you forward, you're essentially throwing punches from a compromised stance, in that the speed, power, and accuracy of your strokes are compromised by your dysfunctional position.

After you've found your body's natural balance point in the water, the next step is to elongate your extremities over that stable point and establish a streamlined position, which can be considered the "swimmer's stance." To do this properly, you should gradually raise your arms toward the surface of the water from the dead man's float position. By extending your arms and supporting your hands on the surface of the water, you change the position of that balance point in relation to the rest of your body, which causes your legs to gradually rise toward the surface. The goal is to straighten your spine and achieve a streamline position with your heels touching the surface before you initiate motion by kicking. It's important to note that a lot of swimmers will not be able to accomplish this because of how their body mass is proportioned. For example, if you have tree trunks for legs or you've got a lot of muscle mass, chances are your feet will remain glued to the bottom (or you may even sink like a rock) despite the fact that your arms are elongated and your back is straight. In such a situation, you'll have to start kicking and moving your arms so that you can stay afloat and achieve the proper streamlined position.

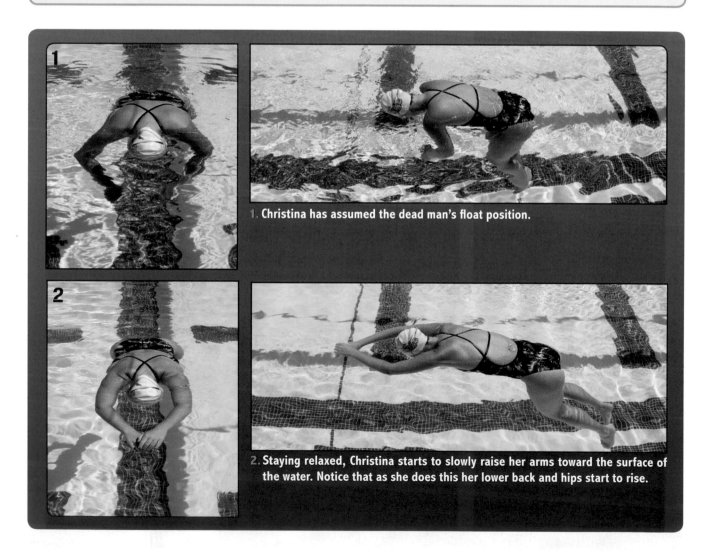

1. Christina has assumed the dead man's float position.

2. Staying relaxed, Christina starts to slowly raise her arms toward the surface of the water. Notice that as she does this her lower back and hips start to rise.

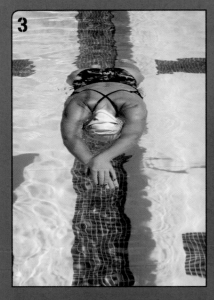

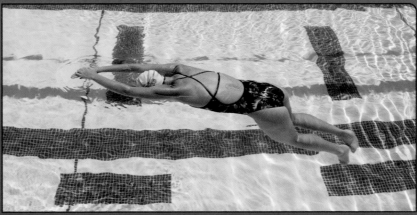

3. As Christina's hands reach the surface, she crosses her right hand over the top of her left hand.

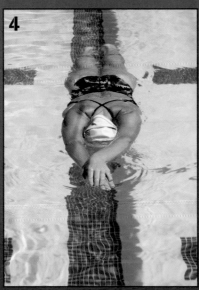

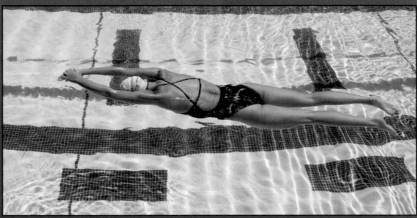

4. Christina extends her arms and stretches out her body and achieves a stream-lined position. Notice that her back is straight and that her body is level.

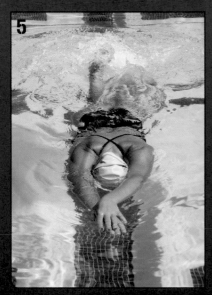

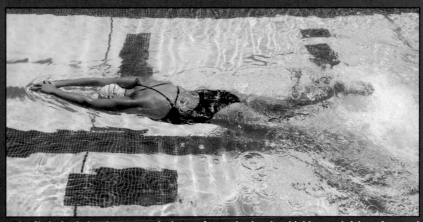

5. As Christina's heels approach the surface, she begins kicking to initiate forward motion.

KICKING TECHNIQUE

The kick is an extension of your streamlined stance. This may seem contradictory to the statement that a strong position dictates your capacity for movement, but it's not. Let me be clear: Although you can achieve the streamlined position while remaining still in the water, you're not in a good position to start swimming freestyle. In other words, even if you can get your body level with the surface, unless you start kicking, you're not going to be able to transition into the swimming stroke. Kicking, in this particular case, is the driving force that allows you to achieve and maintain the ideal streamlined position. For example, a lot of swimmers make the mistake of moving their arms to move forward before they've secured a streamlined position. Going back to the boxing analogy, this is no different than throwing punches from an off-balance stance, in that the speed, power, and accuracy of your movements are compromised. To avoid making the aforementioned mistake, you must achieve your swimmer's stance, or a streamlined position, by raising your arms and kicking your feet before you initiate the swimming stroke.

To execute proper kicking technique, you must move your legs up and down evenly with small kicks. The key is to kick from the hip; meaning that you keep your legs roughly straight with a slight knee bend and keep your toes pointed the entire time. A lot of swimmers make the mistake of kicking from their knees. In other words they pull their heels toward their butt, which is characterized by high kicks that produce large and chaotic splashes. This kicking fault also causes the swimmer to crisscross his or her feet as he or she rotates from side to side, resulting in a loss of power. Another common fault associated with kicking mechanics is to kick only down. Unlike the swimming stroke (or pedal stroke in cycling), there is no relaxation phase to the kick. To generate the most forward propulsion, you have to kick down using the power of your quads and hip flexors and up using the strength of your hamstrings and glutes.

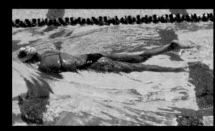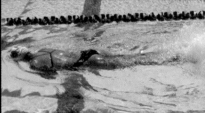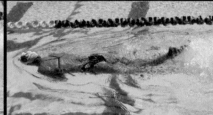

Once you're moving forward under the power of your kick, you should focus on maintaining a streamlined position by keeping your arms extended, your shoulders alongside your ears, and your spine straight in a hollow-tight position. This is your swimmer's stance, which is just like a boxer's stance, in that you can move your arms effectively in combination. The moment you deviate from your stance, you lose power and balance and slow down. In short, you're not going to move as efficiently as you could.

Another way of looking at the streamlined stance is to examine the proper position on a road bike. When you're seated correctly on a road bike, you're in a tight, efficient, and aerodynamic position. The goal is to expose as little of your body as possible to the wind without sacrificing the mechanics of your pedal stroke. If you break your position by lifting your head up, not only do you expose more of your body to wind, which compromises the aerodynamics of your position, but it also affects the efficiency of your pedal stroke: the more wind that hits the front of your body, the more you slow down, and the harder you have to work. The same is true with swimming, in that the more of your body is exposed to water, the more you slow down, and the more energy you have to spend to move forward. By establishing a streamlined position, you not only spread your balance point and increase your buoyancy, but also reduce the water's drag. If you bend at the hips, lift your head up, or compromise your position with faulty kicking mechanics, you're going to have to use a lot more energy to move forward.

Rotation and Reinforcing Midline Stabilization

As I've already mentioned, the moment you attach movement to a position, the weaknesses in an athlete's profile become obvious. It all comes down to midline stabilization and your ability to maintain a flat back position while in motion.

For example, let's say you achieve a perfect streamlined position, but the moment you start to rotate from side to side you relax your core and arch your back. Now everything you do, from kicking to transitioning through the phases of the swimming stroke, is compromised by the weakness of your position. Then you're back to swimming using choppy, awkward, and inefficient strokes. To reduce your chances of executing these faults, you need to keep your trunk engaged and your body fixed in a streamlined position, regardless of whether you're on your side or back or face down. Assuming that you've found your balance and buoyancy in the water and have the core strength to maintain a flat back position while in your streamlined stance, the next thing to address is rotation.

Later in the chapter, I will discuss the phases of the swimming stroke, but it's imperative that you first learn how to maintain a streamlined position while moving forward in rotation. Rotating from one side to another is extremely important in the freestyle stroke, not only for generating forward progress, but also for breathing. If you glance at the photo, you'll notice that the lead arm is extended in front of the body, which is referred to as the hand-lead position, and the shoulders and hips are in line. Aside from being on your side, nothing else really changes. You still want to kick using the same technique, and you're still in a streamlined position. However, when you make the transition from the streamlined position to the rotated position, you must keep your shoulders, hips, and legs in line. As long as your trunk remains tight, the rest of your body will do what it's supposed to do.

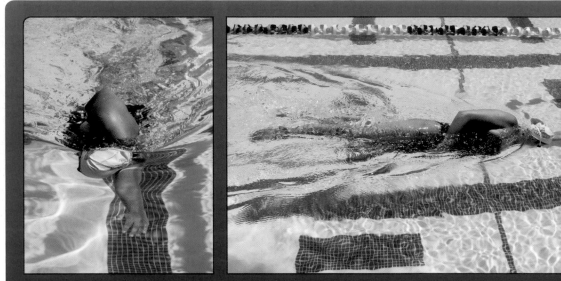

Rudie has established the hand-lead position. Her left arm is extended, with her palm facing the bottom of the pool, and she's using the power of her kick to propel her forward. It's important to notice that her left arm is directly in line with her body, her fingers are relaxed, and she's in the optimal rotated position.

Because rotating onto your side adds an extra level of difficulty, there are a lot of faults associated with this step, all of which can be traced back to the issues of a straight spine and proper midline stabilization. For example, a lot of athletes will turn from the shoulders while keeping their hips square, craning the neck in an attempt to breath, and crisscrossing their feet as they kick. If you've been reading through the checklist sequentially, you already know how to correct these faults: reach full hip extension, keep your midline engaged, maintain a flat back, and kick from your hips and not from your knees. If you have to breathe, remember that your neck is connected to your spine, so if you lift your head up it starts the dominoes falling. To breathe, all you have to do is rotate your head so that your mouth is above the surface of the water. Once you take in a breath of air, you can return to the proper rotated position (see Breathing as a Skill on the next page.)

The bottom line is: If you're unable to balance over your core without using your extremities to keep you afloat, establish a streamlined position, kick from your hips instead of your knees, and rotate onto your side while maintaining a hollow-tight position, then nothing else I show you will work. Swimming is the most technical sport because in addition to trying to move through a medium whose nature is to slow you down, you're also trying to manage a lot of different movements simultaneously. However, if you understand and can implement the guidelines contained within the freestyle checklist, learning each phase of the swimming stroke will be much easier to manage.

BREATHING AS A SKILL

One of the biggest mistakes athletes make when swimming freestyle is holding their breath. With so much to think about—maintaining an ideal position, arm movement, kicking, rotating from side to side, the intensity of the race, etc.—sometimes athletes, even experienced swimmers, forget to breathe. To be more specific, they forget to breathe in rhythm, meaning that they don't take a breath in, slowly exhale until their lungs are empty, and then inhale. Instead, they take a breath in, hold it, and then try to exhale as well as inhale in the brief window when they turn their head to breathe. The result is usually a half-breath of air and a gulp of water. By the time they come up for the next breath, they're swimming out of rhythm, their mechanics are breaking down, and they're choking. In such a situation, they're closer to drowning than to swimming.

To fix this problem, you have to isolate breathing mechanics and master the skill as you layer on the progressions and sequence of drills. This can be accomplished by practicing the following two drills.

The first drill can be done anywhere and simply teaches you the proper breathing mechanics, which is to inhale quickly through your mouth and exhale slowly through your nose. To perform this drill, all you have to do is breathe in through your mouth for a three count, and then exhale through your nose for an eight count. The goal is to take in a full breath of air as you inhale and empty your lungs as you exhale. Although this doesn't directly relate to timing your breath in the stroke, it teaches you how to inhale quickly through your mouth and exhale slowly through your nose and puts you in a relaxed state, both of which are important when you get in the water and try to incorporate the technique while swimming.

Once you're comfortable breathing in through your mouth and out through your nose, the next step is to implement the technique while your head is submerged underwater. The best way to do this is to stand in waist-deep water, keeping your neck and spine in line, and submerge your face. The moment you dunk your head, exhale slowly through your nose until you run out of air. As you empty your lungs, turn your head as if you were swimming freestyle by rotating your upper body and take a breath of air through your mouth as you would when swimming. (You can use the standard three and eight count to make it easy.) Remember, when you're swimming there is only a moment in which to breathe, so you have to make it count. The goal is to take in a full breath of air every time you turn your head to breathe. Once you get comfortable with the stationary breathing drill, you can start incorporating the technique into your swimming stroke.

Another important side note is breathing pattern. A lot of coaches will instruct their athletes to breath every third, fifth, or seventh stroke. The problem with this strategy is breathing on a specific stroke doesn't carry over to every athlete: If I told you to breath every seventh stroke, it may take you 15 seconds before you can take in air, whereas it may take someone else 5 seconds. It's different for every individual, so you have to experiment to find your own ideal pattern. As long as you use proper breathing mechanics as described above, you shouldn't have any trouble finding a rhythm that suits your skill set.

SWIMMING MECHANICS

When you're first learning how to swim freestyle, every stroke is awkward. You thrash your legs with high kicks, crisscross your feet as you rotate back and forth, and push a cupped palm toward the bottom of the pool with a tense arm. As you become more efficient, however, the strokes gradually become more fluid. You shift your body from one support to another with perfect timing, stay in a streamlined position, and kick your legs in a consistent rhythm using the full power of your hips. Staying relaxed is easy when you reach this level because you're not using energy to float on the surface of the water. Instead, the stability of your position coupled with your arms in support increases your buoyancy and keeps you above the water so that you can use your extremities to propel you forward.

Novice swimmers, on the other hand, spend the majority of their energy trying to stay on the surface of the water with only a portion of their energy used to move forward. Pushing an open palm toward the bottom of the pool and executing high kicks are characteristic of someone who has not taken the time to understand the freestyle checklist. As a result, they burn precious energy trying to stay on the surface of the water where they can breathe; rather than use the power of their extremities to move forward.

This is why it's imperative that you follow the checklist in order. First, find your balance and buoyancy in the water. Second, master the streamlined position. Third, attach forward motion to the streamlined position using proper kicking mechanics. And lastly, test the structural alignment of the position by rolling onto your side while continuing to move forward using the power of your kick. Only after you've checked off each item on the checklist should you progress to the next step, which is to master the phases and timing of the swimming stroke.

Quadrant Swimming

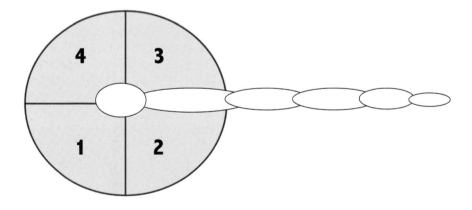

As you will learn shortly, transitioning through the phases of the swimming stroke takes perfect timing and can be a challenge. Quadrant swimming is a simple way of teaching you to be patient in the stroke so that you switch support positions, or transition from one phase of the swimming stroke to the next, at the right moment. If you examine the above diagram, you'll notice that there is a vertical line that bisects the head and a horizontal line that bisects the body. The circle surrounding the head and shoulders is divided into four quadrants. With these four quadrants in mind, let's take a look at the four phases of the swimming stroke: the catch phase, propulsive phase, recovery phase, and entry phase.

Phases of the Swimming Stroke:

Catch Phase

The catch phase is when you are in the hand-lead position (immediately following the entry phase), with your arm extended in front of your body while in a rotated position. The goal is to keep your arm extended and your hand supported on the surface of the water until your opposite arm passes your balance point, which is directly above your lungs. Timing is key. If you retract your supported hand too early, the weight of your opposite arm, which is in the recovery phase, will push you down, forcing you to use extra energy in your next stroke to work your way up to the surface.

As I mentioned before, you want to use the balance and buoyancy of your streamlined position to keep you glued to the surface so that you can use your arms and the power of your kick to keep moving you forward. If you start using your extremities to keep you afloat, you're going to slow down and fatigue at a much faster rate. This is no different than landing out in front of your body when running, in that you're slowing yourself down and then having to accelerate back up to speed with every effort.

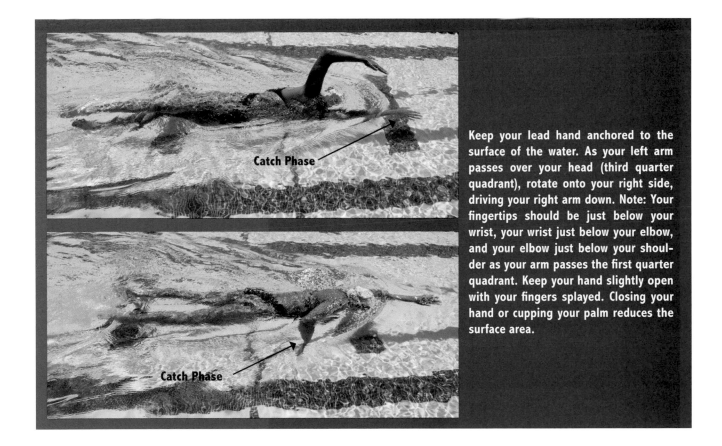

Catch Phase

Catch Phase

Keep your lead hand anchored to the surface of the water. As your left arm passes over your head (third quarter quadrant), rotate onto your right side, driving your right arm down. Note: Your fingertips should be just below your wrist, your wrist just below your elbow, and your elbow just below your shoulder as your arm passes the first quarter quadrant. Keep your hand slightly open with your fingers splayed. Closing your hand or cupping your palm reduces the surface area.

It's worth noting that some coaches refer to this phase of the swimming stroke as the pulling phase. Although pulling is an easy way for the athlete to identify with the movement, the word "pull" is a misnomer in this case because you're not actually pulling against anything. Think about it. Water is a liquid medium. You can't grasp it and pull against it as you would when doing a pull-up on a bar. So how do you pull yourself forward when you have nothing to hold on to? The short answer is you don't. By calling it the pulling phase you're associating a movement to an action that isn't germane. As a result, swimmers will typically implement the fault of pulling their hand down the moment it enters the water, rather than wait for their opposite hand to pass the third quarter of the quadrant.

A much better way of thinking about this phase, which will help you maintain the correct position and properly time the next phase of the swimming stroke, is to imagine that you're grabbing the lane line of a pool. If you were to grab that lane line and pull yourself forward, your hand doesn't change positions in the pool because it's holding on to a stationary object. That is exactly how you should think about your extended hand. It's anchored to the surface as if it were holding on to a solid object, and instead of moving your hand to your body, you're moving your body over your hand. Then, the moment your opposite arm passes the two balloons that are keeping you afloat (or the third quarter), the rotation of your body combined with the kicking of your feet progresses your body over your anchored arm, which is helping support the streamlined position.

It is at this stage that you want to drive your anchored or supported arm down—which is referred to as vaulting. When you execute this step, try to think of your supported arm as a giant paddle that extends from your fingertips all the way down to the inside of your elbow. So instead of vaulting with just your palm, which a lot of swimmers do, you want to create more surface area with your forearm so that you can vault with your fingers, palm, and forearm. The more surface area you have, the easier it is to create support using your opposite arm.

Propulsive Phase

As your vertical forearm passes underneath your body, or the first quarter of the quadrant, you enter the propulsive phase of the swimming stroke. As I mentioned in the catch phase, the pulling of your arm is not a pull; it's a vault. You're using the surface area of your forearm, palm, and fingers to progress you over to your opposite side. For example, if you're vaulting with your left hand, as your right hand enters the water, you're going to drive your arm through and out of the water as you rotate onto your right side. It's this rotation of your body in combination with the vault that allows you to maintain steady progress forward.

An important side note is the bending of the vertical forearm. A lot of athletes misinterpret the vertical forearm as being a vertical arm and will try to keep their arm completely straight as it passes beneath their body. Remember, you want to keep your fingers just barely below your wrist, your wrist just below your elbow, and your elbow just below your shoulder. As your vertical forearm passes underneath your body and you roll onto your opposite side, your arm will naturally bend at the elbow. During this stage you should focus on keeping your forearm vertical to increase the surface area of your arm and maximize acceleration. As your arm bends, your hand will follow a straight path toward your feet and exit near your hip.

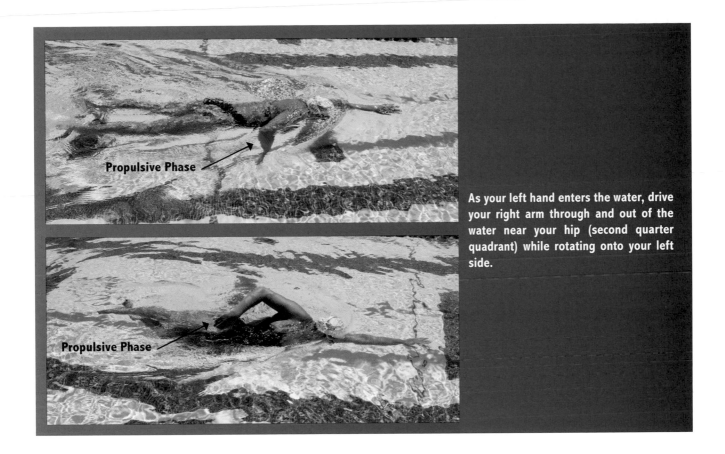

Propulsive Phase

Propulsive Phase

As your left hand enters the water, drive your right arm through and out of the water near your hip (second quarter quadrant) while rotating onto your left side.

Recovery Phase

The moment your hand exits the water as you shift from one support to another, you enter the recovery phase of the swimming stroke. It's important to note that it's called the recovery phase for a reason. A lot of swimmers will remain tense and try to forcefully maneuver their arm over their head as quickly as possible so that they can transition into the next phase. You can tell when someone is doing this because the arm will be curled like a chicken wing and clamped to the side of the body. Another obvious giveaway is when the athlete curls his wrist like a hook or extends his arm straight out of the water as if he were reaching for the sky.

The key is to remain patient and stay focused on keeping your arm relaxed. Think of it like the recovery phase in the pedal stroke when cycling: the moment your foot passes six o'clock, you relax your leg and drive through with the opposite leg. There is zero mechanical advantage to pulling up on the pedal after it passes six o'clock; in fact it can hinder the most important phase of the pedal stroke, which is taking place on the opposite side. It's the exact same thing in swimming, but instead of relaxing your leg as it passes six o'clock, you're relaxing your arm as it passes the second quarter of the quadrant. The moment your hand exits the water you need to pull your elbow over your shoulder and rotate your arm toward your head as if you were waving to your face. As you do this, keep your arm bent with the forearm completely relaxed and your palm facing toward the water.

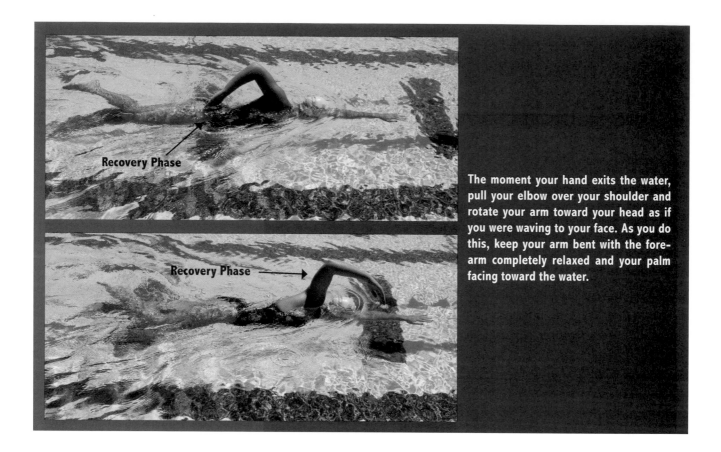

Recovery Phase

Recovery Phase

The moment your hand exits the water, pull your elbow over your shoulder and rotate your arm toward your head as if you were waving to your face. As you do this, keep your arm bent with the forearm completely relaxed and your palm facing toward the water.

Entry

As your hand passes your head in the recovery phase, or passes the third quarter of the quadrant, you start the transition into the entry phase of the swimming stroke. The key with this phase is to remain relaxed, keep your palm facing the water, and penetrate the surface just in front of your head. Because you're simultaneously rotating your body and switching forces as your hand enters the water, it's common for athletes to rotate their palm toward the sky and enter with their thumb down. Such a fault not only increases the water's drag on the hand entering the water, but also prevents you from establishing a strong support with your extended arm. Another fault associated with this phase is to overthink the entry and tense your hand, which again can affect the next phase of the swimming stroke, in this case the catch. A helpful cue that will help with both of these faults is to lead with your fingers instead of the side of your hand. Once you successfully enter the water with a relaxed hand, extend your arm as you continue to rotate your body and transition into the hand-lead position. From there, you establish a support and repeat the process.

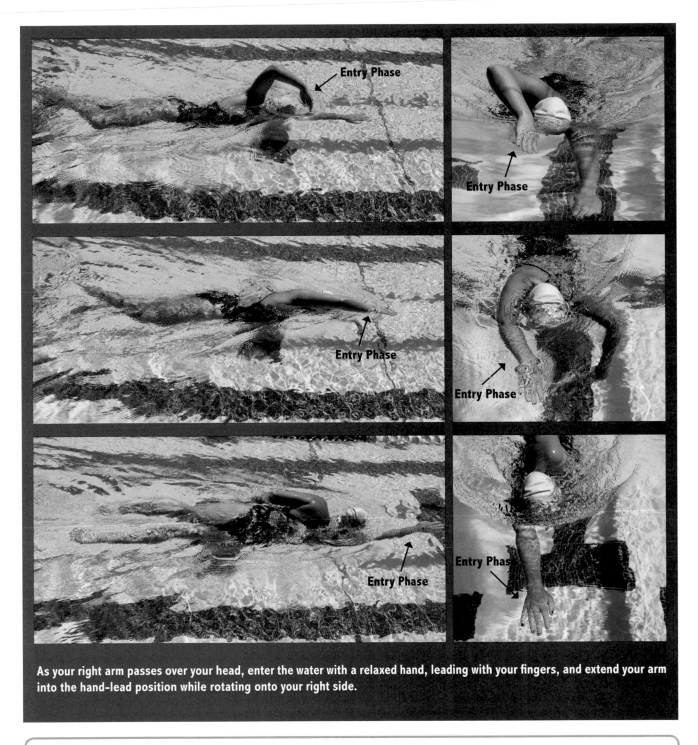

As your right arm passes over your head, enter the water with a relaxed hand, leading with your fingers, and extend your arm into the hand-lead position while rotating onto your right side.

Technical Note: As you know, timing, among other things, is critical to swimming as efficiently as possible. Even if your technique is perfect, a break in rhythm can upset the entire system. For example, if you remove your support before your opposite hand passes over your head—which is the most common timing fault—the weight of your arm combined with the power of gravity will force your body underwater, compromising the velocity and efficiency of your stroke. To help athletes grasp this concept, we often refer to the freestyle stroke as the three-quarter catch-up or three-quarter freestyle. This is just a simple way of reminding the athlete to be patient in the stroke and make sure to keep the lead hand supported until the opposite hand, which is in the recovery phase, passes the head (or passes the third quarter of the quadrant).

SWOLF (GOLF) TEST

Over the years, coaches have developed methods for analyzing stroke frequency or stroke rate, as well as stroke length, as a means of improving swimming efficiency. Although analyzing the measurement of an athlete's stroke length as well as the speed and accuracy of his stroke frequency can be beneficial, it's not necessarily a great gauge because there are countless variables in freestyle swimming. It's not that it's not effective; it's just complicated.

To simplify matters, we've developed what is called the SWOLF test, which not only measures and improves stroke rate and length but is also an important diagnostic drill. Just as Kelly Starrett uses a test/retest to measure improvements with the prescribed mobility exercises featured in his mobility WOD, the SWOLF test is our way of measuring proficiency in the swimming stroke. Usually, we perform the test at the beginning and end of our seminars to illuminate improvements. However, you can implement this test anytime you want to track or measure your progress.

To execute the test, have a friend or coach record your time (to the nearest second) and stroke count as you swim one lap in the pool. It's important to note that a stroke is counted every time a hand enters the water. So if you start from the hand-lead position with your right arm forward, your left hand entering the water is one, your right hand entering the water is two, and so on. Don't make the mistake of counting cycles of left arm and right arm stroke as one.

After you swim one lap, add the two numbers to calculate your score. For example, let's say it takes you 15 seconds and 15 strokes to complete one lap. Your score would be 30. It's important to note that there is no good or bad score; it's just your score. After you complete the test, work through the checklist and spend some time running through the drills featured in this chapter. As you run through the drills, focus on the techniques that give you the most trouble so that you can round out your weaknesses. Once accomplished, you should perform the SWOLF test again to track your progress.

Ultimately, the goal is to lower your SWOLF score by either going faster or taking fewer strokes. But if you lower the stroke count and your time stays the same, it shows that you've lengthened your stroke and swum farther with each effort. Conversely, if your stroke count stays the same but your time improves, that means you're generating more power and getting more velocity per stroke. So if you reduce your time, which is your speed and velocity, or stroke rate, and your distance per stroke, which is your stroke length, it shows that you're getting across the pool faster and with less effort.

INSIDER PERFORMANCE TIPS

BE PATIENT AND PROGRESS AT YOUR OWN PACE

Unless they've had formal lessons or spent a lot of time in the water, learning how to swim touches on people's worst fears and insecurities. It's definitely one of the most technical and challenging sports. A lot of athletes talk themselves out of learning how to swim or learning to be more efficient in the water because they think the learning curve is too slow. This is simply not true. Swimming, although challenging and extremely difficult, does not take a lifetime to learn. In fact, proficiency can be attained in a very short period of time. The key to is to remain patient and focus on the drills that highlight your weakness(es). Also, don't be in a rush to get through the drills. As long as you progress through the sequence of drills at your own pace and spend ample time working on your streamlined stance, you'll be swimming effortlessly in no time.

MASTER THE STREAMLINED SWIMMING STANCE

Streamlined stance and kicking mechanics are universal constants for every athlete. Put another way, they can always be improved and are the quickest way to develop an efficient freestyle stroke. If you can keep your body level and kick properly, everything from timing and rotating to moving your arms through the four phases of the swimming stroke will be much easier to manage.

FOLLOW THE DRILLS SEQUENTIALLY AND FOCUS ON YOUR AREAS OF WEAKNESS

If you're struggling with the movements, or working too hard to move forward, isolate your areas of weakness in the form of a drill until you gain proficiency. That is why we recommend that you go through the drills in order to find the drill or drills that highlight your biggest weakness. If you skip around with the drills in the beginning, you may miss one that highlights one of your weaknesses.

LEARN TO BREATH ON BOTH SIDES OF YOUR BODY

Whether you're an advanced swimmer or brand-new to the sport, you need to be able to breathe comfortably on both sides of your body. That way if you are in an uncontrolled environment like an ocean or lake—which has currents, wakes, and waves—you can adjust your breathing accordingly. This can be practiced a couple of different ways. You can either breathe every odd stroke, or pick an even-stroke count and switch sides every other lap. This doesn't mean that you have to breathe on both sides of your body all the time. Once you're proficient, you can favor one side. The key is to become proficient at breathing on both sides of your body so that you're prepared for any scenario.

SWITCH UP THE STROKE

It's important to mention that the backstroke, which is briefly covered in the drills section, and the breaststroke are still valuable techniques to add to your arsenal if you're just learning how to swim or are competing in a long-distance event such as a 5K or 10K. In such a situation, you can switch up the stroke (assuming you're proficient) to catch your breath and give your muscles a break. If you're an advanced swimmer, the backstroke can be a nice reprieve from the freestyle stroke because you can maintain an efficient streamlined position while keeping your face above water. The breaststroke, on the other hand, is great for beginner triathletes because it allows you to catch your breath and see where you're going. However, neither of these strokes is as efficient as the freestyle stroke, so you want to be mindful to transition to the backstroke or breaststroke only when absolutely necessary.

LEARN TO RELAX AND NOT FIGHT THE WATER

When you watch an experienced swimmer do the freestyle stroke, one of the first things you'll recognize is the fluidity and elegance of her movement. It seems almost effortless. To reach this level, you have to devote time to drilling specific movements. Remember, swimming is like being in quicksand, in that the harder you work, the faster you fatigue, and the lower you sink. You have to remain relaxed, maintain a level body position, and be precise with your movement, which only comes about through hours of practice.

TRAIN IN OPEN WATER

In a pool you can see where you are going and you can breathe more effectively because you're in a controlled environment. In a lake or ocean, on the other hand, you can't see where you are going, the waves are constantly hitting you, and you have to battle currents. This makes everything from timing your stroke to breathing more challenging. For the less experienced swimmer it can also add another level of fear. The only way to conquer this fear and adapt to such an environment is to spend time in open water. Don't wait until the day of the event to test your skills in a lake or ocean. If you know that you have to swim in a lake, go out and swim in a lake. If you're competing in an event that requires you to run into the ocean and swim back, go out and do it. You have to train in the same conditions you're competing in. That goes for running and cycling, as well as swimming.

EMPLOY SWIMMING AIDS AFTER YOU GAIN PROFICIENCY

Although using floatation devices and paddles can help you focus on specific aspects of the stroke, you want to have some level of proficiency with the stroke before you incorporate these tools into your training. Why? Because you don't want to create a crutch that distracts you from proper mechanics, especially when you're first learning. For example, a pull buoy will help raise your legs to the surface so you don't have to kick. This allows you to focus on the swimming stroke while maintaining a level body position. However, if you rely on this tool to maintain a proper streamlined position and never work on kicking mechanics, you're going to have to deal with the consequences come race time. For the best results, gain proficiency with freestyle mechanics, then use swimming aids to isolate specific aspects of the stroke.

KICKING BEATS

Although kicking beats are different for every individual, most triathletes and endurance swimmers have a low kick count, probably two to four beats per stroke cycle. In other words, every time your right arm goes through all four phases of the swimming stroke, you kick your legs only two times. The idea is to get your kicking beat low to reduce your energy expenditure. Your legs are much bigger and tenser than your arms, so if you kick more, you're going to expend more energy. Not only that, but if you're a triathlete, if you kick less, you'll save your legs for the bike and run. However, it's important to note that there is no right or wrong kick count. In the beginning, do what comes natural and whatever it takes to maintain a level body position. Once you're propelling forward without struggle, you can start to experiment with different kicking beats to find your ideal rhythm. The key is to reduce your kicking beat without compromising your streamlined stance or swimming stroke. If reducing your kick count disrupts the rhythm of your stroke or compromises your alignment, revert to your natural kicking pattern.

ROTATE YOUR HEAD AND LOOK FOR YOUR HAND ONLY WHEN YOU BREATHE

A lot of swimmers make the mistake of turning their head in concert with their body every time they rotate from one side to the other. To maintain an efficient body position, your eyes should be looking straight down and you should turn your head only when you breathe. Remember, your head can move independently from your body, so you can rotate or shift from one support to another while keeping your eyes focused on the bottom of the pool. When you need to take a breath, rotate your head as you switch supports and look for the arm that's going through the recovery phase. This will allow you to take in air without having to crane your neck and ruin your neutral spinal alignment.

SKILL TRAINING

Now that you understand the principles and concepts fundamental to learning proper swimming technique, it's time for you to get in the water and start layering on drills. As I've stated throughout the chapter, these drills are designed to strengthen your position and layer on the phases of the swim stroke so that you can learn to relax and move more efficiently through the water. It doesn't matter if you're big, small, tall, short, a beginner, or experienced. What we've done is break down the important universal themes so that all athletes can incorporate the drills into their training. When the drills are carried out correctly, they will improve your swimming mechanics in the shortest amount of time possible, making what used to be an exhausting and unpleasant experience into an effortless, enjoyable one. However, for the best results, it's important that you progress through the drills sequentially, regardless of your experience or skill set. Here's why:

Some of you reading this book may have a ton of experience in the water, while others may have never learned how to swim using proper technique. Although you still want to advance through the drills sequentially, your focus and intent may differ depending on your comfort level and skill set. To help with your understanding, let's use three different examples taken from three different categories to see how a beginner, intermediate, and advanced swimmer would approach the forthcoming sequence of drills.

Novice Swimmer

A novice swimmer is someone with little to no formal training in the water and can barely move forward without drowning. If you fall into this category, you should spend the vast majority of your time working on the beginning set of drills, which focus on balance and buoyancy, midline stabilization, body position, and kicking technique. It takes time to become comfortable in the water, especially if you're new to swimming, so you should be careful not to progress too fast. Learning to swim can be extremely frustrating, scary, and at times embarrassing. The key to progressing up the chain of techniques is to strengthen your position by working your streamlined stance. Just like a boxer, you have to master your stance before you start throwing punches. In swimming that means getting comfortable and proficient in the streamlined stance using good kicking technique before adding rotation or the phases of the swimming stroke.

Intermediate Swimmer

An intermediate swimmer is someone who has had some kind of formal swimming lessons or at least feels comfortable in the water and can move forward using freestyle mechanics. If you fall into this category, the key is to not rush through the beginning drills. You still have to find your balance and buoyancy point (if you haven't done so already) to see where you're weak and what you have to work on.

In addition, you have to spend some time developing a proper streamlined position using proper kicking mechanics before moving on. A lot of athletes who understand basic swimming mechanics skip the beginning drills, thinking that there's nothing in them. Instead, they go right to the arm-lead drills and then wonder why they're having so much trouble.

Although it may take you less time to dial in your streamlined stance, you still need to tune up your position and make sure everything is in line before you tackle the next sequence of drills. Once you transition into the rotation, hand lead, and arm-lead drills, isolate the drill that you struggle with the most so that you can focus your attention on your areas of weakness. Even if you have experience in the water using freestyle mechanics, you will probably need to work on your timing and maintaining a streamlined stance as you progress through the phases of the swimming stroke.

Advanced Swimmer

An advanced swimmer is someone who can swim effortlessly with fluidity and grace. Usually, advanced swimmers have competed on a collegiate level or have spent their entire life in the water. They understand and have probably implemented the drills demonstrated in this chapter at one point or another and understand the importance of body position, timing, and freestyle mechanics. For athletes who fall into this category, running through the drills sequentially still may prove beneficial. Each drill focuses on a specific aspect of the swimming stroke, which is what makes the sequence of drills so effective. While it may take you only one training session to run through the drills, you'll inevitably find one or two drills that expose a hole in your game. For example, you may have no trouble gliding through the water with the freestyle stroke, but the moment you implement the face-wave drill, you start to sink and lose your position. This is an indication that you need to work on your kick, supporting your hand on the surface of the water, and dialing in your body position while in the arm-lead position.

The bottom line is: You're never too good to drill. There is always something that needs work, so find the drill that you're the weakest at and implement that into your skill-training day.

Conclusion

Although refining technique and constantly working to improve movement efficiency is a central theme in this book, nowhere is it more important than in swimming. The biggest mistake that endurance athletes make is to stop implementing fundamental swimming drills once they feel comfortable with a movement. This creates a scenario, just like with running or cycling, in which once you're comfortable with the movement you stop training technique, and focus on volume instead.

Remember that working toward a level body position; building an efficient, powerful, and rhythmic kick; and developing proper timing will remain constants regardless of whether you're a beginner or an Olympic-level swimmer. And while you don't have to master each drill before you start incorporating intervals and tempo training, you do want to remain focused on technique to avoid ingraining dysfunctional movement patterns that will be difficult to undo.

> **Technical Note:**
> *As you will soon recognize, the majority of the skill-training drills are demonstrated on only one side of the body, but every drill should be practiced equally on both sides.*

OPEN-WATER SWIMMING STRATEGIES

If you're swimming in an open body of water such as a lake or ocean, there are a lot of environmental conditions for you to contend with, which include (but are not limited to) currents, waves, and wind. Moreover, if you're competing in a triathlon or long-distance swimming event, there is the added element of athletes trying to overtake your position. In such a situation, you have to employ strategies that not only keep you on course but also capitalize on the advantages you have at your disposal. There are three strategies that will help you deal with the challenges of swimming in an open-water event: spotting, directional swimming, and drafting.

SPOTTING

When you're swimming in open water, conditions often change without warning. For example, a lot of swimmers will make the mistake of checking the current before they get in and formulate a strategy based on that information. The problem is that if the current shifts midrace, which is quite common, you're going to get thrown off course, thus increasing the overall distance you have to swim. To avoid such a situation, you want to constantly spot a marker—whether it's a buoy or landmark such as a tree or mountain—and gain a frame of reference so that you can adjust accordingly. The key is to time your head lift as you bring your arm through the recovery phase of the swimming stroke. Although this breaks the cardinal rule of maintaining a neutral posture and head position, it's necessary so that you can remain on course. Remember that you can also switch to the breaststroke to spot your marker, but this will slow you down and break the rhythm of your stroke. Once you gain a frame of reference, you can use that information to your advantage by employing directional swimming.

DIRECTIONAL SWIMMING

To improve your understanding of directional swimming, let's use the example of an athlete swimming in a lake toward a buoy. The buoy is 50 meters straight ahead, but there is a strong lateral current pushing the swimmer off course. In order to remain on the correct path and maintain the straightest line possible, the swimmer must change the angle of his approach by swimming into the current at a 45-degree angle in relation to the buoy. (The degree of your angle depends on the strength of the current, so it's important to spot frequently so that you position and adjust accordingly.) Although swimming into the current forces you to work harder, it keeps your body in line with the buoy.

If you swim without considering the power of the current, it's going to push you off course. Then you have to switch your direction and swim directly into the current to get back on course. As you can imagine, this is not efficient. In addition to increasing your distance, you have to tackle the current head-on, which slows your progress and increases your energy expenditure.

DRAFTING

When you're swimming in a pool lane lines separate you from other swimmers. In open water, on the other hand, everybody is positioned in uncomfortably close proximity. This can work to your advantage or disadvantage depending on where you are positioned. For example, if you're trailing behind someone, you can position yourself in his or her wake to help pull you forward. If you position yourself in a wake, you're going to be pulled in the direction the person in front of you is swimming and minimize the amount of energy you have to put out. Conversely, if you're leading the pack with other swimmers drafting in your wake, you have to work a lot harder to move forward; it's like carrying an extra weight. Drafting can also get you into trouble if you're behind a group of swimmers who are not spotting or using directional swimming. You might get knocked off course by their lack of skills. You have to know your surroundings and the people you're swimming with, continue to use spotting and directional swimming tactics, and try to keep others from drafting off your wake.

DEAD MAN'S FLOAT

As I mentioned in the introduction to this chapter, you have to understand the importance of body position before you string together a complicated sequence of movements in the form of a freestyle stroke. The purpose of the dead man's float is to help you understand the role of your lungs and how they dictate your natural position in the water. For example, if you look at the photos below, you'll notice that the back and neck are sticking out of the water. Although everyone will look slightly different based on body type, the focus of this drill is to teach you that air trapped in your lungs is what keeps you afloat. In addition, this drill gives you an idea of how your body rests naturally in the water, which is critical in determining kicking pattern.

To perform this drill correctly, take a big breath in using the full capacity of your lungs, relax your arms and legs by letting them dangle directly underneath your body, and keep your head down. A lot of swimmers, when first performing this drill, will make the mistake of tensing their limbs and flexing their neck in an attempt to pull their head out of the water. If you're new to swimming, this step may take a few tries to get right, so be patient.

A helpful hint is to do exactly as the title implies, which is to be dead in the water in a completely relaxed state. When done correctly, as you take a deep breath and dunk your head into the water, your body will rock up and down like a seesaw until it reaches a point where it's completely still. That is your balance point, which can be achieved only if you're totally limp. If you're tense, you'll keep wobbling up and down and never find your natural position in the water before running out of air.

Another critical point, which I mentioned earlier, is that there is no right or wrong result from doing this drill. In other words, don't get frustrated if, say, you sink straight to the bottom. Use whatever information you glean from the drill to determine what you need to work on.

If you attempt to execute the dead man's float, but for whatever reason—whether you have dense muscles or low lung capacity—you sink to the bottom of the pool like a rock, that is an indication that you have to work a lot harder on developing a powerful kick so that you can remain on the surface of the water in a streamlined position. If you bob on the surface effortlessly, on the other hand, you can focus on using your arms to propel you forward.

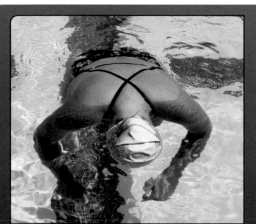 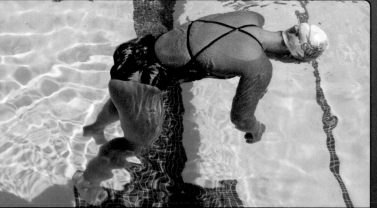

To assume the dead man's float position, Christina takes a big breath using the full capacity of her lungs, completely relaxes her body, and falls forward. As you can see, she's floating on the surface of the water and her back is exposed directly over her lungs. This is her natural position in the water. To get the best results, it's imperative that you stay totally relaxed and avoid tensing your body or extending your neck to pull your head out of the water.

DEAD MAN'S FLOAT WITH ARM RAISE

The dead man's float with arm raise is an extension of the previous drill and should be performed only after you've found your natural position in the water. Assuming that you carried out the previous drill correctly, the next step is to raise your arms up slowly from the dead man's float position. If you glance at the photos, you'll notice that two things happen. As Christina raises her arms, her lower back and the top of her hips come out of the water, and without additional effort her legs start to rise toward the surface. So by simply raising your arms from the dead man's float, you spread your balance point from your lungs to your entire midline, as well as achieve a level body position. The purpose of this drill is to get you to understand that the more elongated your body is, the less drag you have on the surface of the water, and the easier it is to move forward.

An interesting side note to this technique is the difference in body position based on a swimmer's background, muscle density, and body symmetry. For example, if you have a larger upper body than lower body, which is characteristic of a distance swimmer, your legs are going to rise toward the surface and your butt is going to pop out of the water. Conversely, if you're a sprint-distance swimmer or you happen to carry the majority of your weight in your legs, your feet will remain stuck on the bottom and will rise only slightly.

If you fall into that latter category, don't get discouraged. This is just a byproduct of how you are proportioned and means that you will have to use the strength of your kick to keep your body level. Here's a trick: Tucking your chin to your chest may help draw your legs toward the surface. Remember, your spine wants to stay straight. So if you move your head while in the dead man's float arm raise position—whether you move it up or down—your lower body tends to go in the opposite direction.

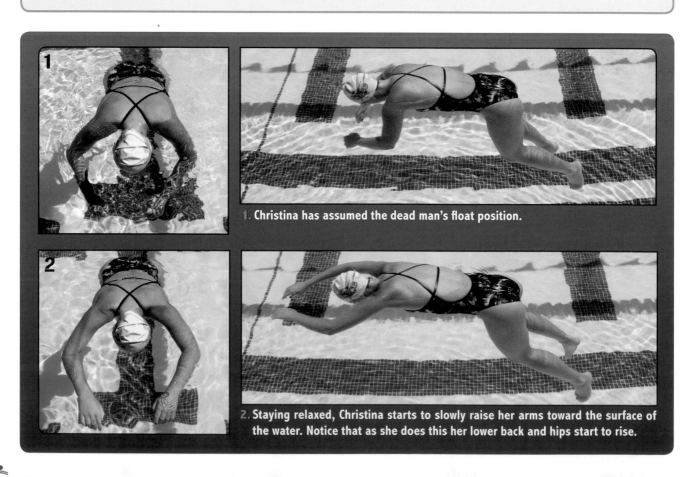

1. Christina has assumed the dead man's float position.

2. Staying relaxed, Christina starts to slowly raise her arms toward the surface of the water. Notice that as she does this her lower back and hips start to rise.

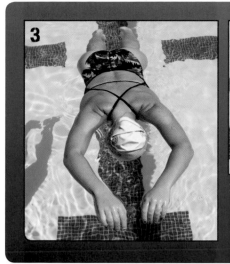
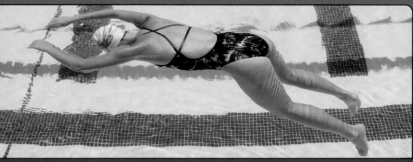

3. As Christina's arms reach the surface of the water, her hips and legs lift, elongating her position. With her body stretched out, her balance point in the water has now extended beyond her lungs into her entire midline. From this position, it is a lot easier to progress forward.

DEAD TO STREAMLINED KICKING

As I mentioned in the introduction to this chapter, the goal of these beginning drills is to teach you how to get into the most efficient position possible before you start moving through the four phases of the swimming stroke. Just like running, cycling, and lifting, if you try to execute a movement without first learning the correct setup position, the subsequent steps will be less effective—you will not move as efficiently as possible. For that reason, it's imperative that you spend time drilling these fundamental techniques, regardless of the drill's simplicity. If you try to skip ahead without ingraining the fundamentals, you not only lengthen your learning curve, but you also increase your susceptibility to fatigue and injury. Taking such an approach is like trying to run in a full sprint without first learning how to walk, or trying to dead lift twice your body weight without knowing how to setup for the exercise.

The goal of this next drill is to teach you how to properly maintain the correct position in the water while adding forward movement. To perform this drill correctly, start from the dead man's float position and slowly raise your arms as demonstrated in the previous sequence. But instead of allowing your arms to float on the surface of the water, you establish the streamlined position by extending your arms overhead and placing one hand on top of the other.

When done correctly, this additional extension of the arms should flatten your body and force your heels toward the surface of the water. The moment your hips reach full extension, or you're as flat as you can get without sacrificing your position, start kicking your legs to initiate forward motion. A common fault that a lot of swimmers make is kicking before they've stopped moving in the water. If you start kicking while still in motion, you will still progress forward, but you have to work a lot harder to achieve the same outcome. Always remember that position dictates your ability to move efficiently, no matter what you're doing. For this drill to be carried out correctly, you have to reach a state of equilibrium, which is a key focus of this drill, before you start to kick.

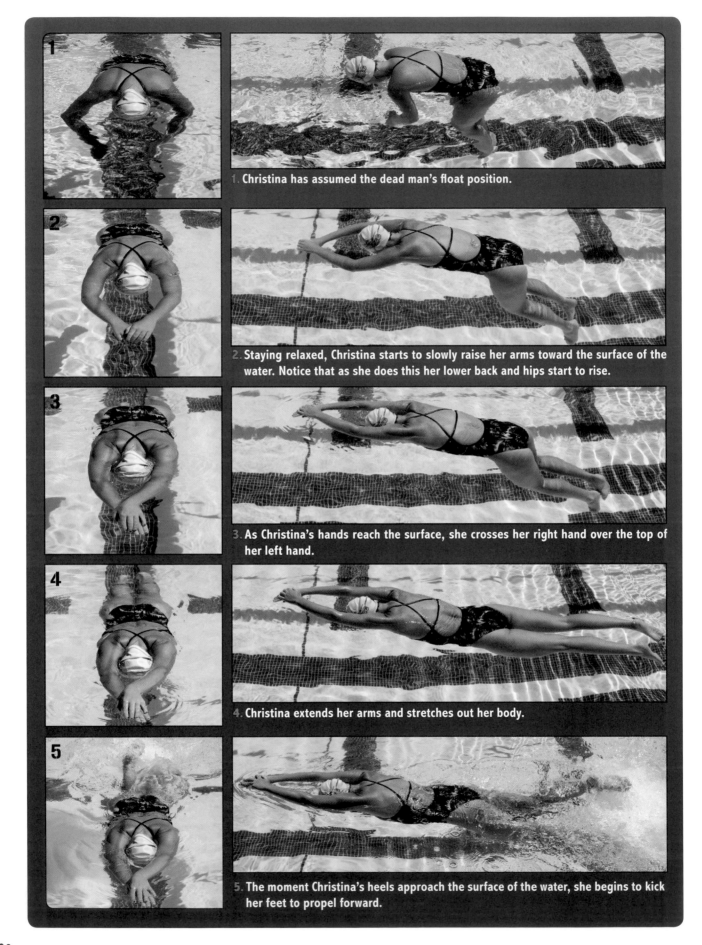

1. Christina has assumed the dead man's float position.

2. Staying relaxed, Christina starts to slowly raise her arms toward the surface of the water. Notice that as she does this her lower back and hips start to rise.

3. As Christina's hands reach the surface, she crosses her right hand over the top of her left hand.

4. Christina extends her arms and stretches out her body.

5. The moment Christina's heels approach the surface of the water, she begins to kick her feet to propel forward.

STREAMLINED KICKING ON THE BACK

Although the focus of this chapter is to layer on drills in sequential order to shorten your learning curve with the freestyle stroke, it's important that you also become well versed in the backstroke, especially if you're a long-distance swimmer or triathlete competing in an endurance event. If you fall into this category, the backstroke is an effective technique to use to catch your breath and give your muscles a momentary break. While the backstroke is not something that is covered in this book, it is important to learn. If you're familiar with the backstroke or you're going through the learning process, then you can incorporate streamlined kicking on the back into the system of drills to help increase your proficiency. Learning and implementing this variation will not only help build symmetry by working different muscle groups, but also give you a strategic advantage in long-distance endurance events.

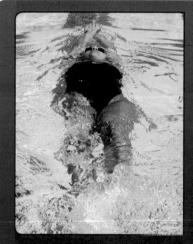
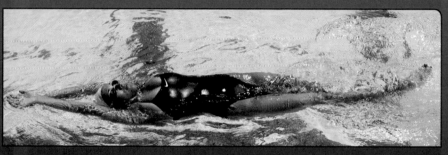

Rudie has achieved a streamlined position on her back and is progressing forward using the power of her kick.

VERTICAL KICKING

The vertical kicking drill is the first step in the next sequence of drills. In addition to developing proper kicking mechanics, it is excellent for testing midline stability. To perform the drill correctly, focus your gaze forward, keep your arms crossed in front of your body, and kick your feet back and forth.

The key is to keep your back flat, your head in a neutral position, and in the same fixed position as you kick your feet underneath your body. Just like the stable-arm drill demonstrated in the running-as-a-skill chapter, vertical kicking should reveal the level of stability required for swimming. For example, if you're wobbling up and down or from side to side (you're unable to maintain a stable position with a flat back), either you're not set in the correct position with your midline properly engaged or your core is underdeveloped. When faced with the former, consider implementing the hollow-rock test on page 26. This test will not only create tension in your midline to the appropriate level, but it will also set your trunk in the correct position. If faced with the latter, you may want to address the strength-and-conditioning exercises to build a stronger midsection and consider spending more time on the fundamental drills outlined in this chapter.

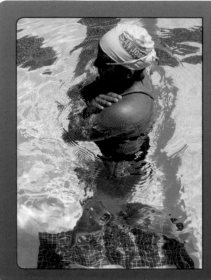
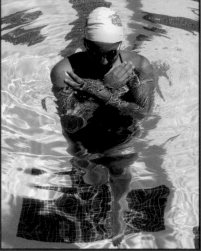

Rudie has established the vertical kicking position and is using proper kicking technique to keep her shoulders above the surface of the water. Her arms are crossed with her hands on her collarbones, her elbows are tight to her body, and her hips are directly under her shoulders. To maintain a straight body, she engages her midline by establishing the flat back position. This tail-tucked position—otherwise referred to as an anterior pelvic tilt—flattens the small of her back and maintains the integrity of her position. Any deviation from this position, whether you're in extension or flexion, will result in excess movement.

VERTICAL KICKING WITH FORWARD LEAN

Once you're able to do the vertical kicking drill with a hollow-tight position, the next step is to fall forward to initiate forward motion. This is challenging, so it's important for you to remain patient and practice, practice, practice. The majority of swimmers attempting this drill for the first time bend at the hips, extend their arms to catch their balance in the water, or lift their neck up to keep their head above the surface. To avoid these faults, keep your head inline with your back, your arms tucked into your body, and your midline engaged. Although this drill is a bit more advanced than the previous drills, it is extremely important to nail because it teaches you how much stability is necessary to maintain a streamlined position as you move forward. If you can perform this drill seamlessly, remaining level as you swim freestyle will be a piece of cake.

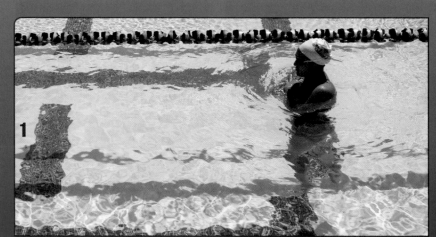
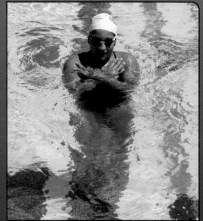

Rudie is executing the vertical kicking drill.

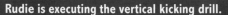

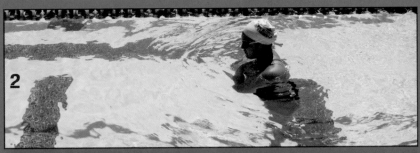
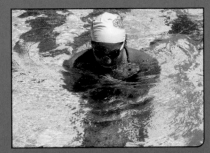

2

Still kicking her legs to keep her shoulders above water, Rudie begins to fall forward to initiate forward movement. It's important to mention that just as when you fall to initiate forward motion in the run, you must avoid bending at the hips or breaking the integrity of your posture in any way.

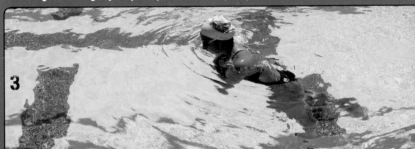
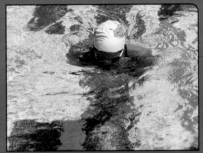

3

Rudie continues to fall forward with a stable body.

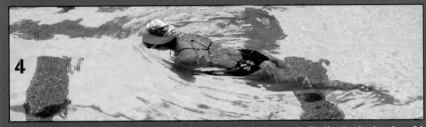
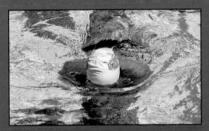

4

Maintaining the integrity of her spine as she falls forward, Rudie dunks her head in the water.

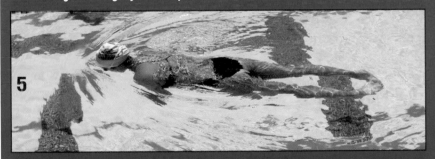
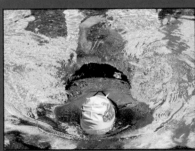

5

Rudie lifts back up so that her body is horizontal to the surface of water.

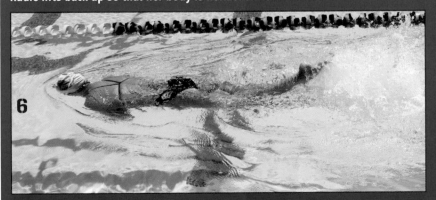
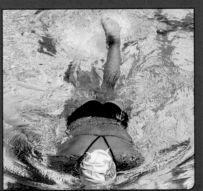

6

The moment Rudie's heels hit the surface of the water; the power of her kick propels her forward.

VERTICAL KICKING WITH BACKWARD LEAN

In addition to giving you a strategic advantage in a long distance event, as the backstroke does, vertical kicking with a backward lean is an excellent way to test midline stability, develop kicking mechanics, and engage different leg muscles to help round out the athlete.

Just as in the previous drill, your body should be straight as you level out, your arms wrapped tight around your chest, and your head in a neutral position. The tendency is to extend the neck and arch the back, which is a break in position. If this happens, don't get frustrated. It takes a ton of tension in the trunk and razor-sharp focus to keep your body straight and your head neutral as you lean backward and level out. The key is to be mindful of your position and keep drilling the fall. With enough practice, you will be able to go from a vertical to horizontal position without compromising your posture, allowing you to move flawlessly across the surface of the water.

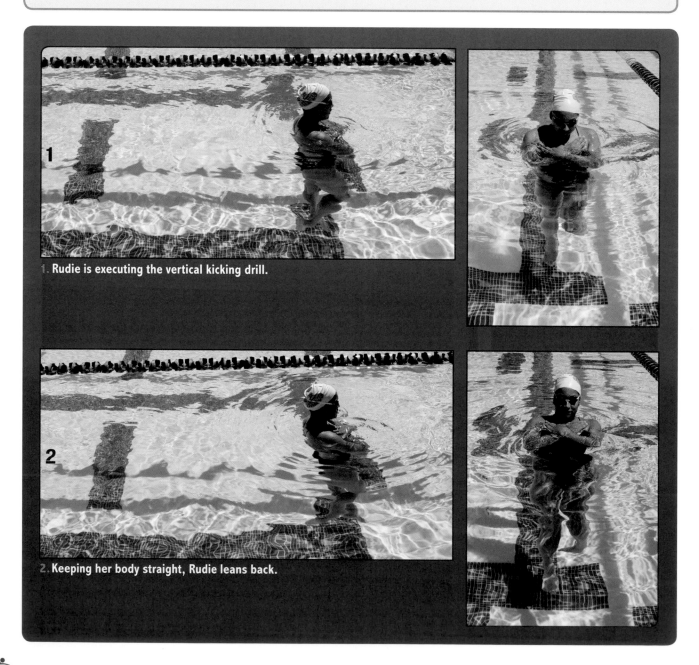

1. Rudie is executing the vertical kicking drill.

2. Keeping her body straight, Rudie leans back.

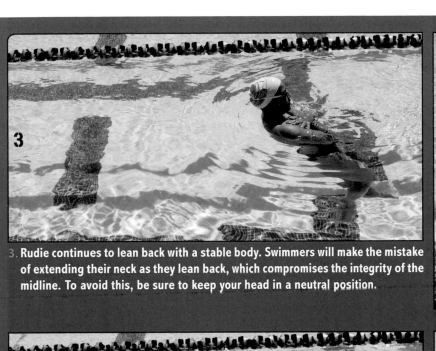

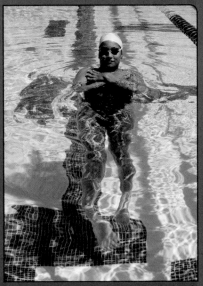

3. Rudie continues to lean back with a stable body. Swimmers will make the mistake of extending their neck as they lean back, which compromises the integrity of the midline. To avoid this, be sure to keep your head in a neutral position.

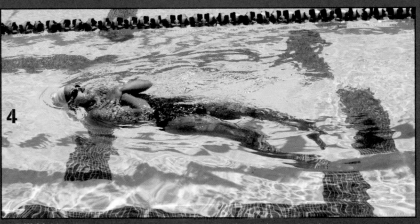

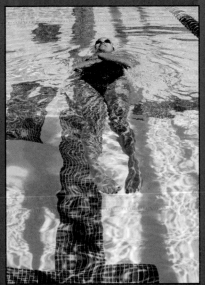

4. Still kicking her feet as she leans back, Rudie begins to level out.

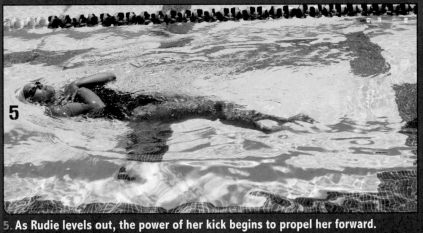

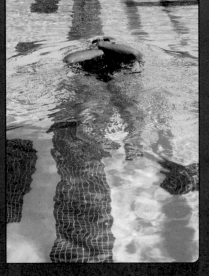

5. As Rudie levels out, the power of her kick begins to propel her forward.

VERTICAL KICKING TO STREAMLINED

As I've repeatedly mentioned, the less drag you have in the water, the faster you go: which is another way of saying that the longer and straighter your body is, the more efficiently you will move through the water. This next drill, vertical kicking to streamlined, puts this concept to work. To get the best results from this drill, execute the same series of steps as before, starting with vertical kicking and transitioning into a forward lean. As you reach your max speed with your hands on your chest, you want to move your hands directly under your face and extend your arms into a streamlined position. The moment you completely flatten out your body, you'll immediately notice an increase in velocity without needing to exert any additional energy. By simply keeping your midline stable and establishing a streamlined position, you reduce the drag on your body, which allows you to progress forward with speed and efficiency.

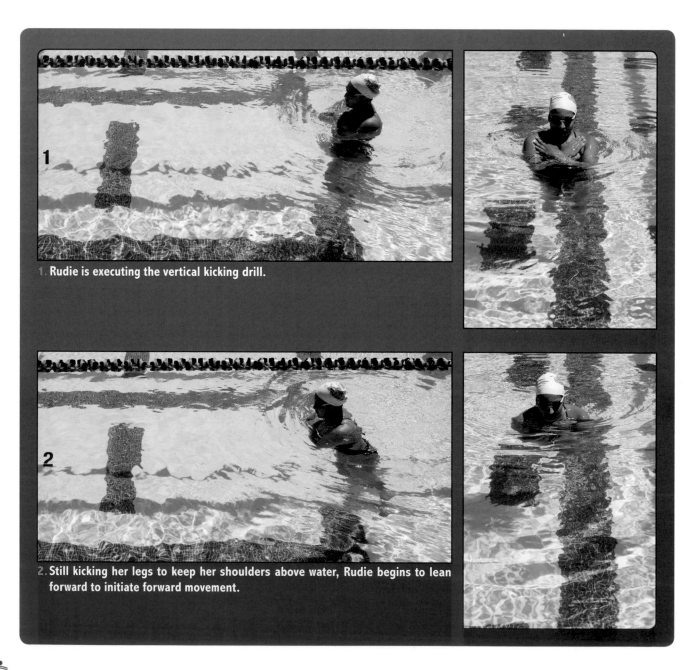

1. Rudie is executing the vertical kicking drill.

2. Still kicking her legs to keep her shoulders above water, Rudie begins to lean forward to initiate forward movement.

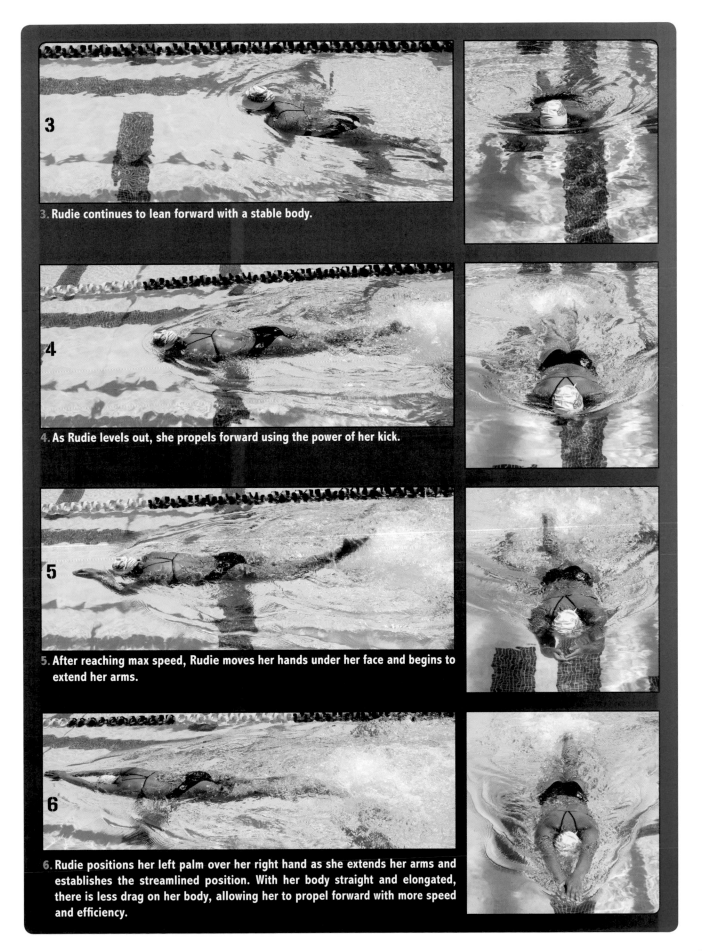

3. Rudie continues to lean forward with a stable body.

4. As Rudie levels out, she propels forward using the power of her kick.

5. After reaching max speed, Rudie moves her hands under her face and begins to extend her arms.

6. Rudie positions her left palm over her right hand as she extends her arms and establishes the streamlined position. With her body straight and elongated, there is less drag on her body, allowing her to propel forward with more speed and efficiency.

HEAD LEAD

Staying on point, we're still working with aligning your body in the most efficient position. Once you've initiated forward motion using the previous techniques, the next step is to roll onto your side while continuing to progress forward by kicking. The goal of this drill is to keep the side of your body perfectly parallel to the surface of the water, with your top shoulder and hip stacked directly over your bottom shoulder and hip. To accomplish this, be sure to keep your eyes down, your top arm tucked as if you were reaching into your pants pocket, and your bottom arm glued to the side of your body.

It's important to remember that your head moves independently and should follow the rotation of your body only when you're coming up for air. A lot of beginners make the mistake of turning their head with their body, or rotating toward their stomach or back as they kick. This will ultimately decrease the efficiency of the stroke. If you're struggling with the rotation, work on the streamlined kick until you're comfortable moving forward with a level body. Then you can incorporate this drill into your training. Although this drill may seem difficult at first, with patience and practice you'll be able to master it.

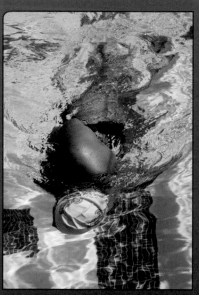
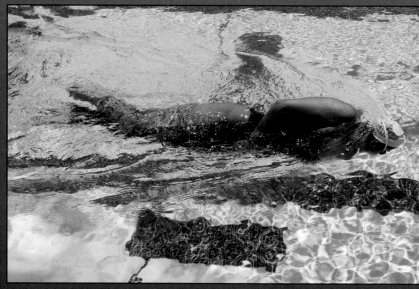

From the streamlined position, Rudie has rotated onto her right side while continuing to move forward using the power of her kick. Notice that her head is pointed down, her right arm is positioned over the top of her right hip as if she were reaching into her pocket, and her left arm is glued to her side.

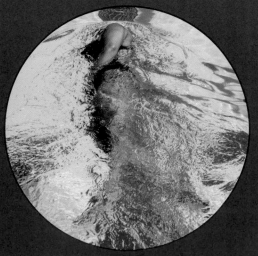

In this photo you can clearly see that Rudie is positioned perfectly on her side with her left shoulder and hip stacked directly over her right shoulder and hip. Remember that this is the exact position you need to assume and maintain when performing this drill.

HEAD LEAD WITH ROTATION

After you can progress forward with the head lead, the next step is to add side-to-side rotation. This drill not only reinforces proper midline stability and kicking mechanics, but also teaches you how to maintain a level body position while rotating from side to side. The key is to rotate your body as slowly as possible while keeping your eyes focused on the bottom of the pool. The only time your head and body should be inline is when you take a breath of air. In addition, if you rotate from side to side too quickly, you compromise the strength of your position and you might bounce up and down, slowing your forward momentum. To ensure proper execution of this drill, focus on maintaining a powerful and rhythmic kick and rotating your shoulders, torso, hips, and legs as a single unit. Done correctly, this will keep you glued to the surface of the water and allow you to control every centimeter of your rotation.

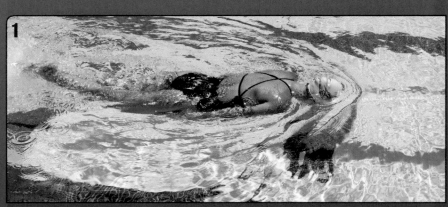

Christina has established the head-lead position. Notice that her head is pointed down, her right arm is positioned over the top of her right hip as if she were reaching into her pocket, and her left arm is tight to her side.

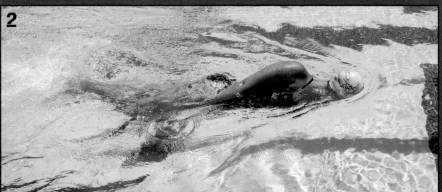

Keeping her head level, Christina slowly rotates onto her left side. Note that she rotates her shoulders, torso, hips, and legs as a single unit.

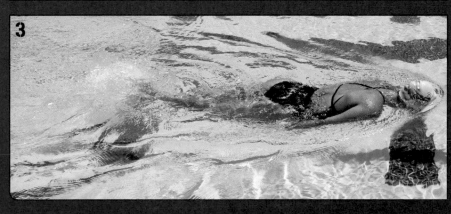

Christina momentarily reestablishes the head-lead position as she rotates toward her right side.

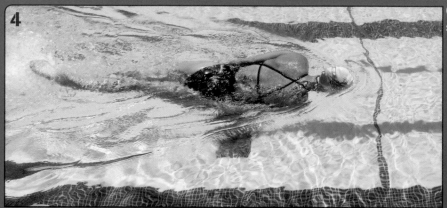

Christina rotates onto her right side.

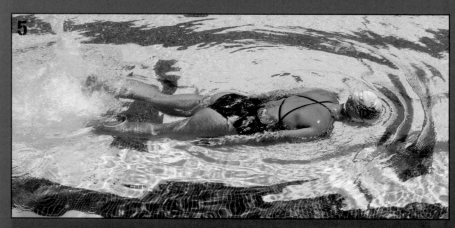

Christina maintains a level body position as she rotates toward her left side and momentarily reestablishes the head-lead position.

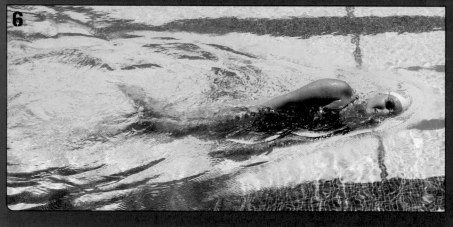

As Christina rotates toward her left side, she turns her head in sync with the rest of her body so that she can take a breath.

HAND LEAD

After you're proficient with the head lead, the next step is to extend your bottom arm while maintaining a rotated position with a straight and level body. Just as in the head-lead drill, you should minimize side-to-side movement, keep your top hand tucked next to your hip, and focus your eyes on the bottom of the pool. When performing this particular drill, remember that your midline is still your balance point. A lot of swimmers will rely on their hand for balance, meaning that they will move their hand up, down, and from side to side in order to maintain the rotated position. This is exactly why the head-lead drill is taught before the hand-lead drill. That way you learn to balance over your core and not through your extremities. If you're using your hand to maintain the proper position—that is, waving your palm from side to side, rotating your arm, or pushing down on the water to keep from sinking—chances are that the integrity of your midline is compromised and your balance point has shifted away from your lungs. In such a situation, take a step back and readdress the previous drills.

To get the best results from this drill, it's important for you to reach max speed with the head lead before extending your bottom arm. As you will inevitably experience, by simply elongating your body, you increase your forward momentum without having to put additional energy into the kick. The takeaway from this drill, aside from teaching the proper rotated position, is that the longer you can extend your body in the water, the faster you go.

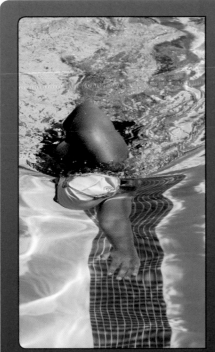
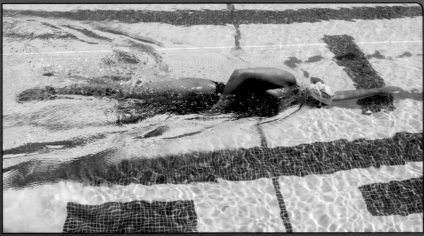

As Rudie reaches max speed with the head lead, she extends her bottom arm with her palm facing the bottom of the pool while continuing to use the power of her kick to propel her forward. With her arm stretched out, she moves faster through the water without expending more energy to kick. It's important to notice that her left arm is directly inline with her body, her fingers are relaxed, and she's in the optimal rotated position.

ARM LEAD

If you've been performing the drills sequentially—as you should!—you already know that each drill builds on the previous one. So, assuming that you're proficient with the previous drills, the next step on this path is to execute the arm lead. If you glance at the photos, you'll notice that the swimmer's top arm is now positioned above the water as if she were going to move into the next swimming phase, which in this case would be the entry phase. With her arm positioned above the water, she now has an added force working against her. To counteract the additional weight, she will have to keep her body in perfect alignment by positioning her top elbow directly over her shoulder. It's also important that the top arm remains in a fixed position. If your body wobbles from side to side or you try to maintain a fully rotated position by moving your extremities, take a step back and address your position. Unless you're an expert swimmer, some of these drills may take a while to master, so it's important to just be patient. If you stick with the protocol and keep doing the drills in sequential order, stringing the four phases of the freestyle stroke together into one fluid motion will become natural and effortless.

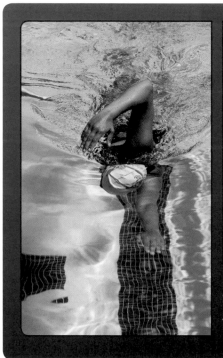

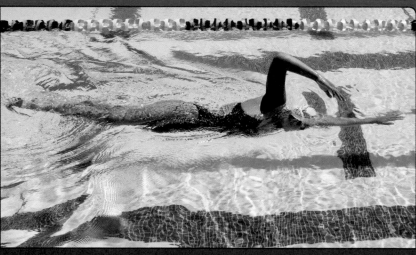

From the hand lead, Rudie lifts her right arm and establishes the arm-lead position. Her elbow is directly over her shoulder, her arm is relaxed, and her hand is just past her head. Just as in the previous drill, she is looking down, her left arm is inline with her body, and she's in the ideal rotated position.

THREE-TOUCH CATCH-UP

I can't say it enough: Keeping your body straight in the water and staying centered over your balance point, which is your lungs, is the primary focus of these drills. However, as you become proficient with each subsequent technique, you must add new elements to challenge the intended focus. For example, if you're able to perform the arm lead without difficulty, the next step is to add movement to simulate the next phase of the freestyle stroke, which is the entry and recovery. To perform the drill correctly, you need to touch the water three times—out in front of your head (entry), at your hip (recovery), and then out in front of your head for the second time (entry)—before switching to your other side. In addition to teaching you how to control your core and maintain rotation, this drill also ingrains the proper recovery and entry mechanics and proper timing. For instance, a lot of swimmers will rotate onto their stomach before they transition into the entry phase, which changes their balance point and reduces their forward momentum. To avoid this, stay on your side until your hand enters the water for the third time, as illustrated in the last photos of the sequence.

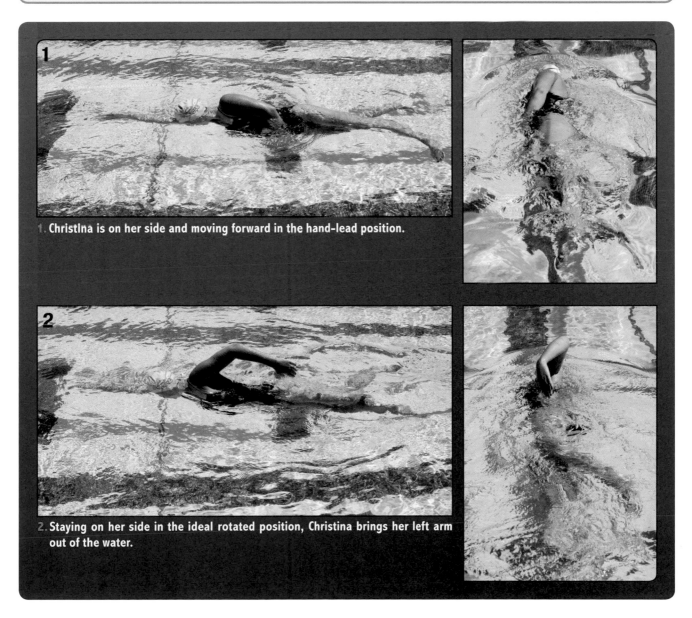

1. Christina is on her side and moving forward in the hand-lead position.

2. Staying on her side in the ideal rotated position, Christina brings her left arm out of the water.

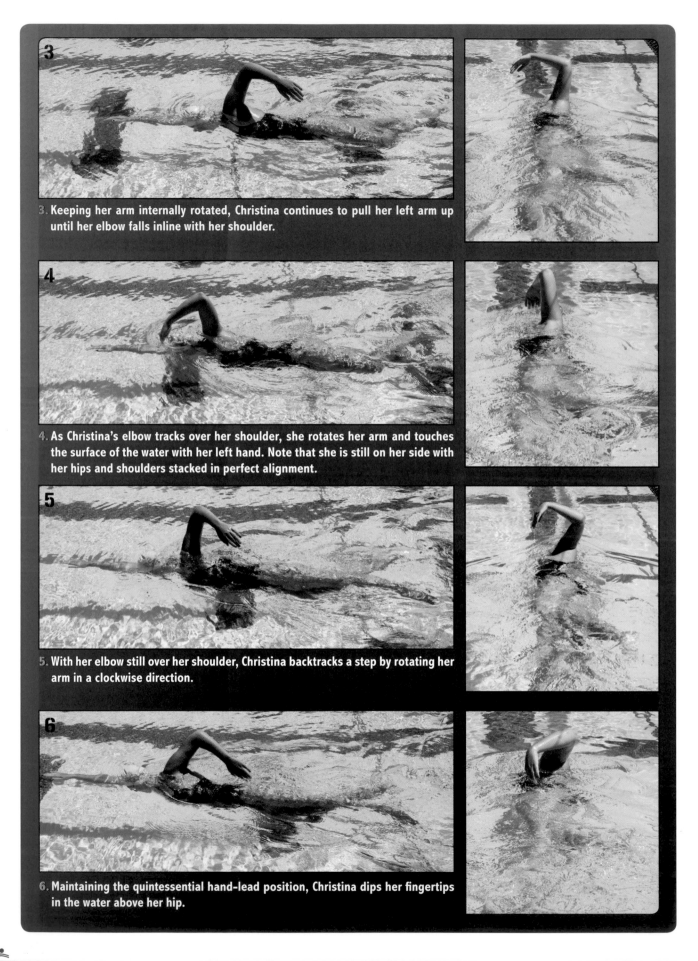

3. Keeping her arm internally rotated, Christina continues to pull her left arm up until her elbow falls inline with her shoulder.

4. As Christina's elbow tracks over her shoulder, she rotates her arm and touches the surface of the water with her left hand. Note that she is still on her side with her hips and shoulders stacked in perfect alignment.

5. With her elbow still over her shoulder, Christina backtracks a step by rotating her arm in a clockwise direction.

6. Maintaining the quintessential hand-lead position, Christina dips her fingertips in the water above her hip.

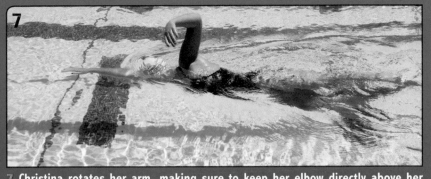

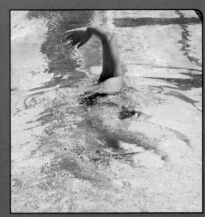

7. Christina rotates her arm, making sure to keep her elbow directly above her shoulder, and transitions through the recovery phase of the freestyle stroke.

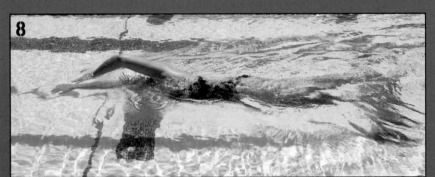

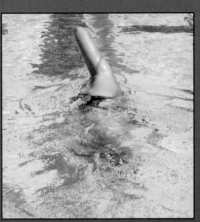

8. Still on her side, Christina enters the water with her hand relaxed and her palm facing the bottom of the pool.

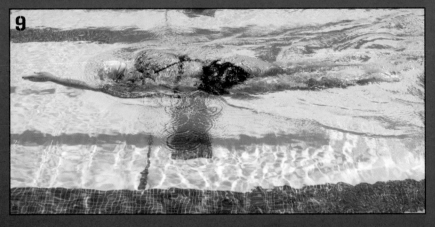

9. As Christina extends her left arm, she rotates onto her left side and momentarily assumes the left-hand-lead position.

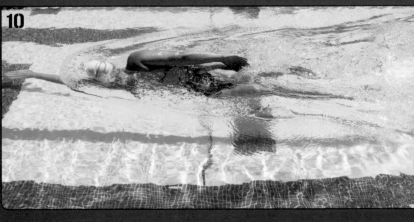

10. Christina will repeat the process on the opposite side.

FACE WAVE

This drill is very similar to the previous one in that you move your arm outside the water while keeping your body in rotation. But instead of touching the water three times, you rotate your arm above the water as if you were waving to yourself, doing a face wave. Moving your arm above the surface of the water challenges your stability, while the face wave—which still challenges core stability to the same degree—emulates the proper mechanics of the recovery phase. To perform this drill correctly, your palm should be facing your body, your arm should be bent at roughly a 90-degree angle, and your elbow should be inline with your shoulder. The key to this drill is to relax your arm, keep your elbow stationary, and remain in a fixed rotated position as you propel forward. Once you complete the face wave—meaning that you raise your elbow out of the water into the arm-lead position, wave your hand back and then forward again—transition into the entry phase of the freestyle stoke and repeat the drill on the opposite side.

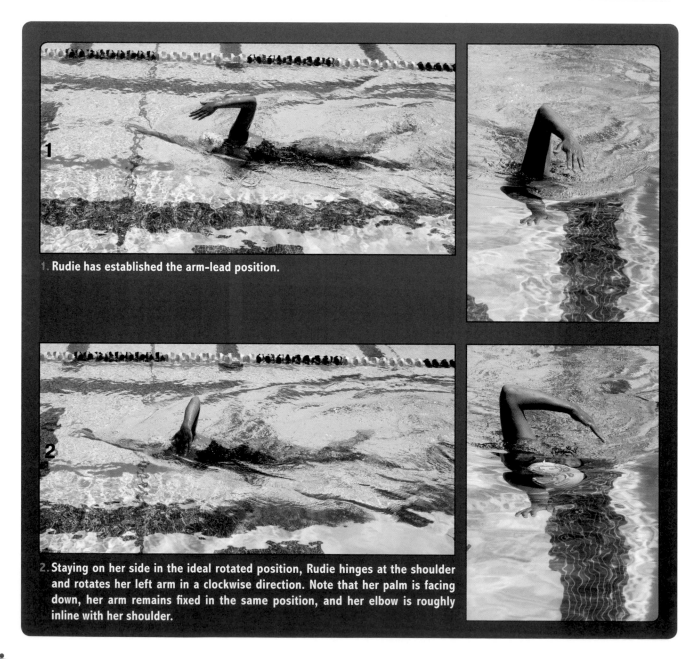

1. Rudie has established the arm-lead position.

2. Staying on her side in the ideal rotated position, Rudie hinges at the shoulder and rotates her left arm in a clockwise direction. Note that her palm is facing down, her arm remains fixed in the same position, and her elbow is roughly inline with her shoulder.

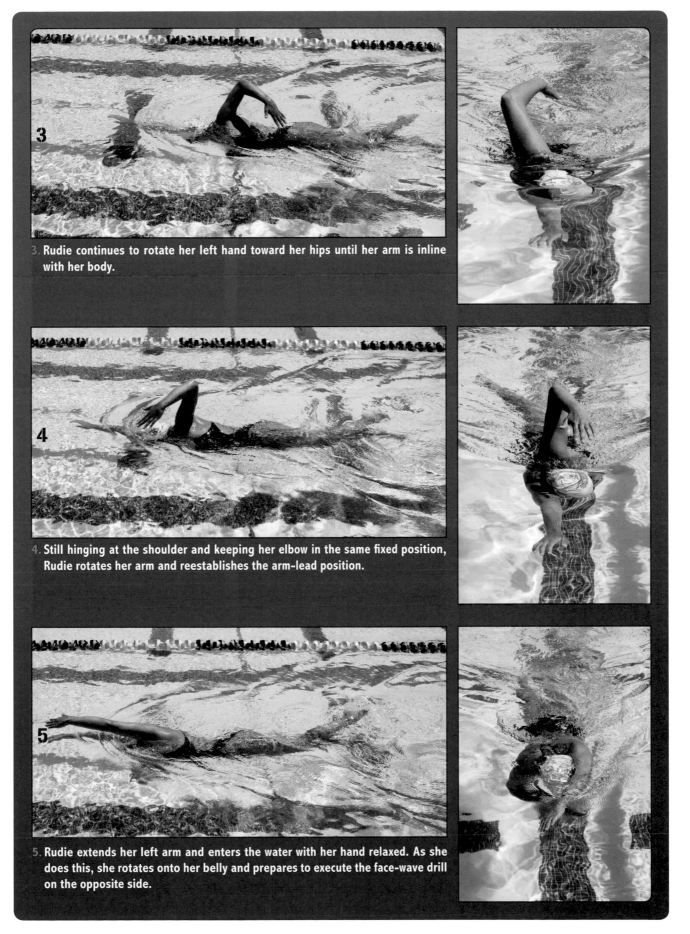

3. Rudie continues to rotate her left hand toward her hips until her arm is inline with her body.

4. Still hinging at the shoulder and keeping her elbow in the same fixed position, Rudie rotates her arm and reestablishes the arm-lead position.

5. Rudie extends her left arm and enters the water with her hand relaxed. As she does this, she rotates onto her belly and prepares to execute the face-wave drill on the opposite side.

THREE-QUARTER CATCH-UP

If you're proficient with the arm lead, the three-touch, and the face wave, you're now ready for the three-quarter catch-up, which is basically the freestyle stroke. Looking at the photos, you may ask, "Why does this have fewer steps than the previous two drills?" While this is an accurate assessment, it's actually not true. Remember, to get to this stage you should already be comfortable balancing over your lungs, keeping the integrity of your midline intact while in rotation, and achieving the arm-lead position. If you can do that, then you're essentially swimming freestyle. The three-quarter catch up combines these drills into one movement, but speeds up the transitions, making the drill more complex. For example, instead of pausing in the arm-lead position and waving your hand back and forth as you did in the previous drills, you pause for only a brief moment (maybe three seconds) before transitioning into the next phase. The whole point of the pause is to exaggerate the arm-lead position before you change sides. After a few rounds of pausing, reduce the amount of time you spend in the arm-lead position, and transition straight into the next stroke. At this point, you'll be swimming freestyle.

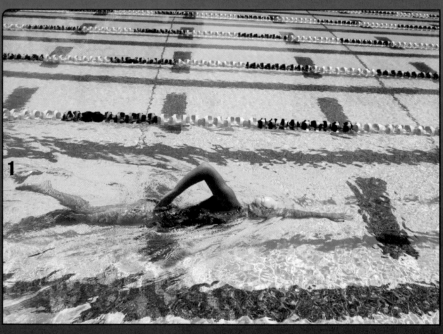

1. To initiate the three-quarter catch-up, Christina establishes the hand-lead position. As she reaches max speed, Christina pulls her right arm out of the water and begins passing through the recovery phase of the swimming stroke. Note that she keeps her left arm stretched out as she pulls her right arm out of the water.

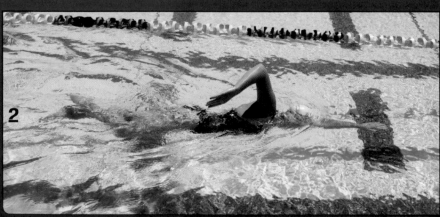

2. Christina pulls her right arm out of the water. It's important to notice that her right arm is bent at a roughly 90-degree angle, her wrist is relaxed, and her elbow is inline with her shoulder.

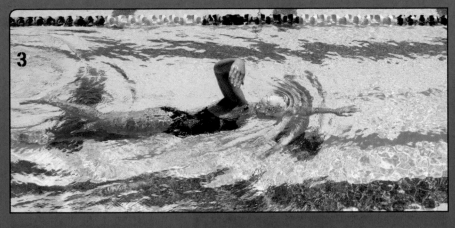

3. Hinging at the shoulder, Christina rotates her arm toward her head.

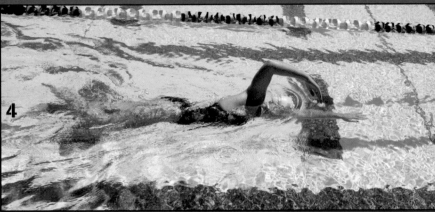

4. Keeping her palm down, Christina momentarily establishes the arm-lead position. It's important to note that if you're performing the three-quarter catch-up, you should hold the arm-lead for at least three seconds before transitioning to the next step in the sequence.

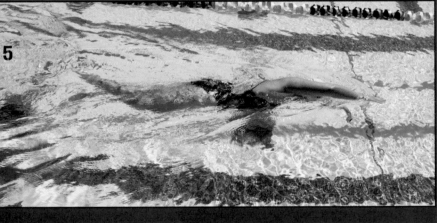

5. After holding the arm lead for three seconds, Christina extends her right arm, enters the water with her right hand, and rolls toward her right side.

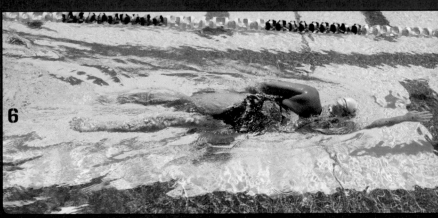

6. Christina establishes the hand-lead position on her right side as she prepares to repeat the sequence on the opposite side.

UNDERWATER FREESTYLE

As you've probably figured out, the underlying theme in all of these drills is to isolate particular aspects of the swimming stroke so that you can focus your attention on a specific area. For example, in the sequence below, we take out the recover phase of the swimming stroke so that you can focus on switching supports using a vertical forearm without worrying about what your arm is doing while it's out of the water. However, to ensure proper technique, it's important for you to carry out the previous drills before attempting the underwater freestyle drill. While this drill is easier, in the sense that it has fewer steps, the previous drills instill the mechanics necessary for performing underwater freestyle properly. In other words, the only way to perform this drill correctly is if you already understand how to switch supports and maintain the hand-lead position. Swimmers who skip over the previous drills won't understand what it feels like to have an external weight bearing down (arm above the water) or how to switch supports at the right time. As a result, the purpose of this drill—which is to time the catch, switch supports using a vertical forearm, and lunge forward as you switch sides—will be lost on them.

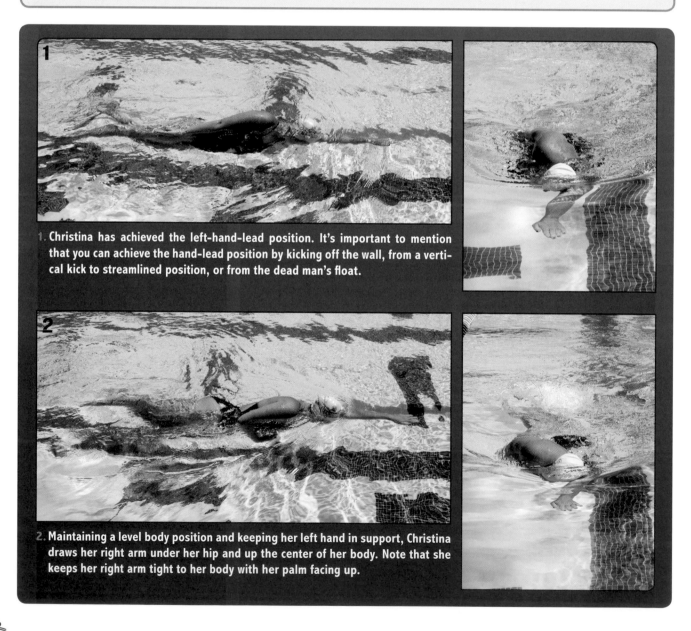

1. Christina has achieved the left-hand-lead position. It's important to mention that you can achieve the hand-lead position by kicking off the wall, from a vertical kick to streamlined position, or from the dead man's float.

2. Maintaining a level body position and keeping her left hand in support, Christina draws her right arm under her hip and up the center of her body. Note that she keeps her right arm tight to her body with her palm facing up.

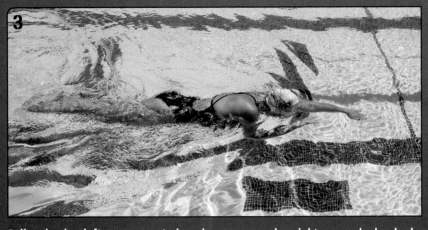

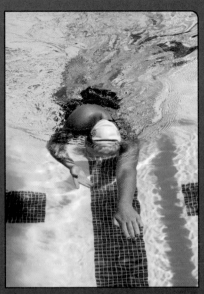

3. Keeping her left arm supported as she maneuvers her right arm under her body, Christina rolls toward her right side and extends her right arm.

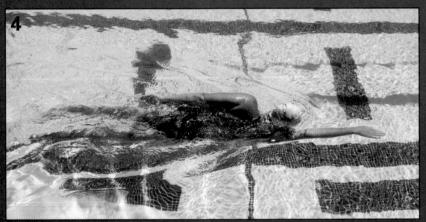

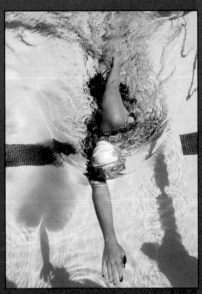

4. As Christina extends her right arm, she turns her palm toward the bottom of the pool and establishes a support with her right hand. As she switches supports, she uses a vertical forearm to propel her body forward. Like all techniques that require you to switch supports, timing is critical to success. To perform this step properly, you should keep your top hand in support until your bottom hand passes under your head. When timed correctly, you should feel a forward lunge as you switch sides.

ACCELERATOR DRILL

Once you've successfully progressed through all the drills in this chapter, you can string the techniques together in the form of the accelerator drill. If you haven't been able to do the previous drills with proficiency, there's no point in doing this one: if you still need to work on properly positioning your body in the water or developing the proper mechanics of midline stabilization and learning the four phases of the freestyle stroke, you will dramatically reduce the benefits of this drill. Remember, the whole purpose of skill-training exercises is to teach you how to move through the water as quickly and as efficiently as possible. If you skip steps or fail to devote time to isolating key stages in the form of a drill, you limit your progression and thwart your performance gains. However, if you're proficient in the drills demonstrated in this chapter, the accelerator drill is an excellent way to train speed intervals, which can be used for conditioning workouts.

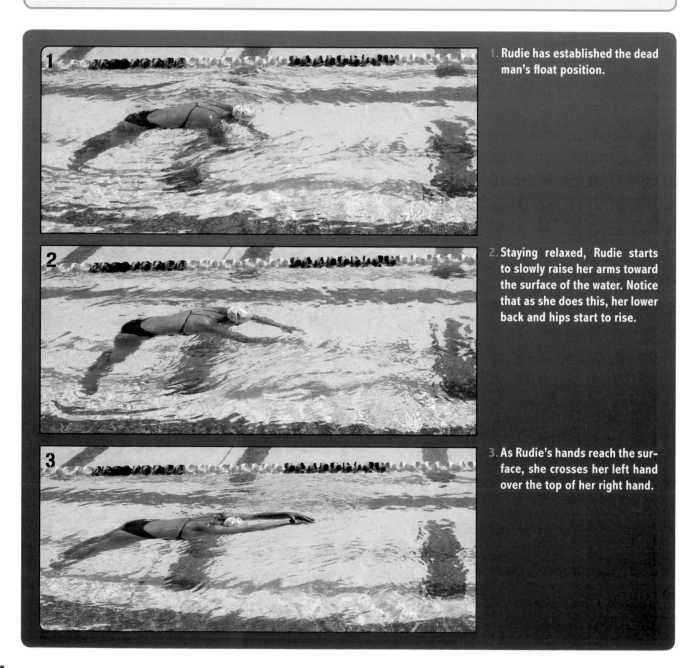

1. Rudie has established the dead man's float position.

2. Staying relaxed, Rudie starts to slowly raise her arms toward the surface of the water. Notice that as she does this, her lower back and hips start to rise.

3. As Rudie's hands reach the surface, she crosses her left hand over the top of her right hand.

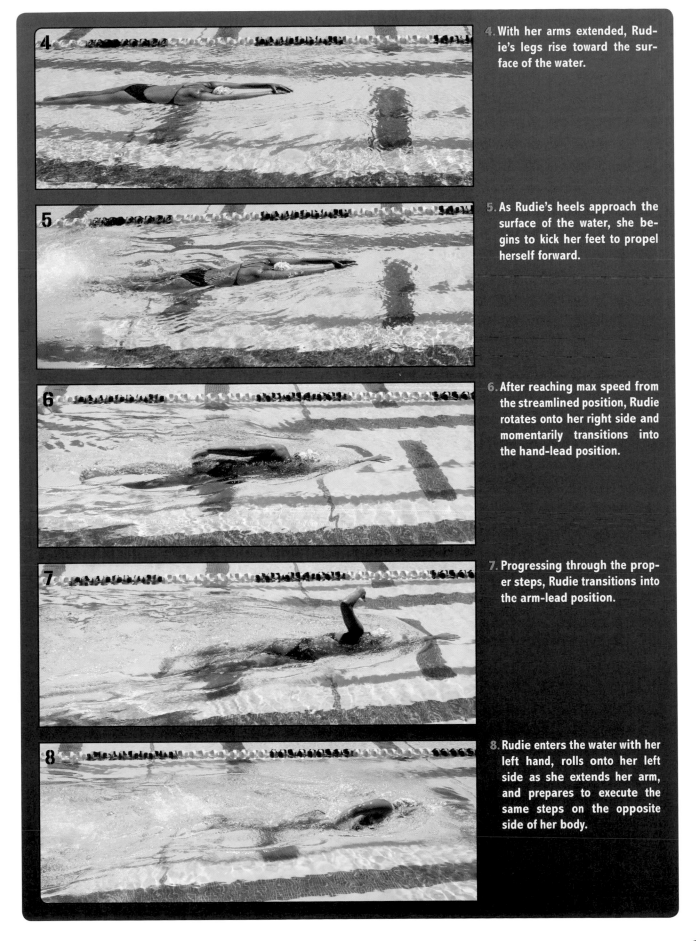

4. With her arms extended, Rudie's legs rise toward the surface of the water.

5. As Rudie's heels approach the surface of the water, she begins to kick her feet to propel herself forward.

6. After reaching max speed from the streamlined position, Rudie rotates onto her right side and momentarily transitions into the hand-lead position.

7. Progressing through the proper steps, Rudie transitions into the arm-lead position.

8. Rudie enters the water with her left hand, rolls onto her left side as she extends her arm, and prepares to execute the same steps on the opposite side of her body.

STRENGTH AND CONDITIONING AS A SKILL

"THE CREW AT CROSSFIT ENDURANCE KNOWS THEIR STUFF. THEIR COMBINATION OF TRADITIONAL PERIODIZED EXERCISE WITH CROSSFIT IS SPOT ON. ANYBODY LOOKING TO MAXIMIZE HIS OR HER ENDURANCE PERFORMANCE WHILE MAINTAINING, OR EVEN IMPROVING, FITNESS MUST READ THIS BOOK."

JOSH EVERETT
CROSSFIT LEVEL 1 AND O-LIFT
COURSE INSTRUCTOR

Success in endurance sports is heavily predicated on your ability to move efficiently. Whether you're running, riding, rowing, or swimming—in fact no matter what activity you do—functional, efficient movement is the key to optimal performance. What's more, learning the fundamental set-up and finishing positions will help you avoid injury. This concept of safe, correct, efficient movement is at the core of the CFE system. However, movement efficiency as it relates to endurance athletics is a teachable and learnable skill. First, you have to learn how to establish stable starting positions for movement (running stance, streamlined position in swimming, ideal seated position on the bike), and then ingrain the proper motor patterns through skill-based drills. Second, you have to develop the strength and capacity to sustain the correct movement pattern by implementing sport-specific high-intensity exercises coupled with a smart strength-and-conditioning protocol.

Although running, cycling, and swimming are the sports you're training to conquer, these activities will not stress your system in a way that promotes strength, speed, power, and mobility. To improve in these areas, you have to incorporate a strength-and-conditioning program that reinforces full range functional movements. Put in another way, in order for your muscles to function the way they're supposed to—meaning that you have full range of motion in all of your joints and that you can go fast, hard, and long without losing form—you have to incorporate a program with movements that express the nature of your physical design: You have to perform full range function movements (squat, lunge, lift, pull, and push), as well as implement weight-bearing exercises that force your body to stabilize at end range positions (bottom of the squat, full hip extension).

The problem with endurance sports is each discipline works within a limited range of motion. Continually working within these limited ranges for extended periods of time is a huge problem, especially if you are a veteran that has done nothing but your respected sport for years on end. If you fall into this category, chances are your muscles and nervous system have adapted to those movement patterns. And while training one-dimensionally has probably made you extremely efficient at your sport (assuming you're performing the movement correctly), it often comes at a cost. Your tissues get stiff and become adaptively short, your muscles become weak and underdeveloped, and injuries become more frequent.

The best way to counter these effects is to 1) treat muscle stiffness and restore normal range to your joints and tissues using the mobility exercises presented in the next chapter and 2) implement a strength-and-conditioning program that requires a synchronized action of more than one muscle and joint at a time (compound movements). These can include (but are not limited to) power lifts, Olympic lifts, full-body-weight movements (gymnastics), and core-specific exercises.

CATEGORIES OF MOVEMENTS

In this chapter, I provide a breakdown of proper lifting and movement mechanics to all the exercises utilized in CFE training system, which includes:

POWER LIFTS:

Power-lifting incorporates basic barbell movements in the form of a squat, dead lift, and bench press. These lifts, along with overhead-pressing movements and other variations of the dead lift and squat, are primarily used to develop strength and power.

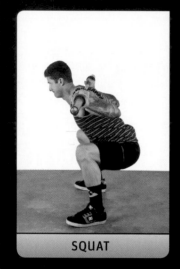

SQUAT

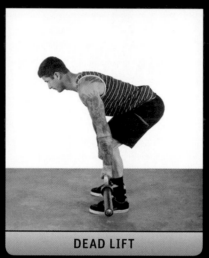

DEAD LIFT

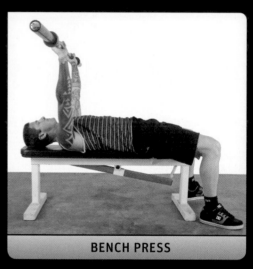

BENCH PRESS

OLYMPIC LIFTS:

An Olympic lift can be defined as a ballistic weightlifting movement that requires you to lift a barbell from the ground to overhead in one continuous movement (snatch), or up to your shoulders (clean), and then, after a momentary pause, pressed overhead (jerk). These lifts can be broken up into specific variants, which will be described in detail over the following pages. When used correctly, the Olympic lifts and their variations build explosive power, speed, and strength.

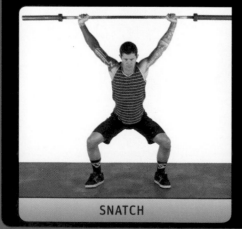

SNATCH

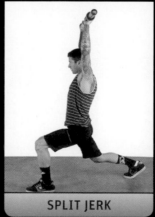

SPLIT JERK

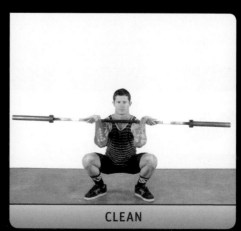

CLEAN

FULL-BODY MOVEMENTS:

Full-body movements can include everything from dumbbell, barbell, or kettlebell exercises such as thrusters and swings to body-weight movements like push-ups, burpees, and box jumps. These movements not only help build strength, speed, power, and increased mobility, but also develop cardiovascular endurance, muscular endurance, and anaerobic and aerobic capacity.

Although full-body movements can include the Olympic and power lifts, for the purposes of this book, full-body movements refer to exercises that are used in conditioning circuits (CrossFit WODs).

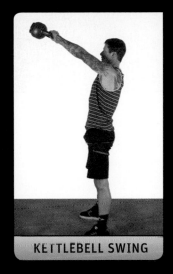

KETTLEBELL SWING

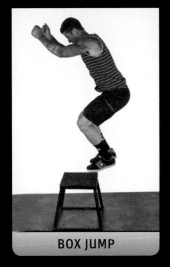

BOX JUMP

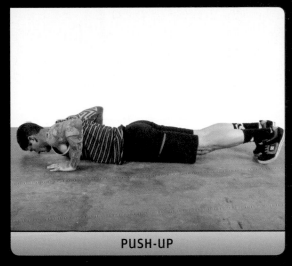

PUSH-UP

TRUNK/STABILITY EXERCISES:

Although all of the lifts or movements help develop the stabilization muscles of the trunk, these exercises focus exclusively on developing midline stability and abdominal strength, which as you already know play a key role in running, cycling, swimming, and lifting mechanics. These exercises can be part of a conditioning circuit or a finisher to a workout.

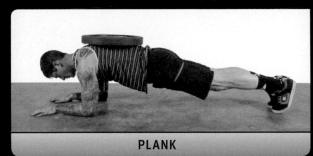

PLANK

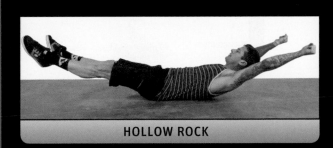

HOLLOW ROCK

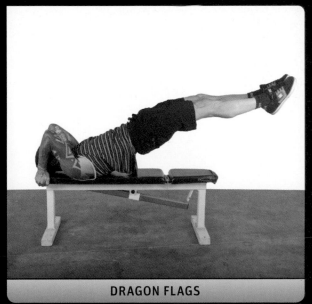

DRAGON FLAGS

Each group of exercises is important because they build and develop an athlete in different ways. For example, the power lifts and Olympic lifts primarily build strength and explosive power, while the conditioning exercises (full-body movements) help develop anaerobic and aerobic capacity, muscular endurance, and speed. As you will see in the programming chapter, these categories are interwoven into strength-bias CFE WODs and CrossFit WODs that are constantly varied to develop the athlete's complete profile. In addition to promoting strength, power, and speed, which in turn allows you to run harder, swim faster, and conquer grades on your bike in record time, the CFE strength-and-conditioning model allows athletes to develop areas of weakness as well as train movements that are directly related to their sport.

I'll use the dead lift as an example. It is a full-range exercise that utilizes the same muscle groups and joints as cycling. In fact, the setup for the dead lift is very similar to your position on a bike. But instead of keeping your hips locked in place as you would on a bike, effectively restricting your joints and muscles by the pedal stroke, you maximize the potential of that range by firing multiple joints and multiple muscles at the same time. You're still using the same muscles as when you drive your foot down into the pedal, but you increase the power range by opening up the hips and extending the legs. This not only makes you more powerful within that limited range and teaches you how to recruit more muscle into that movement, but also strengthens your position by forcing midline and back stabilization and mobilizes joints that don't get expressed through normal ranges of motion on the bike.

To enhance performance in any sport, you have to incorporate a strength-and-conditioning program aimed at developing strength, power, speed, and increased mobility. Endurance as a sport is no different. If you've had exposure to CrossFit, the movements presented in this chapter will look very familiar. However, even if you're proficient with CrossFit skills, it's important that you continue to dedicate time and practice to each technique. Lifting weights or performing body-weight movements incorrectly is no different than running, riding, or swimming with bad form, in that it ingrains dysfunctional motor-control patterns that are inefficient, unsafe, and difficult to reverse.

Strength-and-Conditioning Checklist

To help you navigate through all the lifts and exercises in this chapter, I've provided a checklist to highlight the key factors of this program. The goal of this chapter is to illuminate the movements commonly used in the CFE system. Although I breakdown each movement and provide useful tips, I recommend that you find a coach and sign up at the nearest CrossFit gym if you are seriously interested in the CFE program. There is no way you can learn all of the intricate skills introduced in this chapter, especially the more complex movements like Olympic lifts, without a coach. A good coach will also help you perfect key movements used in the CFE system, as well as provide useful cues* that will allow you to effectively perform or execute these movements.

*"Cues": Helpful verbal tips aimed at correcting a movement fault. For example, if someone is squatting and he is rolling forward onto the balls of his feet, the coach may say something like, "Keep your weight on your heels." A coaching cue can also be used to help remind the athlete of proper movement pattern. Using the same example of a squat, the coach may say something like, "Stabilize your trunk before taking the weight out of the rack."

STRENGTH-AND-CONDITIONING MOVEMENT CHECKLIST

☑ **Scale Movements**

☑ **Master the Setup**

☑ **Create a Position of Stability**

☑ **Build a Symmetrical Athlete**

Scale Movements

If you've never had a strength-and-conditioning program or have no exposure to the functional exercises presented in this chapter, you need to take it slowly and learn how to scale the movements to suit your skill set and strength base. Remember, the goal is to build your muscles and increase work capacity so that you can increase strength, power, speed, and stamina without impeding your recovery or causing injury. To accomplish these goals, you have to start from the beginning and progress steadily up the ladder. For some of you, that means mastering body-weight movements (air squats, push-ups, supine body rows), and then gradually working your way up to the more advanced techniques (back squats, bench press, pull-ups). For those of you with a CrossFit base, working on the dynamic lifts and perfecting gymnastic movements is the best way to continue to make performance gains.

As you will see shortly, almost every movement can be modified and scaled down to suit your strength, skillset, and mobility. To shorten your learning curve, I've provided several progressions and detailed dialogue that highlight specific performance tips. For instance, if you're unable to perform a strict dead-hang pull-up, you can do a supine body row on the rings, or perform the downward motion of the pull-up by slowly lowering yourself down from the bar. As you get stronger and more proficient with the technique, you can progress up the ladder of exercises until you reach your goal. However, it's up to your coach to figure out what you can and can't handle.

The simple fact is: scaling down a movement is difficult to do on your own. As I've mentioned, to get the best results you need to enlist the help of an experienced coach that understands how to modify exercises based on your strengths and weakness. For example, some of you may have the strength to execute a body-weight squat but lack the mobility to perform the movement correctly to its end range, while others may have the flexibility to drop below parallel but lack the strength to perform the movement under load. The adjustments are subtle and complex. Having an experienced outside eye will make scaling weight and movements much easier to manage.

Master the Setup

If you've read through the previous chapters, you know that the most important aspect of any movement is the setup. For example, in the running chapter, you learned the importance of stabilizing your trunk and pulling your arms into the correct position before falling forward to initiate movement. In the cycling chapter, you learned that a strong position on the bike dictates your ability to generate power in the pedal stroke and effectively steer and control the bike. In the swimming chapter, you learned that finding your balance and buoyancy point and arriving at a level body position before moving your arms reduces the water's drag, increasing speed.

Lifting or performing functional exercises is no different. You want to be methodical in your approach and always use the same setup sequence. For example, if I'm setting up for a dead lift, I'll always walk my shins to the bar, hinge forward from the hips with my back flat, assume my grip on the bar, and then pull my shoulders back and raise my hips to get as tight as possible. Only then will I start the pull. Performing the same sequence of steps every time you lift will ingrain proper mechanics and establish movement patterns needed to perform the task safely and efficiently.

It's also important to understand your limitations and make sure that you can perform the movement accurately. For example, if you're unable to set up properly for a dead lift because your hamstrings are too tight, don't avoid that issue by rounding your back. Instead, elevate the dead lift weight off the ground using blocks so that you can set up into an ideal position. Although this shortens your range of motion, it allows you to set up correctly, which not only increases the efficiency of the movement but also reduces your chances of getting hurt.

This idea of reducing range to cater to your mobility restriction also applies to movement. For example, most people can setup correctly for a squat but don't have the mobility to squat below parallel without defaulting into a poor position (knees caving inward, ankles collapsing, back rounding). Although performing the squat to its end range is ideal, that doesn't mean you execute a full range of motion at the expense of technique. In other words, performing the technique correctly always takes precedence over range. In such a situation, scale the range of the movement by squatting down to a box. By executing the movement properly, you will load the right muscle groups, and you will eventually increase your mobility. With enough practice and attention to skill, you will slowly but surely inch your way to a full-range movement. While this may be frustrating and at times embarrassing, it's much better than setting up or performing a movement incorrectly and getting injured or developing dysfunctional motor patterns.

Create a Position of Stability

In addition to providing progressions and variations for the more difficult movements, I've also noted common faults associated with some of them. The vast majority of these faults stem from a weak core and failing to create a position of stability before, during, or at the end of the prescribed movement. It's important to remember that strength-and-conditioning exercises are no different than running, cycling, or swimming in that they all start and end with the trunk.

The only way you can perform any of these movements correctly is if you stabilize your spine and maintain a neutral posture before you start moving through your extremities. If your midline is not engaged and your spine is not stabilized before executing a specific movement, you will never be able to reclaim a strong and safe position once motion is created. Not only that but your body will find stability in weaker positions and make up for the lack of stability by compensating in other areas: that could mean your knees tracking in on a squat, your shoulders rolling forward and elbows flaring out in a push-up, or your head tilting up to the ceiling in a dead lift.

To avoid these and similar faults, keep your core engaged and stabilize your spine in a neutral position before executing any of these exercises. In addition to preventing injury, strengthening and building your midline through functional exercise will increase your ability to maintain form while running, cycling, or swimming for prolonged periods of time. The weaker your core, the faster you lose form, causing you to lose power, speed, and stamina. Unless you build strength and develop capacity under load, your midline will never reach its full potential. In other words, simply going out and running, riding, or swimming is never going to test or develop your core strength like lifting heavy weight!

Build a Symmetrical Athlete

A symmetrical athlete is an efficient and powerful athlete. To make the most of your strength-and-conditioning program and address the problems that stem from sport-specific training, you have to identify your weak areas and work on building a better body, one whose muscles are equally developed, whose frame is thus symmetrical. Because every individual is unique, you and/or your coach have to determine where your imbalances lie, and then target those areas. For example, if you've done nothing but run and bike in terms of training, chances are good that you rely on your quadriceps to perform most movements.

Once this imbalance has taken hold, the powerful muscles in your posterior chain, such as your glutes and hamstrings, take a nap. As a result, power and speed, which is provided by the posterior-chain muscles, is lost, injuries become more frequent, and because you're relying on one major muscle group when you could be relying on three, you fatigue quicker. If you fall into this category, you need to focus on exercises that target your hamstrings and glutes, such as the dead lift. As you round out your frame, you will begin to run, bike, and swim more effectively. Along these same lines, you don't want to overwork or focus on muscles that are already overdeveloped. This will only impede your ability to perform the correct mechanics in your sport and limit your gains. It's also important to note that those fortunate few who already have a well-balanced frame shouldn't neglect strength- and conditioning. Whether you're imbalanced or perfectly symmetrical and strong, everyone has weaknesses, and it's up to you to target them so you can become stronger, faster, and more efficient.

SKILL TRAINING

As I previously stated, the goal of this chapter is to introduce CrossFit Endurance movements as well as properly demonstrate how to perform them. As you study the photos, it's important for you not to make the mistake of thinking that you have to move exactly as illustrated in the sequences. We all have different frame sizes (trunk lengths, arm and leg lengths). As a result, the way you set up for the dead lift may look totally different from how I do it. My intention is to briefly outline why we perform the movement, as well as provide universal how-to cues so that you can coach and perform the exercise more effectively. In addition, these universal cues will equip you with the load order sequencing for each exercise, which is another way of addressing the step-by-step process to correctly performing the movement.

Here's an example of load ordering for the back squat:

1. As you find your grip on the bar, engage your midline and stabilize your spine by achieving a neutral posture before lifting the weight out of the rack.

2. With the bar resting in the meat of your upper back, just above your scapula, drive your elbows up to pin the bar in place.

3. Lift the weight out of the rack and step back with your trunk tight. Don't look down to check your foot position! This will compromise the strength of your position. You should already know how far to space your feet before setting up for the lift.

4. Keeping your head neutral and your back flat, drive your hamstrings back and slowly lower into the bottom-squat position. As you do this, drive your knees out. Your big toes should remain on the floor and your weight should be in your heels. The combination of these actions loads the hamstrings and the glutes and unloads the quadriceps.

5. After your hips drop below parallel, extend your hips and knees to stand tall. Your trunk should still be tight, your back flat, and your head in a neutral position. Like the descent, your hips and torso rise at the same speed.

6. As you reach full extension, squeeze your glutes and lock out your hips. Repeat steps 4 to 6 to execute another repetition.

As you will come to understand, a lot of the load sequencing is the same for most exercises. You will be given the same cues over and over again: stabilize your midline, maintain a level body position, keep your back flat, drive your knees out, keep your head in a neutral position. Although this may seem redundant, it's important for you to grasp these concepts because prioritizing these movements is the best way to ingrain proper position. Remember Kelly Starrett's mantra: "Position is power." The only way you're going to learn the correct way to perform the exercises, develop proper motor patterns, and get stronger, faster, and prevent injury is to know what position you need to maintain regardless of the exercise.

If you're interested in learning more about these movements or want to see videos of them being performed, visit www.CrossFit.com: there are hundreds of videos in the exercise archive. In addition to visiting the CrossFit website, I highly recommend that you attend a CrossFit Level 1 or CrossFit Endurance Trainer course. As I've repeatedly stated, although you can extract a lot of information from these pages and be a self-trained endurance athlete, you'll get only so far. At some point, you have to find a coach and surround yourself with like-minded people. This will not only help to shorten your learning curve, but also help you identify and correct faults that may have been going unnoticed.

SQUAT: PROPER SETUP

In this sequence, I demonstrate how to remove the barbell from the rack to execute a back squat. Since midline stabilization is the prerequisite for all movement, engaging your abdominals before stepping under load is priority one as you approach the barbell. (For the goods on proper midline stabilization, flip back to Chapter 2.)

With your midline firm and your spine protected, the next step is to secure your grip on the bar. You can use a thumb-under grip, as demonstrated below, or a thumb-over grip. Because the grip doesn't necessarily affect the technique of the squat, grip is a matter of personal preference. Once you assume a comfortable grip, step under the weight, position the bar in the meat of your upper back, just above your shoulder blades, and then drive your elbows back to pin the bar in place. Note: Avoid placing the bar on your neck to prevent injury and discomfort. With your midline still stabilized, lift the bar off the rack, step back, and assume your squatting stance—see narrow stance and wide stance back squat.

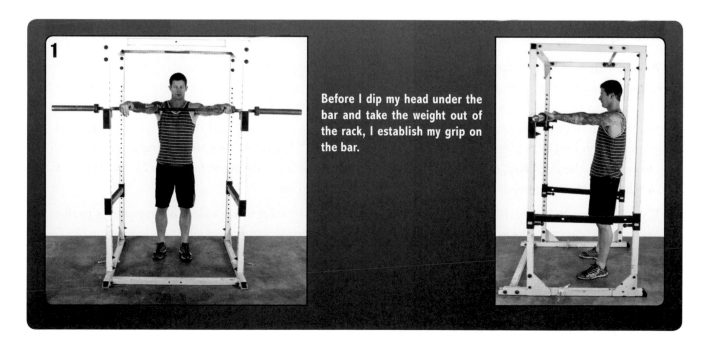

Before I dip my head under the bar and take the weight out of the rack, I establish my grip on the bar.

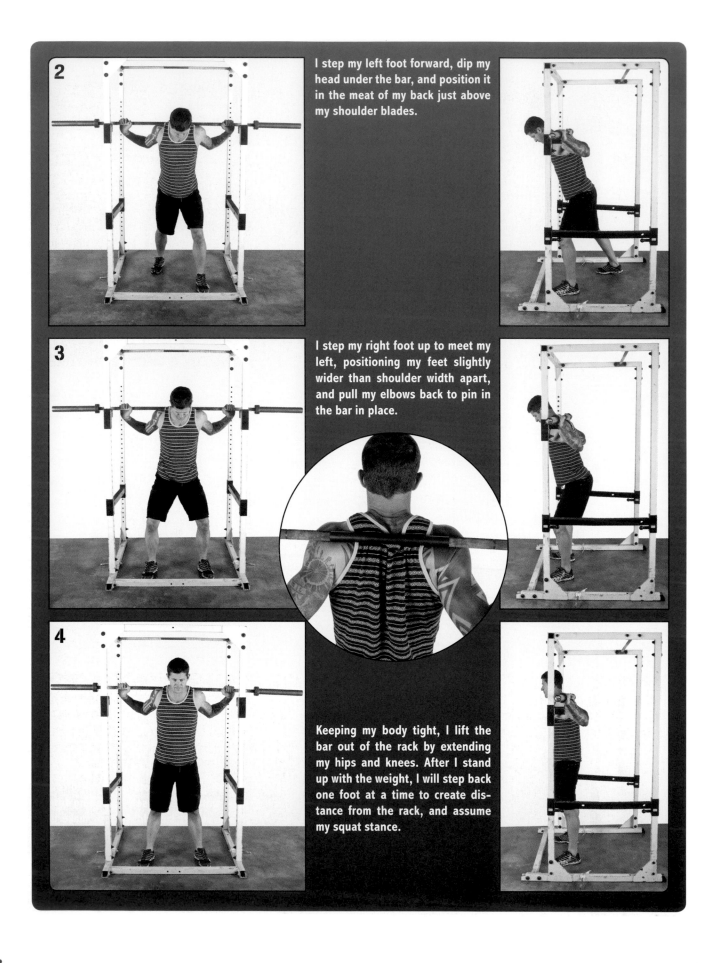

2 I step my left foot forward, dip my head under the bar, and position it in the meat of my back just above my shoulder blades.

3 I step my right foot up to meet my left, positioning my feet slightly wider than shoulder width apart, and pull my elbows back to pin in the bar in place.

4 Keeping my body tight, I lift the bar out of the rack by extending my hips and knees. After I stand up with the weight, I will step back one foot at a time to create distance from the rack, and assume my squat stance.

Common Fault: Broken Midline

Whether you're running, cycling, or performing a strength exercise, you always have to stabilize your spine by contracting your abdominals first. If you initiate a back squat with a broken midline, the load will force your back into flexion, which compromises the integrity of your spine and will inevitably cause injury. In addition to being unsafe, the weight on your back prevents you from reclaiming a strong position. That means you'll never be able to stabilize your midline to protect your spine or assume the correct position once you're under load.

If you make the mistake of lifting the weight out of the rack without engaging your core, you must immediately re-rack the weight and start from square one. Another problem, which is not illustrated in the photos below but is nevertheless important to address, is overextension. A lot of athletes will tilt the top of their pelvis forward, driving their butt into the air, and pushing their chest up. This overextended position not only puts stress on your spine, but the weight bearing down on your shoulders compresses your disks, which can lead to back injuries.

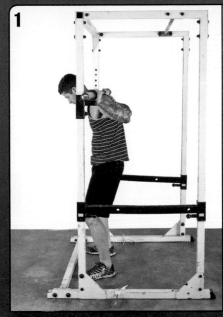

I'm preparing to take the weight out of the rack to do a back squat. Note: I've forgotten to stabilize my midline before stepping under the bar.

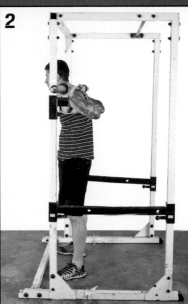

I stand up with the bar by extending my hips and knees.

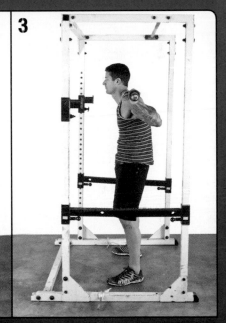

I step back to create distance from the rack. Notice how my back is rounded forward into flexion and how my belly is soft. Unable to reclaim a solid position while under load, I will have to re-rack the weight and start the process again with a tight core. Note: If I were to continue with the exercise by dropping down into a squat, I would have to make up for the lack of stability by losing form in another area, whether it's my head, feet, knees, or hips, which can lead to a host of injuries.

Wide-Stance Back Squat

If you've taken the bar out of the rack and stepped back with a stable midline, the next step is to assume your squat stance. Depending on your preference, you can assume either a wide stance, as demonstrated below, or a narrow stance, as demonstrated in the next sequence. I prefer a wide-stance back squat with my feet just wider than shoulder width because it requires more activation from my glutes and hamstrings. As I've already mentioned, the vast majority of runners and cyclists are quad-dominant. If you fall into this category, assuming a wide stance is probably more beneficial. Not only will it help build the muscles that have been neglected from years of cycling and running, but it will also balance out your frame, turning you into a more efficient athlete.

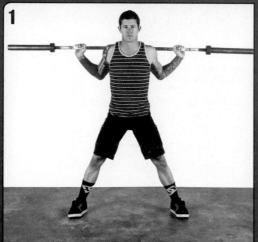

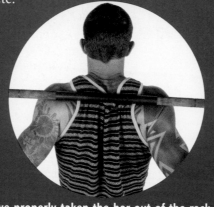

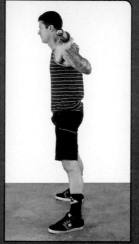

1

I've properly taken the bar out of the rack, and assumed a wide-stance back squat by positioning my feet just wider than shoulder width apart.

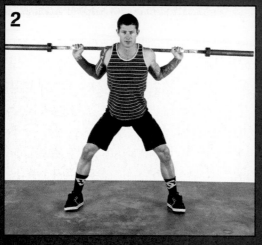

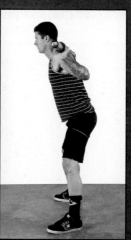

2

Keeping my midline engaged, elbows back, and head neutral, I focus on driving my hamstrings back and shoving my knees out laterally as I lower down. The combination of these actions loads my hamstrings and glutes. A lot of coaches will cue their athletes to pull their butt back as they initiate the squat, which typically puts them into an overextended position. In my experience, cuing athletes to drive their hamstrings back gets much better results.

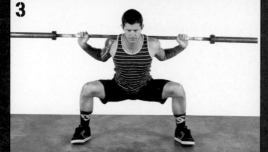

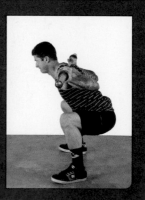

3

With my weight in my heels, I continue to lower myself until my thighs are parallel to the floor.

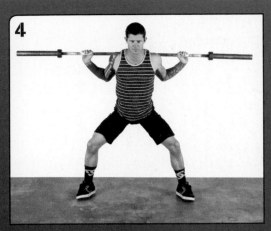

4

To push myself up, I extend my legs. It's important to note that I'm driving my knees out laterally and that my weight is in my heels. Again, this allows me to keep my posterior chain active by keeping my hamstrings and glutes loaded.

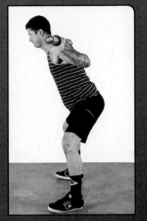

5

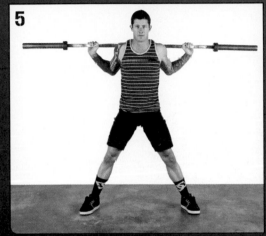

I stand up with the bar by extending my hips and knees. It's important to notice that the bar remains level throughout the squat. If the bar swerves or dips to one side, you'll lose form and have to shift your weight to make up for the deviation.

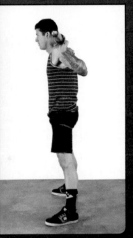

Narrow-Stance Back Squat

Although the narrow-stance back squat offers a broader range of motion from the hips when compared with the wide-stance back squat, it encourages you to engage the quads in order to stand up from the bottom of the squat. Targeting the quadriceps in a strength exercise is less than ideal for an endurance athlete who has spent years developing nothing but his quads. However, if your hamstrings are tight or you lack the hip mobility to perform the wide-stance version, the narrow-stance variation is an excellent option.

1

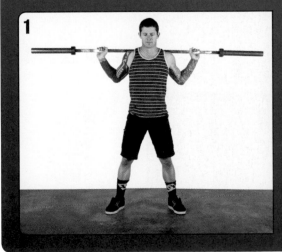

I've assumed a narrow-stance back squat stance with my feet positioned just shoulder width apart.

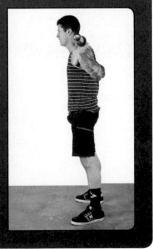

2

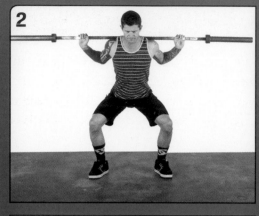

Driving my knees out laterally, I pull my hamstrings back and lower myself.

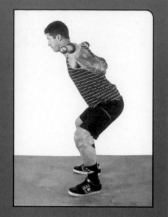

3

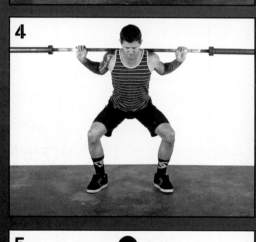

I drop down into the full squat, with my thighs below parallel.

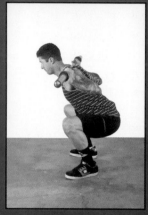

4

Keeping my weight in my heels and driving my knees out laterally, I raise my hips and extend my legs.

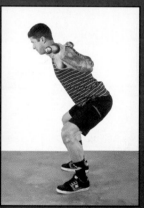

5

I stand up with the bar by extending my hips and knees.

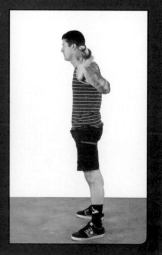

BOX SQUAT

If you're a quad-dominant athlete who struggles to engage the glutes and hamstrings in back squats, the box squat is an excellent exercise for you. If you look at the photos, you'll notice that I slowly lower myself onto the box, finding the seat with my butt. It's imperative that you keep your midline stabilized to protect your spine. If you relax your core, the load bearing down on your back will compress your disks, which is a mechanism for injury.

Once you find the box, immediately drive your heels into the ground, shove your knees out laterally, and lift your hips off the box. In addition to bringing your posterior chain online and decreasing the chances of your quads dominating the lift, the box squat is highly versatile in that you can increase or decrease the elevation of the squat based on your level of flexibility. For example, if you have tight hips and are unable to drop down into a full squat (or below parallel), you can opt for a higher box to suit your level of mobility. As your hip mobility increases, you can drop down to lower and lower boxes until you've achieved the full squat.

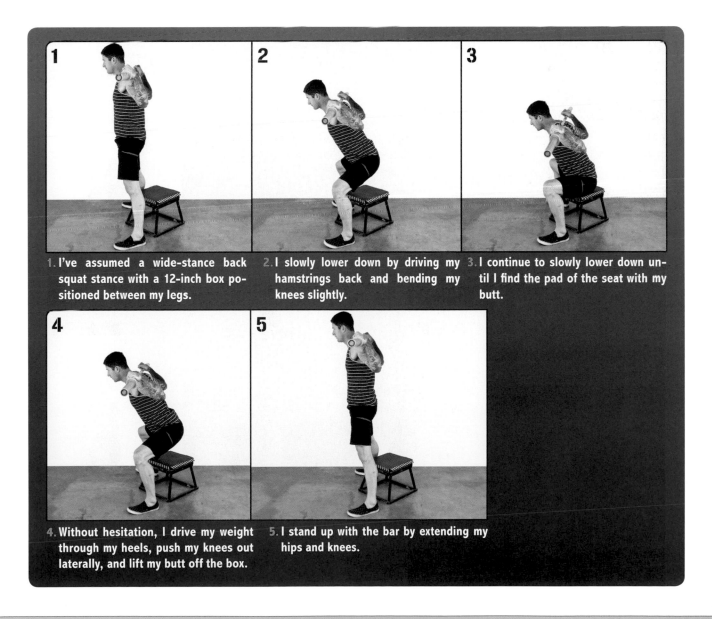

1. I've assumed a wide-stance back squat stance with a 12-inch box positioned between my legs.

2. I slowly lower down by driving my hamstrings back and bending my knees slightly.

3. I continue to slowly lower down until I find the pad of the seat with my butt.

4. Without hesitation, I drive my weight through my heels, push my knees out laterally, and lift my butt off the box.

5. I stand up with the bar by extending my hips and knees.

GOOD MORNING

Good mornings will increase your hamstring flexibility, build your posterior chain, and develop midline stabilization. If you look at the photos, you'll notice that the setup is exactly the same as for the back squat in that I take the weight out of the rack and position the bar in the meat of my back just above my shoulder blades. However, instead of dropping down into a squat, I pull my hamstrings back, creasing from the hips with a straight back.

Once I reach my end range of motion, I extend my hips and knees and use the power of my lower back, glutes, and hamstrings to pull myself back into the standing position. The goal is for your upper body to become parallel to the ground, but you never want to force the movement past your end range. When this exercise is performed correctly, you will engage your distal (lower) hamstrings, glutes, and lower-back muscles, which is not only important in running and cycling but also aids in the back squat.

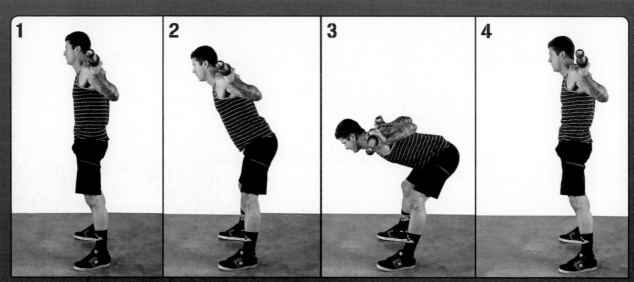

1 I've taken the weight out of the rack with the bar positioned in the meat of my back just above my shoulder blades. My midline is tight, and my elbows are pulled back to pin the bar in place.

2 Keeping my back flat and my legs as straight as possible, I pull my hamstrings back.

3 I keep creasing at the hips until my upper body is parallel to the ground. It's important to note that this position looks very similar to a bad squat. For example, if you lift your hips the bottom position in a back squat without keeping your chest up, chances are you're going to look a lot like me in this photo. With your hips on the same horizontal plane as your shoulders, you have no choice but to extend your legs, and use the power of your hamstrings and lower back to pull yourself back up to the standing position. By working good mornings specifically, you not only reap the benefits that the lift has to offer, but you also build the capacity and strength needed to pull yourself out of a squat-gone-bad situation should that worst-case scenario occur.

4 I extend my hips and use the strength of my hamstrings and lower back to pull me upright. I squeeze my glutes to stabilize my back and lock out my hips.

FRONT SQUAT

Although I've been preaching the importance of developing your posterior chain through back squatting, it is still important to build strength in your quads and inner thighs. After all, you're still using them in endurance efforts. To continue to build strength, power, speed, and muscle in these areas, it's important for you to incorporate the front squat into your strength-training regimen. With the weight in front of your body, balancing on your fingertips and shoulders, you're still engaging your glutes and hamstrings, but you're also recruiting your quads and abductors, both of which play a vital role in endurance athletics. The key to executing this lift is to keep your elbows high and your chest up as you drop into the squat. If your midline breaks or your elbows drop, you're likely to round forward and flex at the spine, which compromises the lift and increases your chances of getting hurt.

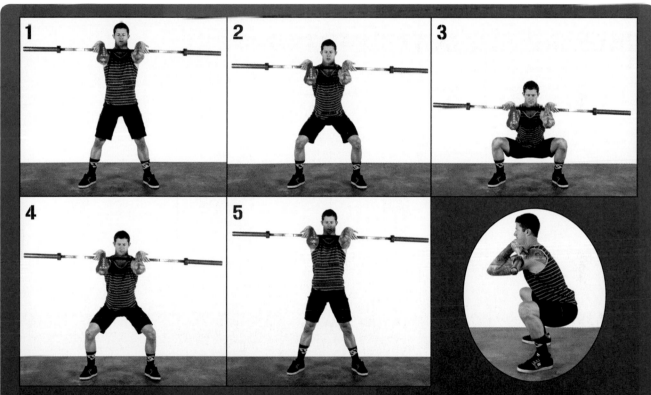

1) I've lifted the barbell out of the rack to begin the front squat. My midline is tight, my arms are up at a 90-degree angle, and the bar is balancing on my fingertips and the front of my shoulders. Note that my fingers are simply a balancing point to keep the barbell level and my elbows up. It's also important to note that you can assume a wide or narrow stance based on your preference. Here my feet are just wider than shoulder width.

2) Keeping my chest lifted, my elbows up, and my head neutral, I pull my hips back and drive my knees out laterally as I lower down.

3) I sink my hips below parallel. It's important to note that I'm fighting hard to keep my elbows up and my chest lifted. If you relax your core or allow your arms to drop, you'll round forward into flexion.

4) Driving through my heels, I press my knees out laterally, elevate my hips, and extend my knees to stand up.

5) I stand up by extending my hips and knees.

DEAD LIFT GRIP

There are two grips that you can use when setting up for the dead lift: an over-under grip (flip grip), or a double-over grip. While deciding which grip to use is a matter of personal preference, I favor the former because it offers superior control. With one hand over and one hand under, you can counteract the spin of the bar, which prevents the weight from slipping out of your hands as you pull it off the floor. The double-over grip is safe and highly effective, but it doesn't offer the same element of control as the flip grip, especially as you increase weight. It's also important to mention that you can secure a hook grip on the bar using either the over-under or double-over grip to help maintain your hold. Using the hook grip is also a matter of personal preference. I suggest that you experiment with various grips until you find one that feels comfortable and allows you to safely and effectively execute the lift.

Over-Under Grip (Flip Grip)

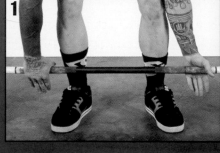

1. Positioning both of my hands at about a thumb's distance from my shins, I wrap my right hand over the bar with my palm facing toward me, and wrap my left hand under the bar with my palm facing away from me.

2. I curl my fingers around the bar, hooking my thumb over the top of my index and middle fingers.

Double-Over Grip

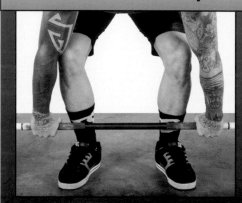

To secure the double-over grip, I wrap both hands around the bar with my palms facing toward me. Note: You can use a traditional grip or a hook grip.

Over-Under Hook Grip

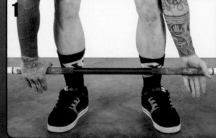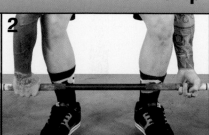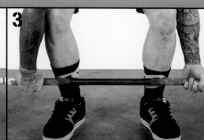

I secure a flip grip with both hands about a thumb's distance from my shins.

I hook my thumbs around the bar.

To secure the hook grip, I wrap my index and middle fingers over the top of my thumbs and curl my pinky and ring fingers around the bar.

DEAD LIFT

The dead lift is one of the most important exercises for an endurance athlete because in addition to strengthening the posterior chain, developing midline stabilization, and increasing flexibility, it teaches an athlete how to generate power from the hamstrings. This is especially important if you're a cyclist. For example, if you're charging up a hill, you need to keep your back flat and use your hamstrings to generate watts through the pedal stroke. The better you are at keeping a solid position and using your hamstrings to generate power, the faster you'll climb. Cyclists who are not effective in the climb are ones that round forward at the back and use their quads to generate power through the pedal stroke. The same is true with the dead lift.

The athletes who struggle to get into the correct setup position are more likely to round forward from the back and use their quads to pull the weight off the ground. Not only is this inefficient, but it also wastes energy and increases your chances of injury. To engage your hamstrings in the dead lift, you have to set up with a flat back, position your shoulders over the bar, drive through your heels, and lift the weight off the ground without rounding forward.

If you're unable to achieve the correct dead lift setup position due to mobility restrictions, stop what you're doing and immediately find a solution. Setting up or lifting with a rounded back is not an option! In addition to risking injury, rounding forward forces you to lift with your back muscles and quads instead of your hamstrings, which is exactly the opposite point of the dead lift. If you're an endurance athlete who has never performed the dead lift or you're unable to get into the correct setup position, elevating the bar on boxes, bumper plates, or a platform to a comfortable height is advisable. As you increase your range of motion, lower the starting position until you can set up on the ground without restriction.

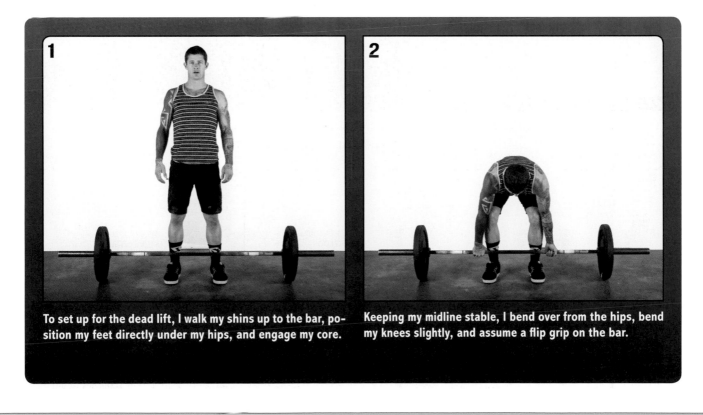

1 To set up for the dead lift, I walk my shins up to the bar, position my feet directly under my hips, and engage my core.

2 Keeping my midline stable, I bend over from the hips, bend my knees slightly, and assume a flip grip on the bar.

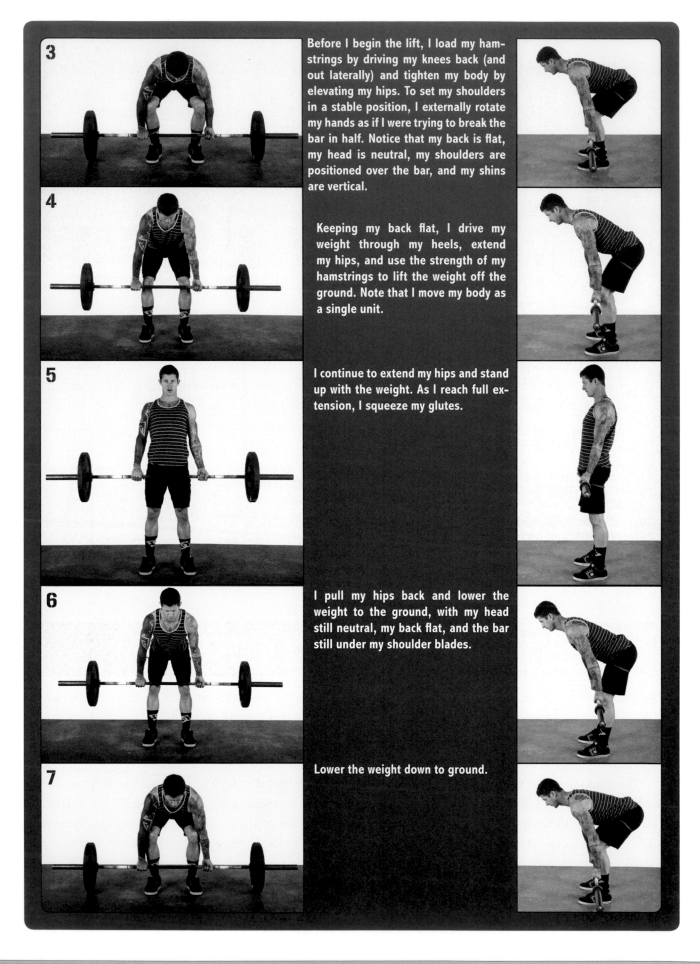

3

Before I begin the lift, I load my hamstrings by driving my knees back (and out laterally) and tighten my body by elevating my hips. To set my shoulders in a stable position, I externally rotate my hands as if I were trying to break the bar in half. Notice that my back is flat, my head is neutral, my shoulders are positioned over the bar, and my shins are vertical.

4

Keeping my back flat, I drive my weight through my heels, extend my hips, and use the strength of my hamstrings to lift the weight off the ground. Note that I move my body as a single unit.

5

I continue to extend my hips and stand up with the weight. As I reach full extension, I squeeze my glutes.

6

I pull my hips back and lower the weight to the ground, with my head still neutral, my back flat, and the bar still under my shoulder blades.

Lower the weight down to ground.

7

The Romanian/Stiff-Legged Dead Lift

The Romanian, or stiff-legged dead lift is very similar to the dead lift, in that you're simply pulling the weight from the ground to mid-thigh. But instead of setting up with your knees slightly bent and your hips back, you bend forward from the hips with your back flat and keep your legs as straight as possible. Unlike the traditional dead lift, which engages the entire posterior chain, the Romanian dead lift isolates and targets the lower and upper hamstrings. For that reason, it's important that you remain conservative in the amount of weight you load on the bar. Although this exercise is an excellent way to increase strength and range of motion, it puts a lot of stress on your hamstrings and can leave you seriously sore. Not only that, but the heavier the weight, the more likely you are to lose form and get hurt. If you round your back, or break in any way, immediately drop the bar and lower the weight.

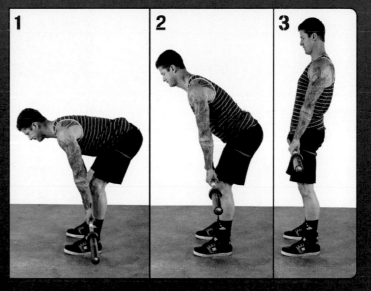

1. To set up for the Romanian dead lift, I walk my shins up to the bar, with my feet directly under my hips, and tighten my core. Next, I bend over from the hips with a flat back, keeping my legs as straight as possible, and take a double-over grip on the bar with my shoulders over the bar. Note: Using a double-over grip gives you a little extra range of motion, making it the preferable grip for this lift.

2. Keeping my back flat and driving my weight through my heels, I extend my hips and use the power of my hamstrings to pull the bar off the ground.

3. I extend my hips and stand up. From here, I will lower the weight to the ground, keeping my legs as straight as possible and my back flat.

SUMO DEAD LIFT

Sometimes your anatomical makeup hinders your ability to perform certain lifts. For example, if you have long legs and a short torso, positioning your feet directly under your hips and gripping the bar wider than your hips to set up for the traditional dead lift can be difficult. In such a situation, assuming a wide stance and securing a flip grip between your legs as demonstrated is an excellent alternative.

The Sumo dead lift stance is also a great option if you lack mobility in your hips and hamstrings. The wide stance will not only allow you to get your back flat, but also reduces the distance you have to pull the bar, which significantly decreases your chances of rounding forward into flexion. It's important to note that even if you can set up easily for the traditional dead lift, randomly incorporating a sumo dead lift into your strength routine offers several advantages: in addition to hitting all the same muscle groups as the dead lift, the sumo stance forces you to engage your hips (more than the traditional dead lift) and recruits your adductors, both of which are key for endurance sports.

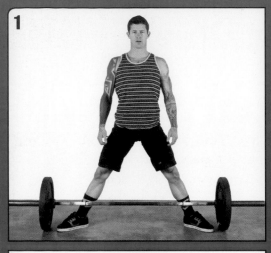

1

To set up for the sumo dead lift, I walk my shins up to the bar, take my feet wider than my shoulders with my toes angled out, and tighten my core to stabilize my midline.

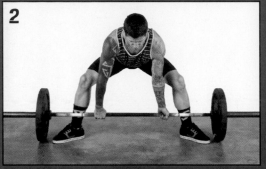

2

I pull my hips back, bend forward from the hips, and assume a flip grip on the bar. Once accomplished, I tighten my body and take the slack out of my hamstrings by lifting my hips, getting my shins vertical, and flattening my back.

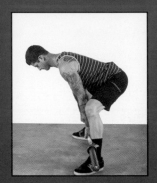

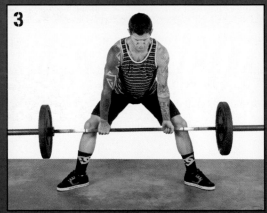

3

Keeping my back flat, I drive my weight through my heels, extend my hips, and drag the bar up my shins to knee level.

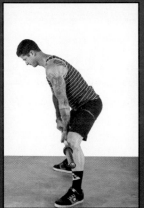

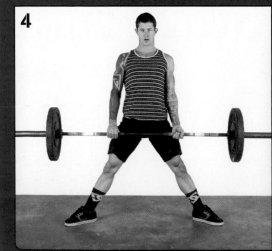

4

Continuing to extend my hips, I stand up with the bar and squeeze my glutes as I reach full extension.

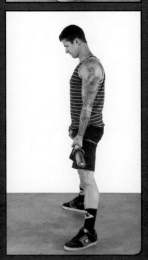

BENCH PRESS

Although I don't prescribe the bench press that often, it's still important to randomly incorporate this lift into your strength-training routine, especially if you're a cyclist. The goal of this exercise is to bring balance to an athlete who has an underdeveloped chest by strengthening his chest and triceps.

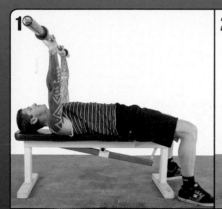 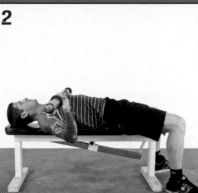 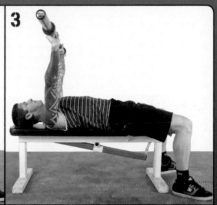

1 I've taken the weight out of the rack and positioned the bar directly over my shoulders. Notice that my back is flush with the bench and that the bar is in the center of my palms.

2 I pull my elbows back at a 45-degree angle and lower the bar straight down to my chest.

3 I press the weight straight up using the power of my chest and triceps.

FLOOR PRESS

Other than the fact that you're lying on the ground and stopping once your elbows and arms touch the ground, the protocol for the floor press is the same as the bench press. You still want the bar positioned over your shoulders and you're still lowering your elbows at a 45-degree angle. As in the box squat, keep the load low and focus on controlling the descent of the weight to avoid injury. If your chest and triceps are underdeveloped or you simply want to increase your strength and muscle coordination, this is an excellent exercise to add to your strength-training program.

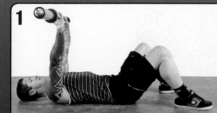 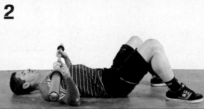 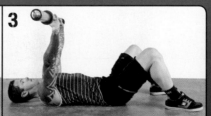

1 I'm holding the bar above my shoulders in preparation for the floor press. To set my shoulders in a stable position I squeeze my shoulder blades and externally rotate my hands as if I were trying to break the bar.

2 I lower the weight slowly by pulling my elbows back at a 45-degree angle.

3 I press the bar straight up and lock out my arms to complete the movement.

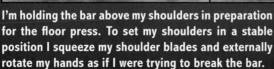

STRICT PRESS (SHOULDER PRESS):

Setting up for the press is similar to setting up for the back squat and front squat, in that you want to stabilize your midline before you take the bar out of the rack to initiate the lift. Once your core is engaged, grip the bar with your hands just wider than your shoulders, making sure to lock your thumb around the bar, and step in with your chest up. With your back flat, your chest under the bar, and the weight resting in the center of your palms, lift the bar out of the rack and get your forearms as vertical as possible.

Proper Setup

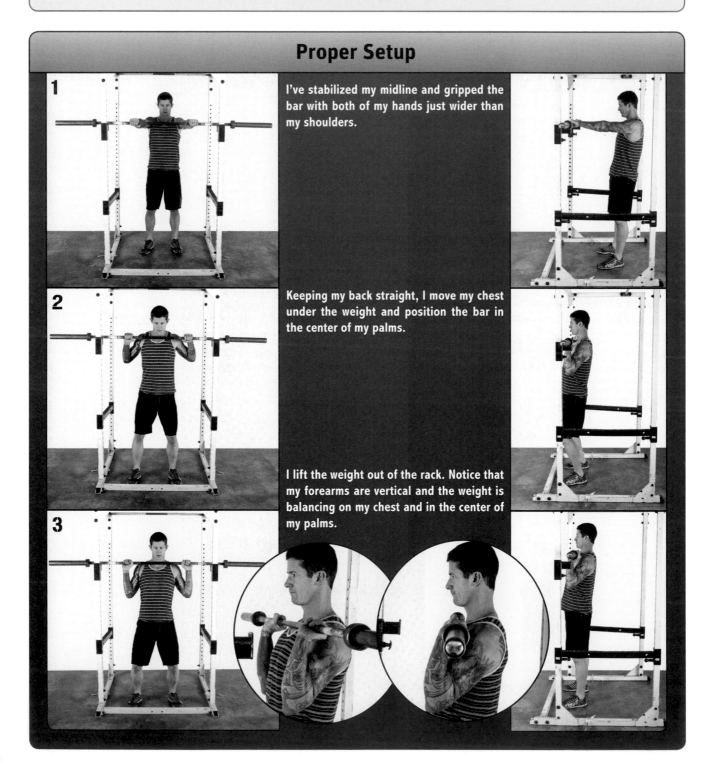

1 I've stabilized my midline and gripped the bar with both of my hands just wider than my shoulders.

2 Keeping my back straight, I move my chest under the weight and position the bar in the center of my palms.

3 I lift the weight out of the rack. Notice that my forearms are vertical and the weight is balancing on my chest and in the center of my palms.

Strict Press (Shoulder Press)

Whether you lift the barbell out of the rack or pull it from the ground and take the weight onto your chest in the form of a clean, your forearms should always be vertical, with the bar balancing on your chest and in the center of your palms. Once you achieve this position, you can initiate the press by shrugging your shoulders and lifting the weight directly overhead. It's very important to keep your elbows tight to your body. If your arms flare out to the side or your shoulders roll forward, you will sacrifice power and increase your chance of injury. It's important to mention that because you're initiating the movement from a dead-stop position, you have to engage your shoulders, triceps, and traps to heave the weight up off your chest. Although this prevents you from lifting as much weight as you could when executing a push press (next exercise), it develops core stability and raw strength as opposed to the explosive power characteristic of the push press.

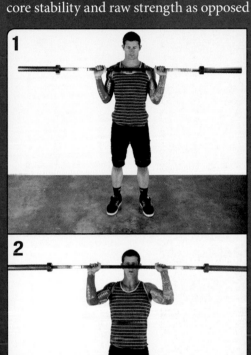

1

The bar is positioned on my chest and in the center of my palms. My head is neutral, my feet are directly under my hips, and my forearms are vertical.

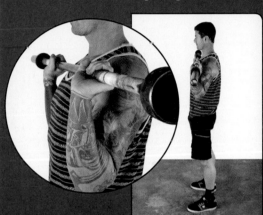

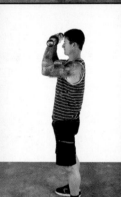

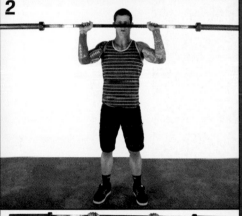

2

Drawing my head slightly back, I shrug my shoulders and press the weight straight up. It's important to move your head behind the bar's path to avoid having to move the bar around your head. If you do the latter, you'll lose power in your press and compromise the lift.

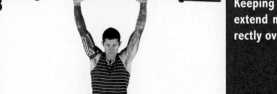

3

Keeping my elbows in and my core tight, I extend my arms and press the weight directly overheard.

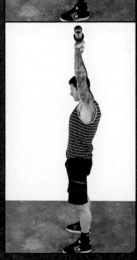

Dumbbell Shoulder Press

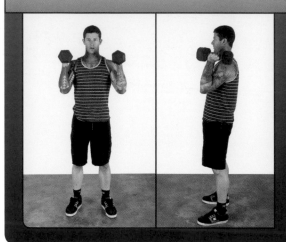

It's important to note that the pressing elements can also be performed with dumbbells. The movement is performed in the exact same manner as the barbell press, but you don't have to move your head out of the way from the bar path, making it easier to maintain an upright torso. If you're new to the pressing movements and you haven't lifted weights before, the dumbbells are an excellent option because it corrects strength imbalances and places a higher stability demand on your shoulders and midline.

PUSH PRESS

The push press is another component of the overhead press that you can add to a workout or strength-training session. To execute this technique correctly, you need to drop down by bending your knees slightly and then immediately straighten your legs and extend your hips. The key is to drive your knees out and maintain an upright torso as you lower down. This upward momentum generated by your legs and hips accelerates the bar off your chest, making it easier to lock out your elbows and shoulders to complete the press. As a result, you will be able to lift roughly 30 percent more weight than you can in a strict press. It's important to note that this exercise puts more emphasis on explosive power than on raw strength. To get the best results from your strength-training regimen, you have to constantly mix in new exercises to keep your body guessing. For example, one week you can focus on the strict press to develop raw power, and then switch it up the following week by incorporating the push press to build your explosive power. By constantly varying your workouts, your body is forced to adjust to new challenges, which not only helps build a well-rounded athlete, but also maximizes the benefits of the strength-and-conditioning program.

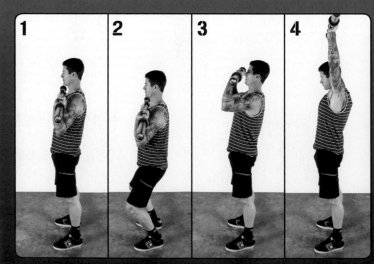

1. I've got the bar positioned on my chest and in the center of my palms. My head is neutral, my feet are directly under my hips, and my forearms are vertical.

2. Keeping my weight in my heels and my back straight, I drop down by bending my knees slightly. As I lower down, I drive my knees out laterally and keep my torso upright.

3. I extend my knees and hips violently, using the upward momentum generated by my legs and hips to press the weight overhead. Notice how I draw my head back slightly to clear the bar's path.

4. Keeping my elbows in tight, I extend my arms and press the weight overhead.

Olympic-Lifting Techniques

HOOK GRIP

If you read the section on power lifting, you know how to set up for the dead lift using a hook grip. The same grip is used for the clean and snatch. The hook grip is not as prevalent in the power-lifting community because the lift is slow and requires minimal body movement. The power clean, on the other hand, requires you to pull the bar from the ground to your shoulders in one explosive movement. That means you have to hang on to the bar for much longer and pull faster. The hook grip allows you to do that because it is a sturdier and more reliable grip. One caveat: The hook grip can be uncomfortable and even painful when first starting out. With enough practice, though, you'll callous your thumb and develop the hand coordination to assume the grip comfortably and without pain.

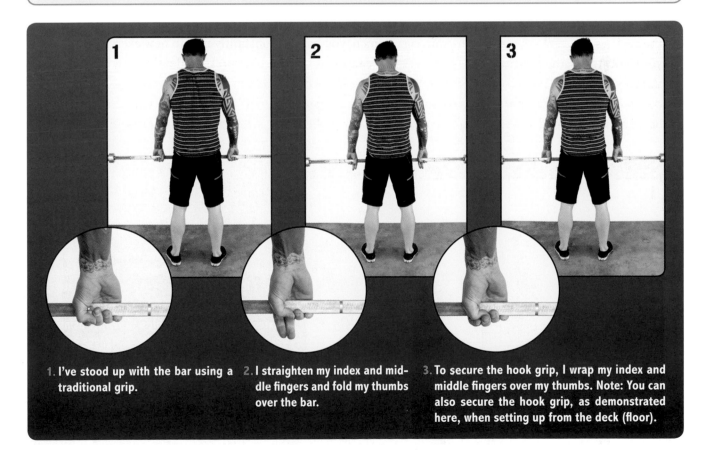

1. I've stood up with the bar using a traditional grip.

2. I straighten my index and middle fingers and fold my thumbs over the bar.

3. To secure the hook grip, I wrap my index and middle fingers over my thumbs. Note: You can also secure the hook grip, as demonstrated here, when setting up from the deck (floor).

POWER CLEAN

The power clean is a variant of the clean in which the lifter pulls the weight off the ground to shoulder level in one explosive movement. Unlike the clean, which requires you to receive the bar in the bottom of the full front squat, in the power clean you catch the bar above parallel.

If you're new to Olympic lifting, starting out with a light weight and learning the power variant, as demonstrated below, is the way to go. In addition to building explosive power, you'll develop technique and gain experience with the movement. The majority of beginners don't feel comfortable dropping under a heavy load in the full-front-squat position. If you fall into this category, I suggest you practice the front squat and execute the power clean in your early stages of development. As you get stronger and become technically proficient with the movement, you can start adding weight and practice receiving the bar in a quarter- and half-squat positions. Once you're comfortable pulling your body under the weight, you can progress to the full clean. It's important to mention that even if you're proficient with the full clean, the power clean is still an excellent variant to include in your routine, especially if your quads are blown from a previous workout or event.

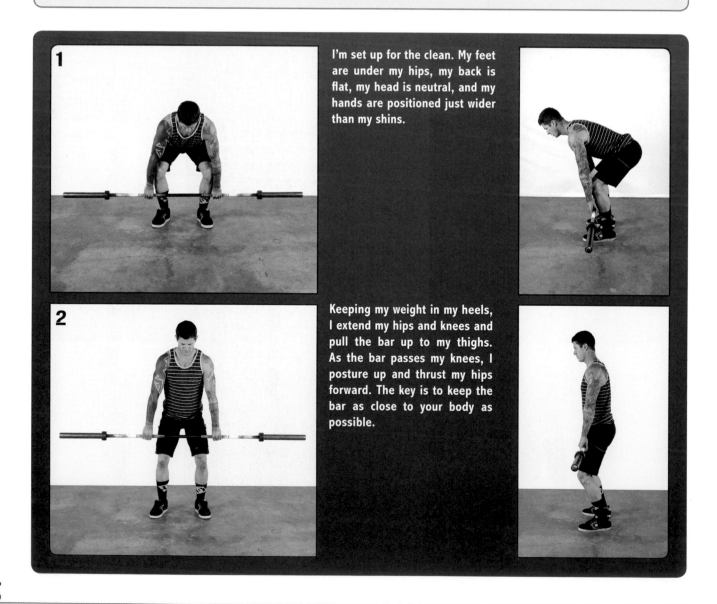

1 I'm set up for the clean. My feet are under my hips, my back is flat, my head is neutral, and my hands are positioned just wider than my shins.

2 Keeping my weight in my heels, I extend my hips and knees and pull the bar up to my thighs. As the bar passes my knees, I posture up and thrust my hips forward. The key is to keep the bar as close to your body as possible.

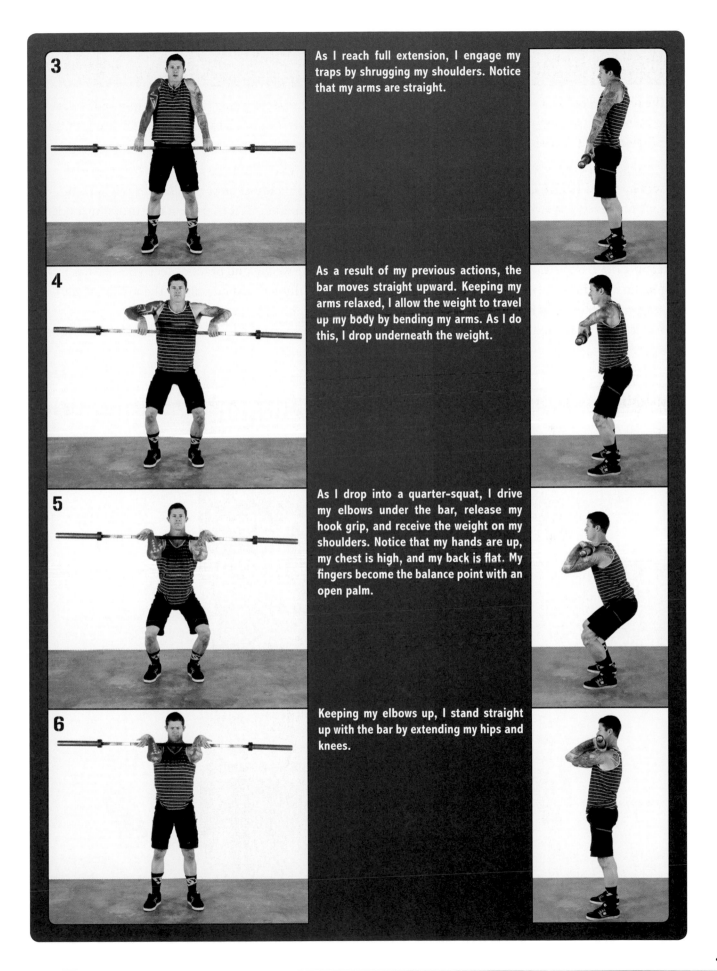

3

As I reach full extension, I engage my traps by shrugging my shoulders. Notice that my arms are straight.

4

As a result of my previous actions, the bar moves straight upward. Keeping my arms relaxed, I allow the weight to travel up my body by bending my arms. As I do this, I drop underneath the weight.

5

As I drop into a quarter-squat, I drive my elbows under the bar, release my hook grip, and receive the weight on my shoulders. Notice that my hands are up, my chest is high, and my back is flat. My fingers become the balance point with an open palm.

6

Keeping my elbows up, I stand straight up with the bar by extending my hips and knees.

HANG POWER CLEAN

To get the most out of your strength-training routine and improve your technique with an Olympic lift, you have to not only mix up the exercise, but also work on specific extensions of the movement. For example, in the previous sequence I demonstrated a variant of the clean, the power clean, which removes the front squat from the equation, allowing the practitioner to focus on the catch, as opposed to the drop.

In this next sequence, I break down the technique even further. The hang power clean is the same as the power clean, in that you pull the weight up to shoulder level and receive the bar in the standing, quarter-squat, or half-squat position. But instead of pulling the weight off the floor and using the upward momentum of your pull to accelerate the bar up to your shoulders, you initiate the movement from your thighs. With the momentum of your pull seriously reduced, you have to explode into the movement by extending your hips and knees while violently shrugging your shoulders. This hang variation not only builds speed and explosive power, but also allows you to focus on the second aspect of the movement, which is getting your elbows under the bar and receiving the weight on your shoulders.

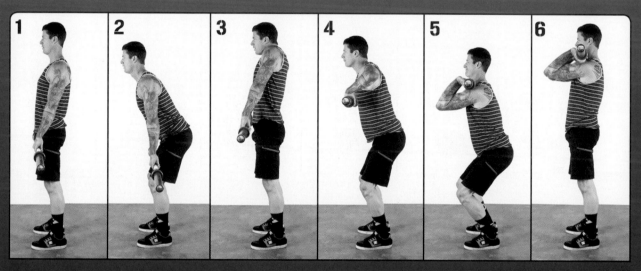

1. I've dead lifted the bar up to the standing position. Note: You can secure a hook grip from the deck or while standing, as demonstrated in the beginning of the chapter.

2. Keeping my weight in my heels, I pull my hips back, bend my knees slightly, and lower the bar to mid-thigh level.

3. I extend my hips and knees and engage my traps by shrugging my shoulders.

4. The bar accelerates up my body as a result of my previous actions. Keeping my arms relaxed, I allow the weight to travel upward by bending my arms. As I do this, I drop down slightly by pulling my hips back and bending my knees.

5. As I drop into a quarter-squat, I drive my elbows under the bar with lightning-quick speed, release my hook grip, and receive bar on my shoulders and fingertips. Notice that my chest is up, my back is flat, and my elbows are positioned at a nearly 90-degree angle.

6. Keeping my chest and elbows up, I stand straight up with the bar by extending my hips and knees.

CLEAN

In this sequence, I demonstrate a full clean by receiving the bar in a deep front-squat position. As a rule of thumb, the more weight you attempt to lift—whether you're executing a clean or snatch—the shorter your pull, and the shorter your pull, the lower you have to squat to catch the weight. If you look at the photos below, you'll notice that although I demonstrate the technique using only the bar, it doesn't travel much higher than my bellybutton, which is characteristic of a heavy clean. It's important to note that I'm still extending my hips and knees and shrugging my traps to accelerate the weight upward, but because of the (hypothetical) load, I can't pull the bar higher than my abdomen. To receive the bar, I have to pull myself under it with lightning-quick speed and razor-sharp accuracy before it begins its descent toward the ground. If your timing is off by a fraction of a second or you're unable to stabilize yourself in the bottom front-squat position, you'll miss the lift. If you're a novice lifter or you lack the mobility to get into a good squat position, practice the power variant and become proficient with the front squat, using light weight until you can comfortably drop under the bar.

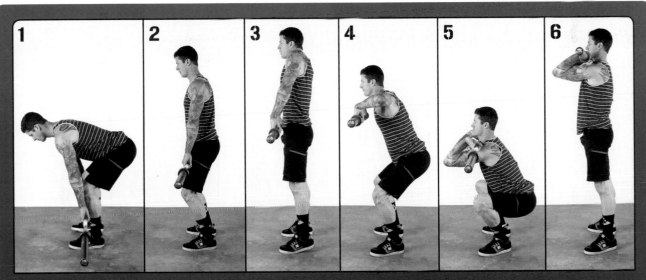

1. I'm set up for the clean. My feet are under my hips, my back is flat, my head is neutral, and my hands are just wider than my shins.

2. In one fluid motion, I extend my hips and knees and pull the bar up to my thighs. It's important to note that as the bar passes my knees, I pull my torso upright and thrust my hips forward.

3. As I extend my hips and knees, I engage my traps by shrugging my shoulders. Notice that my arms are straight.

4. As the weight travels past my hips, I begin pulling myself under the bar.

5. To receive the bar at its peak height, I drop my hips just below knee level, drive my elbows under the bar, release my hook grip, and catch the weight on my shoulders.

6. Keeping my weight driving through my heels, my chest up, and my elbows high, I front-squat the weight up to the standing position.

NOTE: The hang clean is the same as the hang power clean, but instead of receiving the bar in the standing position, you pull yourself under the bar and receive the weight in the bottom-front-squat position. Just like the hang-power variant, the hang clean allows you to focus on the secondary pull, which is the extension of your hips and knees, and the catch.

PUSH JERK

The setup for the push jerk is mechanically very similar to the one for the push-press, in that you dip down into a quarter-squat and then extend your hips and knees so you can generate enough upward momentum to accelerate the bar off your shoulders. But instead of locking out your knees and pressing the weight directly overhead, you drop under the weight in a half- or quarter-squat and receive the bar with your elbows locked out. The push jerk not only allows you to lift more weight overhead, but it's a more explosive dynamic movement, which helps to develop speed and accuracy.

It's important to note that you can execute the push jerk as an independent movement or as an extension of the clean. If you're doing the former, you want to assume the press position as you prepare to take the weight out of the rack, as demonstrated in the previous section. If you're doing the latter, you have to readjust your position before you progress to the next stage of the lift. For example, if you glance at the first photo in the sequence, you'll notice that I've received the bar on my shoulders and fingertips. To assume the correct press position, I drop my elbows and readjust my grip so that the bar is balancing in the center of my palms. Once my forearms are vertical and my grip is set, I bring my feet directly under my hips and assume a solid pressing stance. From here, I can effectively execute the push jerk.

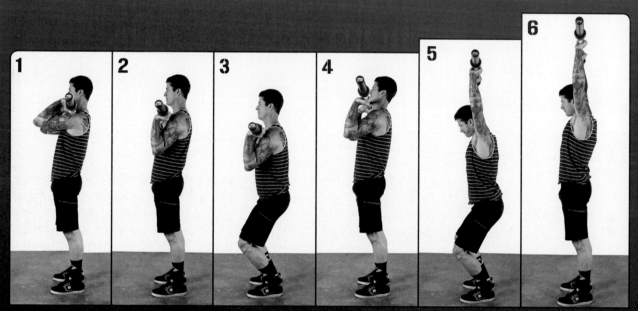

1. I've received the bar on my shoulders after successfully completing a clean. My elbows are up, and the bar is balancing on the front of my shoulders and my fingertips.

2. To set up for the push jerk, I drop my elbows until my forearms are vertical and reposition my grip so that the bar is balancing in the center of my palms. It's important to note that the more vertical you get your forearms, the more drive you'll get out of the press.

3. Keeping my posture erect, I drop myself down slightly by bending my knees.

4. I extend my knees, engage my traps by shrugging my shoulders, and use the upward momentum generated by my legs to press the weight off my chest. Notice how I pull my head back slightly to clear the bar's path.

5. As the weight travels upward, I drop down by bending my knees, lock out my arms, and catch the weight overhead in a half-squat position.

6. Keeping my arms fully extended, I stand up with the bar overhead.

SPLIT JERK

If you're trying to press a heavy load overhead, sometimes it can be difficult to get under the weight using the push jerk. In such a situation, the split jerk is an excellent option: for the vast majority of people it's faster to drop into the staggered stance of a deep lunge. To correctly execute the split jerk, you dip down slightly, just as you would to execute a push press, and then extend your knees and use the power generated by your legs and hips to raise the weight off your shoulders. As the weight is lifted up, move under the bar by sliding one foot back and one foot forward and lock out your arms before the weight starts to come down. If you're soft in the shoulders or your split is too shallow, you'll miss the lift. After you've successfully received the weight and stabilized your position, slide your front foot back, and then your rear foot forward, putting you in a square stance. Keeping the bar in the same fixed position overhead and centering your body under the weight as you slide your feet into position is mandatory.

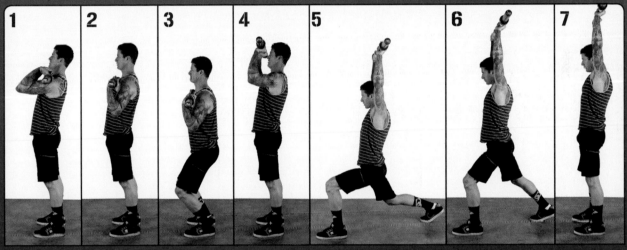

1. I've received the bar on my shoulders after successfully completing a clean. My elbows are up, and the bar is balancing on the front of my shoulders and my fingertips.

2. To set up for the push jerk, I drop my elbows until my forearms are vertical, and reposition my grip so that the bar is balancing in the center of my palms. It's important to note that the more vertical you get your forearms, the more drive you'll get out of the press.

3. Keeping my body erect, I drop down slightly by bending my knees.

4. I extend my knees, engage my traps by shrugging my shoulders, and use the upward momentum generated by my legs to press the weight off my chest. Notice how I pull my head back slightly to clear the bar's path.

5. As the bar accelerates upward, I drop into a deep lunge by sliding my left foot forward and my right foot back and lock out my arms. It's important to notice that my left shin is vertical, my right foot is turned in slightly, and my weight is centered directly under the bar. If your knee tracks over your lead foot or you externally rotate your back leg, you not only compromise the lift, but also increase your chances of injury.

6. Keeping my weight centered under the bar, my midline stable, and my arms locked out overhead, I slide my front foot back and stand up. It's important that you always transition into a standing square stance by moving your front foot first. If you slide your back leg forward as you stand up, you risk losing control of the bar overhead and dumping the weight behind your back.

7. To finish the sequence, I slide my rear foot up to my left foot, squaring my stance, and stand up.

POWER SNATCH

Other than the spacing of your hands and the distance the bar has to travel, the setup and extension for the snatch is exactly the same as for the clean. Assume a hook grip on the bar, position your feet directly under your hips, keep your back straight, and pull your chest up with your hips slightly elevated. To initiate the pull, rise up by extending your hips and knees and shrugging your shoulders. But unlike the clean, which requires you to catch the bar on your shoulders, drop into a quarter- or half-squat as the bar moves upward and receive the weight with your arms locked out overhead.

Just as I mentioned in the power clean introduction, there are two reasons you might want to do a power snatch instead of the full snatch. Either you want to work on speed and explosion by isolating the movement, or you're a beginner who doesn't feel comfortable dropping under a heavy load in an overhead squat. If you fall into the latter category, work on the power variant to dial in your technique. In the meantime, build strength and capacity with the overhead squat and work the snatch balance to develop your timing and confidence. Once you feel comfortable dropping under the bar in a full over-head squat, start increasing the weight and working on your full snatch.

Note: you can also perform the power stanch or full snatch from the hang position. The hang snatch shares all the same principles as the hang power clean, in that you start standing, dip down slightly, and then initiate your pull from mid-thighs. But instead of receiving the weight on your shoulders, you pull the weight above your head and catch the bar with locked-out arms. Because the bar has to travel a greater distance, you have to execute a more violent extension of the hips and knees to get the weight overhead.

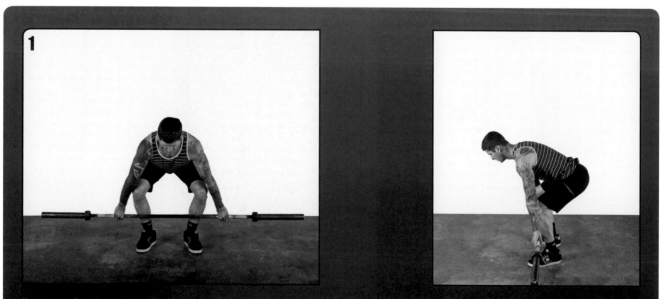

1

I'm set up for the snatch. My feet are under my hips, my back is flat, my head is neutral, and my hands are just wider than my shins. Note: finding the right placement of your hands for the snatch is different for everybody and often takes time to figure out. However, if you're new to the lift and you have no idea where to position your hands, place the bar (or a PVC pipe) on the top of your head and then put a 90-degree bend in your elbows. Wherever your hands are, that's where they should go to start: as you become more experienced with the snatch, you'll figure out if it's more comfortable to widen or narrow your grip.

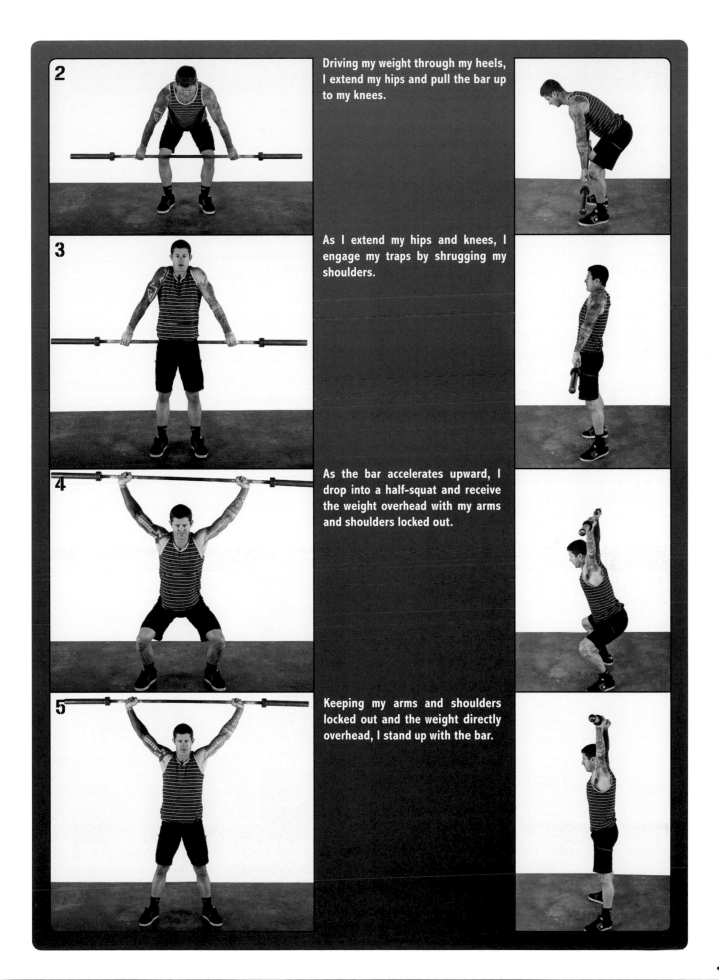

2

Driving my weight through my heels, I extend my hips and pull the bar up to my knees.

3

As I extend my hips and knees, I engage my traps by shrugging my shoulders.

4

As the bar accelerates upward, I drop into a half-squat and receive the weight overhead with my arms and shoulders locked out.

5

Keeping my arms and shoulders locked out and the weight directly overhead, I stand up with the bar.

OVERHEAD SQUAT

The overhead squat is an excellent lift to execute, because in addition to enforcing a rock-solid midline, increasing strength, and improving shoulder and hip mobility, it will build up your confidence and co-ordination in receiving the bar overhead to complete a full snatch. To get the best results from this lift, follow these guidelines:

First, keep your shoulders engaged by drawing your traps up and externally rotating your arms. This not only protects your shoulders from injury, but also helps keep the weight locked in a fixed position overhead.

Second, you want to control your descent by lowering yourself into the bottom-squat position slowly. As a rule, the faster you lower yourself, the harder it is to control the weight. By descending slowly, you reduce the bounce out of the bottom position and keep the weight in the same fixed position overhead as you stand back up with the weight.

Third, keep your chest up as you pull your hips back to lower down. Just as with the front squat, if you lean forward or round forward into flexion, you'll loose control of the weight and dump it to the ground before you can complete the lift.

Finally, keep your core engaged. Although a tight midline is mandatory for just about every movement I demonstrate, there are few lifts that are more demanding on the midline than the overhead squat. If you're brand new to the strength lifts, it's important that you develop technique and capacity with the back squat and shoulder press before executing this particular lift. If you already have a good base in those lifts, and you want to build strength, as well as improve your full snatch, the overhead squat is an excellent lift to incorporate into your strength-training routine.

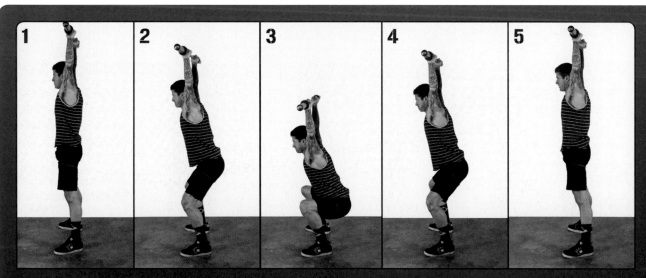

1. I've pressed the bar directly overhead using a snatch grip. Notice that my feet are just wider than my shoulders.

2. Keeping my shoulders engaged and arms locked out, I pull my hips back and start to lower myself slowly.

3. I ease down into the bottom-squat position. Notice that my chest is up, my back is flat, my arms are locked out, and my weight is centered directly under the bar.

4. Driving my weight through my heels and pushing my knees out laterally, I engage my glutes and hamstrings, extend my hips and knees, and begin to stand up.

5. With my shoulders still engaged and arms locked out, I stand straight up with the bar.

SNATCH

Once you're proficient with the power snatch and overhead squat, and you feel somewhat comfortable receiving the bar overhead, you can begin increasing the weight and executing the full snatch. As you already know, the more weight you lift, the shorter the distance you'll be able to pull the bar. So if you're working toward your one-rep max, chances are you'll be able to pull the weight up only to your stomach. Just as in the clean, you have to drop under the weight with lightning-quick speed and receive the weight before it starts to travel downward. It's important to note that if you're performing the hang snatch, you won't have the same momentum because you're initiating your pull from the mid-thighs. As a result, you have to decrease the weight to increase your efficiency and be extremely aggressive in pulling yourself under the bar.

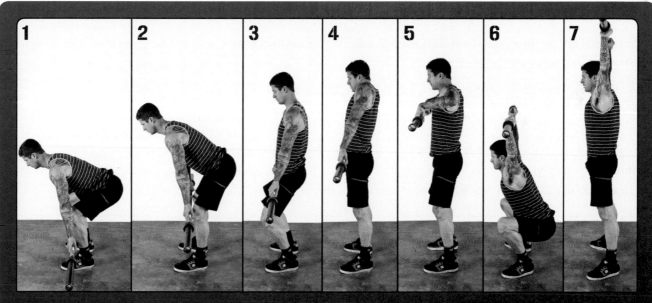

1. I'm set up for the snatch. My feet are under my hips, my back is flat, my head is neutral, and my hands are just wider than my shins.

2. Driving my weight through my heels, I extend my hips and pull the bar up to my knees.

3. As I extend my hips and knees and pull the bar up to my thighs, I lift my torso up to vertical and drive my hips forward.

4. Still extending my hips and knees, I engage my traps by shrugging my shoulders.

5. As a result of my previous actions, the bar flies straight upward. Keeping my arms relaxed, I allow the bar to keep accelerating upward by bending my arms.

6. As the bar passes my hips, I drop into a bottom-squat position, engage my shoulders and lock out my arms, and receive the weight directly overhead.

7. After stabilizing the weight in the bottom-overhead-squat position, I stand straight up with the bar.

PUSH-UP

While there is an endless variety of exercises and tools for building your chest and triceps, nothing is more functional or beneficial than the classic push-up. Unlike the bench press or other upper-body exercises, you don't need anything besides a flat surface to perform this exercise. Although the push-up has been around for about 2,500 years, most people still don't know how to do it properly: despite its simplicity, there is a lot of technique involved. To do it right, position your arms just wider than your shoulders, screw your hands into the ground and externally rotate your shoulders to lock out your arms, and engage your core and glutes to stabilize your midline. Common faults include overextension (hips elevated in a near pike) and being stingy with the range of motion (by not touching chest and legs to the ground). Note: If you want to increase your range of motion, use parallettes, but instead of placing your feet on the ground, place them on a box.

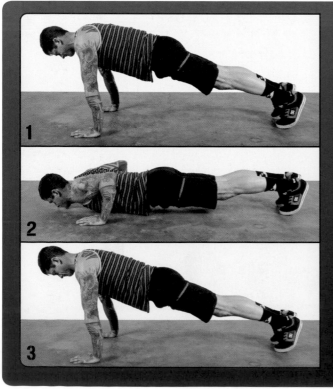

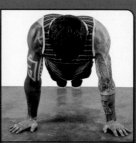

I've assumed the top push-up position with my hands just wider than my shoulders. My back is flat and my arms are externally rotated (eyes of my elbows forward).

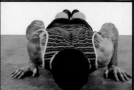

I draw my elbows back at a 45-degree angle and lower myself to the ground. Notice that I touch my chest and thighs to the ground.

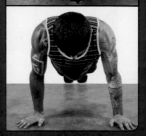

Keeping my elbows tight to my body and my back flat, I press myself back up, lock out my arms, and reestablish the starting position.

INCLINE PUSH-UP

If you're unable to perform a classic push-up properly because you lack enough strength, you can increase your elevation using parallettes. If you don't have parallettes at your disposal, then a chair, bench, or wall will work. By performing this movement from an elevated position, you transfer a portion of your weight to your feet, which decreases the load on your arms and makes the push-up easier. As you build strength and master the technique, work your way down toward the ground until you can perform multiple full-range repetitions, as demonstrated in the previous sequence. If you're using parallettes, there is an added advantage in that you increase your range of motion by dropping your chest between the two bars.

1

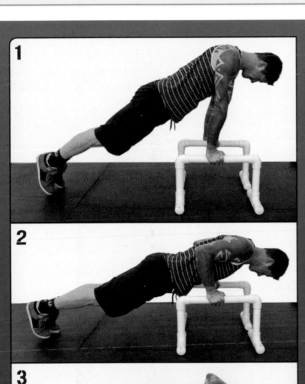

I've assumed the push-up position on the parallettes. My back is flat, my shoulders are externally rotated, and my arms are locked out.

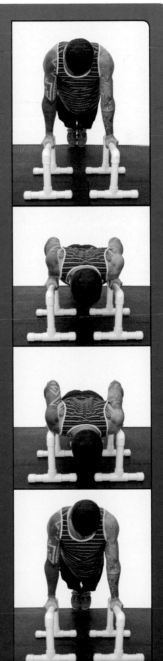

2

I draw my elbows back at a 45-degree angle and lower myself between the parallettes. Note: If you're new to this exercise or have an undeveloped chest and triceps, this is as far down as you should go.

3

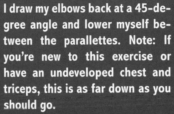

To increase my range of motion, I keep lowering down until my shoulders are parallel with the parallettes.

4

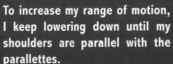

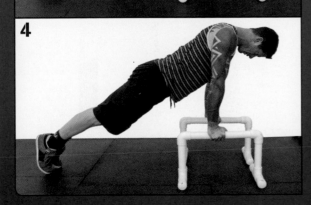

Keeping my elbows tight to my body and my back flat, I press myself up, lock out my arms, and reestablish the starting position.

CLAPPING PUSH-UP

There are thousands of variations on the classic push-up. In fact, you could probably write an entire book devoted just to the subject. But the goal of this manual is to provide you with functional strength and conditioning movements so that you can run, bike, and swim faster, longer, and with less pain. Once you've mastered the push-up technique and you're strong enough to sequence multiple full-range reps, try adding a ballistic element in the form of a clapping push-up. Just like the classic push-up, most of you have probably seen or performed the clapping push-up at some point in your life. To execute this technique correctly, you have to extend your arms with such force that your upper body lifts off the ground. As you go airborne, clap your hands and then return them to the ground to absorb your body's impact. It's important to mention that this exercise is about building explosive power. The moment you fail to achieve full extension from your arms with enough velocity to clap your hands, either take a break to recover, or revert to the classic push-up.

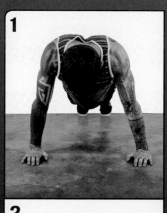

1 I've assumed the top push-up position with my hands just wider than my shoulders.

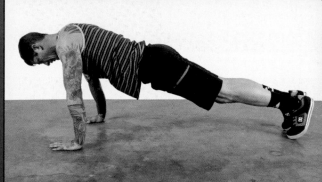

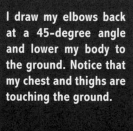

2 I draw my elbows back at a 45-degree angle and lower my body to the ground. Notice that my chest and thighs are touching the ground.

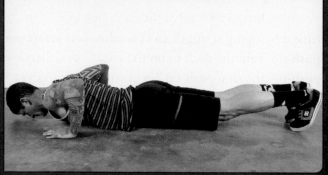

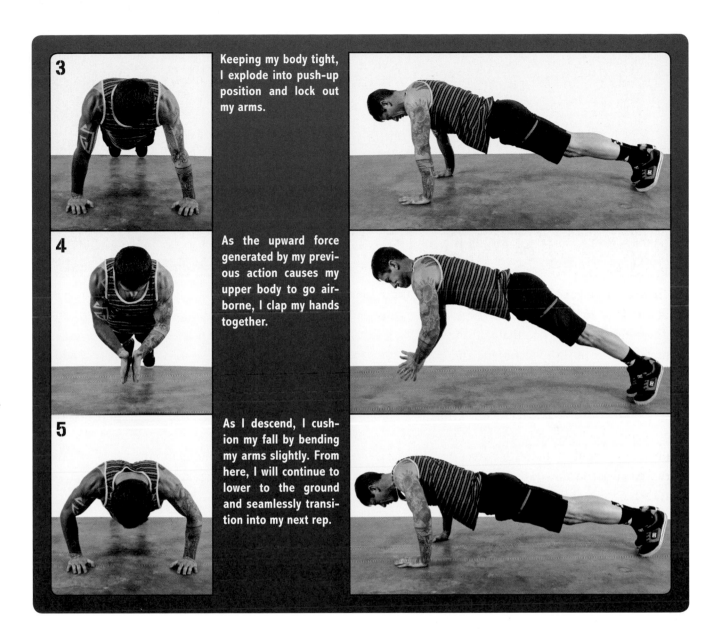

3 Keeping my body tight, I explode into push-up position and lock out my arms.

4 As the upward force generated by my previous action causes my upper body to go airborne, I clap my hands together.

5 As I descend, I cushion my fall by bending my arms slightly. From here, I will continue to lower to the ground and seamlessly transition into my next rep.

RING PUSH-UP

The ring push-up adds a new dimension of difficulty to the classic push-up or parallette push-up. With your body suspended in the air, you have an element of instability to overcome. If you've never performed this movement, chances are your body and arms will shake furiously as you struggle to maintain a rigid position. Just as with all of the complicated or demanding variations demonstrated, you must put in your time developing strength and coordination before performing this exercise. If you can't perform a perfect push-up from the deck or on the parallettes, then avoid this exercise. However, if you can nail the classic push-up, the ring push-up is a great way to progress your strength.

To execute this technique correctly, secure a plank position with your arms locked out, lower yourself until your chest dips below the rings, and then extend your arms. Just as in the classic push-up, your arms should be straight, shoulders externally rotated, and back flat. If you overextend or your elbows flare out, you'll lose power and increase your chances of getting hurt.

1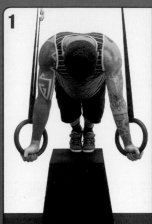

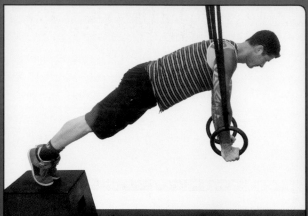

I've achieved the upright push-up position on the rings. Notice that my back is straight and my arms are externally rotated.

2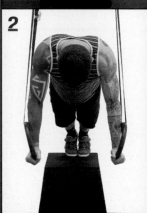

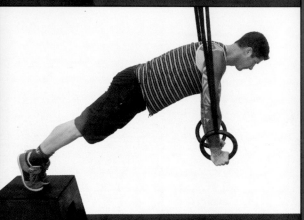

Keeping my shoulders externally rotated, I internally rotate my hands so that my palms are facing each other.

3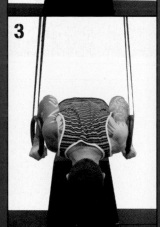

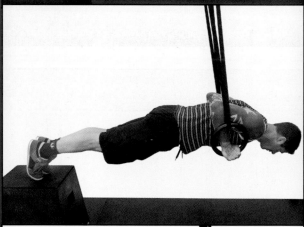

I draw my elbows back at a 45-degree angle and lower myself until my chest is on the same horizontal plane as my hands.

4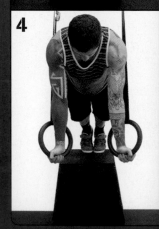

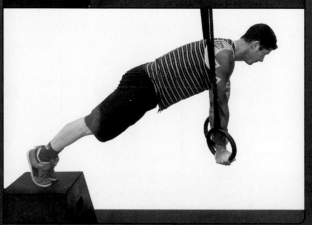

Keeping my arms close to my torso and my body tight, I extend my arms and press myself up. To complete the sequence, I lock out my arms and externally rotate my hands.

DIP

The dip is another pressing exercise that helps strengthen your triceps, deltoids, pecs, and abs. You can perform this movement on a dip bar, parallettes, or, if you're proficient with the movement, on the rings (see next sequence). To increase the intensity of this exercise, you can add weight by using a weight vest or weight belt or by squeezing a dumbbell between your legs. If you're unable to perform this movement accurately, you can take it down a notch by hooking a resistance band around the dip bars and under your feet.

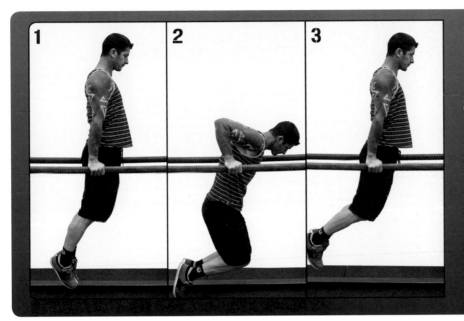

1. I've achieved a neutral spine position on the parallel bars. Note that the bars are just wider than shoulder width.

2. Keeping my back perfectly vertical, I draw my elbows back at a 45-degree angle and lower myself until my chest is parallel with the bars.

3. Keeping my chest up and my back flat, I press myself back up, and lock out my arms and complete the sequence.

Ring Dip

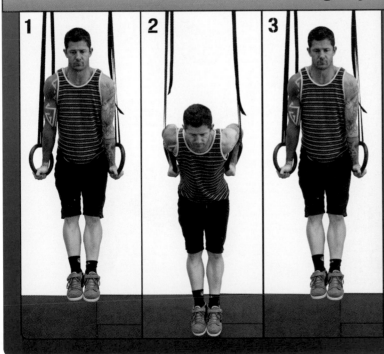

Once you can execute multiple reps of the dip effortlessly, you can progress to the ring dip to increase the challenge. Just as with the ring push-up, you have to engage your core and stabilize your shoulders to keep your arms from flaring out as you drop into the bottom position and press yourself out.

1. I've achieved a neutral spine position on the rings. Notice that my back is straight and my arms are externally rotated.

2. I lower myself into the dip position by internally rotating my hands so that my thumbs are facing forward and then drawing my elbows back.

3. Keeping my arms in tight to my body, I press myself up.

HANDSTAND PUSH-UP (HSPU)

The handstand push-up (HSPU) is an extremely demanding exercise for the core, shoulders, and triceps. Unless you have an extensive background in gymnastics and can perform a freestanding handstand, you will have to use a wall to maintain balance and form. If you glance at the photos below, you'll notice that as I kick up into the handstand I find the wall with my left foot. Once I stabilize myself, I straighten my legs and avoid falling backward by keeping my heels on the wall.

It's important to note that overextension can be a huge problem. So keep your core engaged, your arms locked, and your shoulders externally rotated. If this is your first time and you're unable to execute the exercise because of a lack of strength, start by kicking up to a handstand and holding the position, or just do the second half of the exercise by lowering yourself from the handstand into the bottom position and then allowing your legs to drop to the ground. You can also reduce the range of motion by lowering your body a quarter of the way down and then pressing yourself back up; as you get stronger, work to lower your body farther down until you can achieve a full range of motion by touching your head to the ground. It's important to note that if you can execute this movement with ease, you can increase the challenge by doing it on the parallettes.

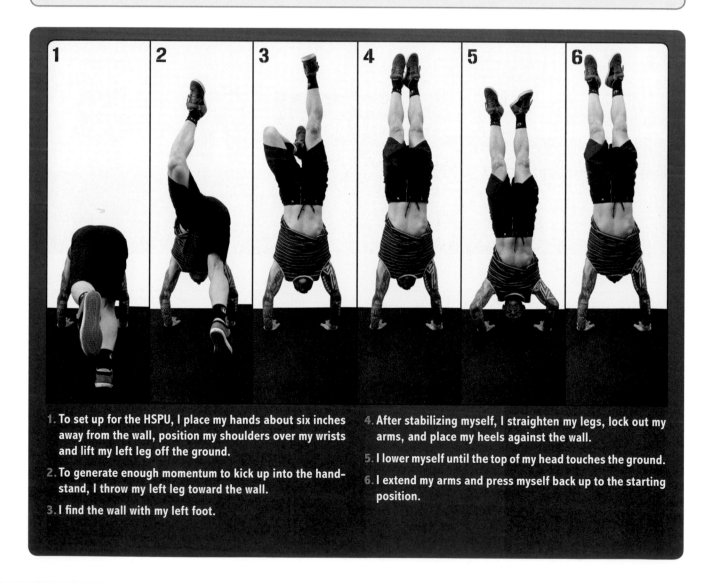

1. To set up for the HSPU, I place my hands about six inches away from the wall, position my shoulders over my wrists and lift my left leg off the ground.

2. To generate enough momentum to kick up into the handstand, I throw my left leg toward the wall.

3. I find the wall with my left foot.

4. After stabilizing myself, I straighten my legs, lock out my arms, and place my heels against the wall.

5. I lower myself until the top of my head touches the ground.

6. I extend my arms and press myself back up to the starting position.

HOLLOW POSITION

Before you initiate the pull-up, you have to know how to set up on the bar. Most athletes simply jump up on the bar and then initiate their pull without really engaging their muscles. Just as in setting up for a squat, a press, or any other exercise for that matter, you have to stabilize your midline before you execute the movement. As I've mentioned, reclaiming a solid position once you're in motion is extremely difficult, if not impossible. If you glance at the photos, you'll notice that I engage my core and achieve a hollow-tight position while hanging from the bar. In addition to protecting my spine and locking my shoulders in the correct position, it's much easier to initiate a pull up than when overextended in a dead hang.

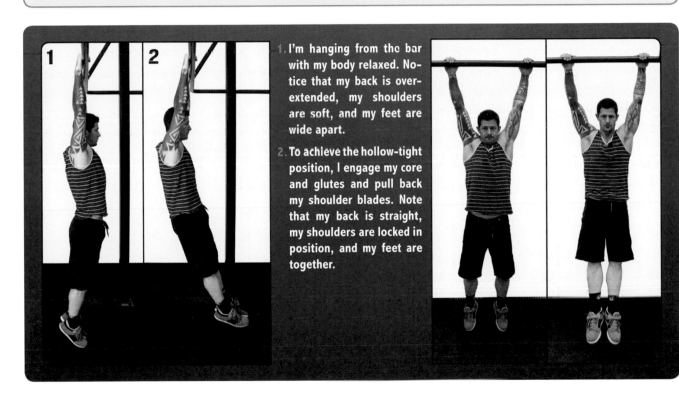

1. I'm hanging from the bar with my body relaxed. Notice that my back is overextended, my shoulders are soft, and my feet are wide apart.

2. To achieve the hollow-tight position, I engage my core and glutes and pull back my shoulder blades. Note that my back is straight, my shoulders are locked in position, and my feet are together.

Bar Grips

Although choosing which grip to utilize is mostly a matter of personal preference, I always recommend the false grip (Figure A) over the thumb-under grip (Figure B) because it provides more stability and gripping power. If you look at the photos, you'll notice that the false grip allows me to wrap my palm over the top of the bar. This sets my wrist and forearm in a strong position and makes it easier to position my knuckles over the bar, which increases the strength of my grip. While the thumb-under grip may seem stronger, it places the wrist and arm directly under the bar, which makes pulling and kipping extremely difficult. In addition to making for an awkward pulling position, the thumb-under grip places more stress and demand on your fingers, which have to hold all of your weight. With a tremendous amount of demand being placed on your forearms, most people won't last for more than a few seconds, which can make doing multiple full-range pull-ups difficult.

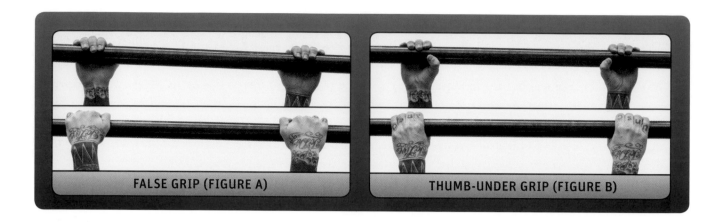

FALSE GRIP (FIGURE A)

THUMB-UNDER GRIP (FIGURE B)

DEAD HANG PULL-UP

The dead hang pull-up develops strength in your back and the anterior chain (biceps) of your arms. Obviously, the pull-up benefits swimmers because it targets the lats and biceps, both of which are used in the freestyle stroke. But it's also great for runners and cyclists because it strengthens the back muscles, which help to maintain your form. As I've mentioned before, form is everything. If your back is weak or underdeveloped, maintaining a tight position with your back flat is extremely difficult. The moment you compromise your posture by overextending or rounding forward, your muscles have to work harder to compensate for the weaker position, which not only increases fatigue, but also your chances of injury.

If you're unable to perform a pull-up for lack of strength or technique, work the upright (supine) rows (see next sequence) to develop strength in your back. In the meantime, spend time hanging on the bar and pulling yourself as high as you can to develop technique and coordination. You can also step on a box, position your chin over the bar, and slowly lower yourself down. Hooking a resistant band around your feet can also be effective. If you can perform multiple full-range reps of the dead hang pull-up, you can increase the challenge by using a weight belt or weight vest.

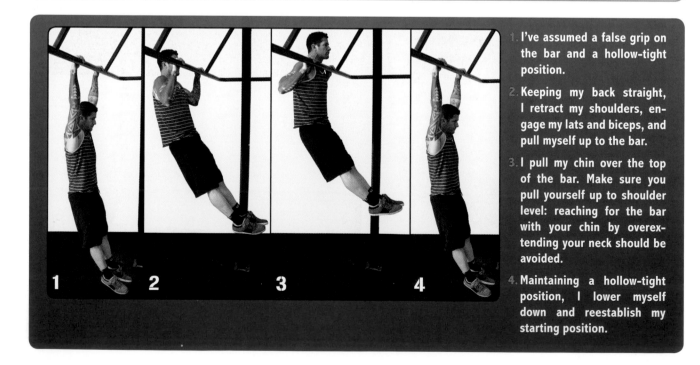

1. I've assumed a false grip on the bar and a hollow-tight position.

2. Keeping my back straight, I retract my shoulders, engage my lats and biceps, and pull myself up to the bar.

3. I pull my chin over the top of the bar. Make sure you pull yourself up to shoulder level: reaching for the bar with your chin by overextending your neck should be avoided.

4. Maintaining a hollow-tight position, I lower myself down and reestablish my starting position.

UPRIGHT (SUPINE) ROW

The upright, or supine, row also strengthens the back and biceps. As I mentioned in the previous technique, the upright row is an excellent progression for the pull-up because you can dictate the challenge by adjusting the angle of your body: the more upright you are, the easier it is, and vice versa. So you may want to begin with your body closer to vertical, at a 45- to 90-degree angle, and then walk underneath the rings as you get stronger. It's important to mention that how close your body is to the ground determines which muscles are recruited. For instance, if you're in a more vertical position, you're probably going to feel it more in your lats and biceps. As you lower the rings, the demand will shift to your upper back. Even if you can already perform a perfect dead hang pull-up, doing a full-range supine row from an extreme angle (with your back nearly parallel to the ground) is an excellent way to develop your upper-back muscles. Note: If you're trying to progress to a dead hang pull-up you may want to consider supplementing with some assisted pull-ups so that you can work on the technique and recruit the correct muscles into the movement, specifically your lats.

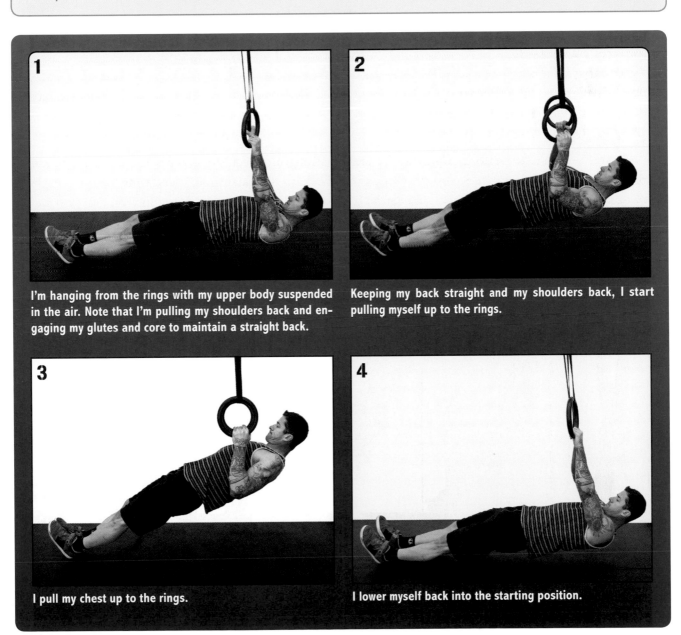

1 I'm hanging from the rings with my upper body suspended in the air. Note that I'm pulling my shoulders back and engaging my glutes and core to maintain a straight back.

2 Keeping my back straight and my shoulders back, I start pulling myself up to the rings.

3 I pull my chest up to the rings.

4 I lower myself back into the starting position.

KIP

The kip is a brilliant way to generate momentum so that you can pull yourself up to the bar using less energy and strength than you would when starting from a dead hang position. If you glance at the photos, you'll notice that I start in a hollow-tight position, pull myself under the bar, and then pull my shoulders back. This back-and-forth rocking motion takes the initiate phase of the pull-up, which is the most difficult, out of the equation. It's like the strict press compared with a push press, in that you generate enough momentum to accelerate the barbell, or in this case your body, out of the starting position, making the rest of the movement easier to manage.

If you're new to the kip, I suggest spending some time perfecting the technique before moving on to the kipping pull-up. A lot of athletes make the mistake of breaking in the midline by spreading their feet, overextending, and bending their legs as they pull themselves under the bar. This is no different running with sloppy form and saying it's o.k. It's not.

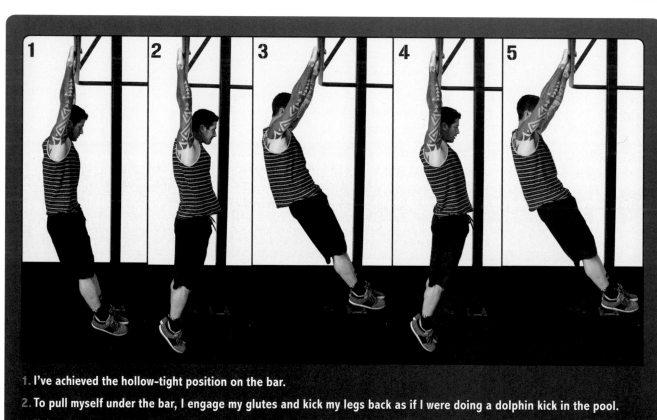

1. I've achieved the hollow-tight position on the bar.

2. To pull myself under the bar, I engage my glutes and kick my legs back as if I were doing a dolphin kick in the pool.

3. Using the momentum of my previous actions to my advantage, I kick my feet forward and pull myself away from the bar.

4. Maintaining momentum along a horizontal plane, I pull myself under the bar for the second time.

5. Once again, I use the momentum generated by my previous action to pull myself away from the bar. Note that you can use this exercise as a warm-up, going back-and-forth as demonstrated, or to develop the strength for a kipping pull-up.

Kipping Pull-Up

In this sequence, I demonstrate how to use the momentum of the kip to perform a pull-up. To reiterate, the kip allows you to generate momentum so that you can execute a full-range pull-up with less effort. In most cases, I'll prescribe the kipping pull-up for a conditioning workout, so that more reps can be performed in a shorter span of time, and program strict or dead hang weighted pull-ups for a strength circuit. If you want more challenge from this exercise, you can increase the range of motion by bring your chest up to the bar (chest to bar pull-up)

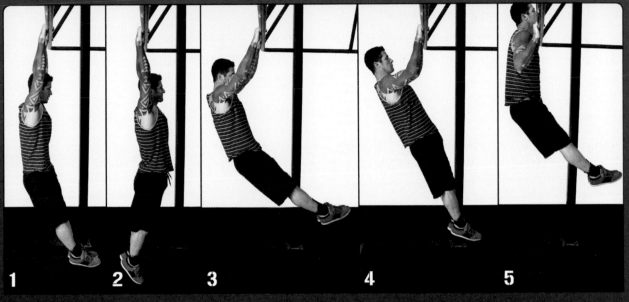

1. I've achieved the hollow-tight position on the bar.

2. To pull myself under the bar, I engage my glutes and kick my legs back as if I were doing a dolphin kick in the pool.

3. Using the momentum of my previous action to my advantage, I kick my feet forward and pull myself away from the bar.

4. As I swing back, I use the momentum generated by the kip to accelerate my body upward.

5. Keeping my body tight, I pull my chin over the bar.

CHIN-UP

While this is an important exercise for all endurance athletes, it is especially beneficial for runners, who need to keep their arms bent at a 90-degree angle for long periods of time. I suggest substituting the chin-up for the strict pull every so often to strengthen your biceps and back.

1. I've assumed a supinated grip (palms facing me) on the bar. To set up for the pull-up, I've achieved a hollow-tight position by engaging my abs and glutes.

2. Staying tight, I pull my chin over the bar.

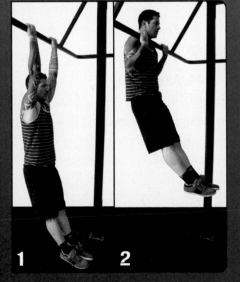

L-SIT PULL-UP

The L-sit pull-up is an advanced exercise that challenges your core, hip flexors, back, and arms. To effectively perform this exercise, you must be able to hold an L-sit, either on the ground or on the parallettes, as well as be able to perform a dead hang pull-up with relative ease. If you're unable to do so, you should practice the two individual exercises to develop strength and technique. It's important to note that some athletes can perform both movements but struggle to put them together to complete one L-sit pull-up. This is primarily because of a lack of coordination. If this happens to you, work a progression of the L-sit by keeping your knees bent at a 90-degree angle, which places less demand on your core and hip flexors. As you develop strength and coordination, try straightening your legs until you can fully extend your legs, as demonstrated below.

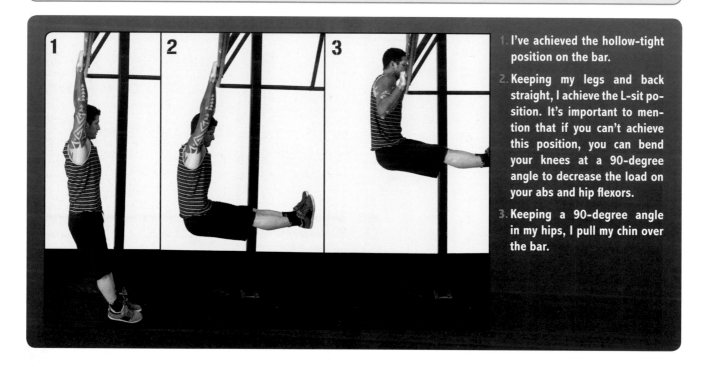

1. I've achieved the hollow-tight position on the bar.

2. Keeping my legs and back straight, I achieve the L-sit position. It's important to mention that if you can't achieve this position, you can bend your knees at a 90-degree angle to decrease the load on your abs and hip flexors.

3. Keeping a 90-degree angle in my hips, I pull my chin over the bar.

ROPE CLIMB

The rope climb is an excellent full-body pulling exercise that develops grip, arm, back, and core strength. If you've never climbed a rope before, I suggest starting with one of the "foot lace" techniques (Sequence A and B). In addition to lightening the load on your upper body, you can stabilize your position and use the power of your legs to ascend the rope. There are two foot-lock variations: experiment with both, and then choose the one that feels the most natural. Even if you can climb up the rope without using your legs, you should still spend some quality time becoming proficient with the leg-lacing techniques, primarily for safety reasons. If your grip falters during your ascent, using your legs to support your body weight not only reduces the eccentric load on your arms, but also decreases your chances of falling off the rope as you descend.

Sequence A: Rope Climb Option 1

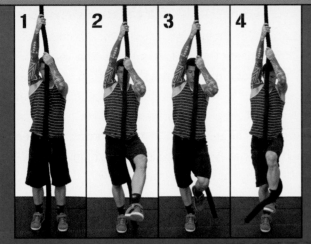

1. I've got a firm grip on the rope.
2. I wrap my left leg around the front of the rope.
3. I hook the rope in the crook of my left leg.
4. Circling my left leg in a clockwise direction, I hook my left foot under the rope.

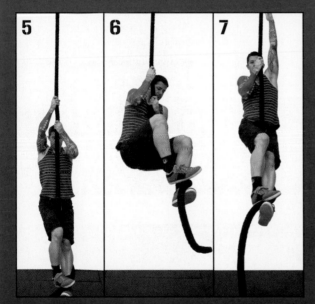

5. Pulling myself up with my arms, I step my right foot over my left foot and pin the rope between my feet. Note that I'm flexing my left foot to keep the rope from slipping off my leg.
6. Using my arms to support my weight, I pull myself up and slide both of my feet up the rope.
7. I reestablish my foot clamp on the rope. With my feet supporting the weight of my body, I reach my left arm up the rope and secure a tight grip. From here, I will repeat the sequence until I reach the top of the rope. It's important to note that you use the same technique going down and going up.

Sequence B: Rope Climb Option 2

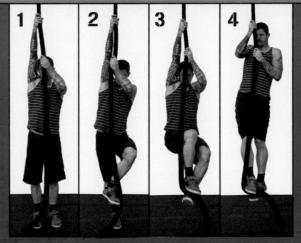

1. I've got a firm grip on the rope.
2. I maneuver my left leg across my body and hook my left foot around the front of the rope. Notice that unlike in the first option the rope is not wrapped around my leg.
3. Using my arms to support the weight of my body, I maneuver my right knee to the inside of the rope and my left leg and step my right foot over my left foot, pinning the rope between my feet.
4. I use my legs and arms to ascend the rope.

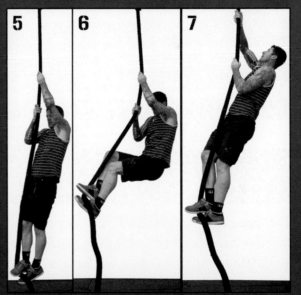

5. I reach my left arm up the rope and secure a tight grip.
6. Pulling myself up with my arms, I slide both of my feet up the rope. Notice that I keep the rope clamped between my feet.
7. I pin the rope between my feet and momentarily take the load off my arms. As I do this, I reach my right arm up the rope and prepare to repeat the sequence.

MUSCLE-UP

The muscle-up is a gymnastics technique that combines a pull-up with a dip. While being able to perform a strict dead hang pull-up and ring dip with precision is mandatory before attempting this exercise, I'm sorry to say that it doesn't ensure your success. The transition between the two movements is very technical and requires a specific skill set. To begin, you have to secure a false grip on the rings. If you've never used this grip, you should lower the rings to chest level to familiarize yourself with the hold. If you scan the photos in Sequence A, you'll notice that my wrist is folded over the ring. Although this grip may seem awkward at first, it not only provides a strong pulling position, but also makes transitioning to the dip easier.

Once you understand how to achieve a false grip, the next step is to work on the transition from the pull-up to the dip. The best way to accomplish this is to start in a kneeling position (Sequence B). With the power of your legs taking the stress off your upper body, you can focus on pulling the rings to your chest using the false grip, keeping your arms in tight, and transitioning to the dip with less effort. After dialing in your technique, you can attempt the full-range muscle-up (Sequence C).

The key is to keep the false grip intact as you pull, keep your arms in tight to your body, and then lever forward by driving your elbows up and shifting the weight of your upper body over your hands the moment you pull your chest to the rings. You can make the full-range muscle-up easier by adding a kip, which is common, and often necessary, when first learning the progression. When this movement is done correctly—whether you perform a strict or kipping muscle-up—you'll not only develop your coordination, but you'll build total upper-body strength.

Sequence A: False Grip

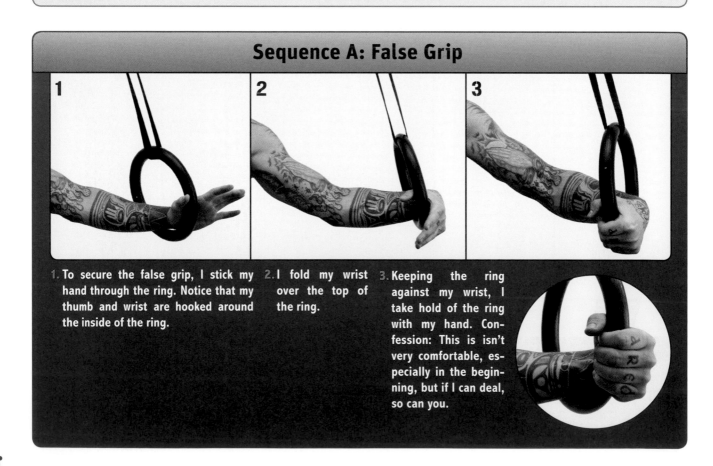

1. To secure the false grip, I stick my hand through the ring. Notice that my thumb and wrist are hooked around the inside of the ring.

2. I fold my wrist over the top of the ring.

3. Keeping the ring against my wrist, I take hold of the ring with my hand. Confession: This is isn't very comfortable, especially in the beginning, but if I can deal, so can you.

Sequence B: Muscle-Up Progression

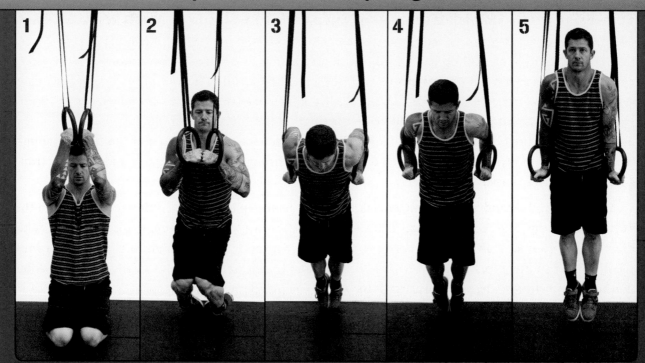

1	2	3	4	5
I've secured a false grip on the rings from the kneeling position.	Using my legs to help lift me, I pull my chest up to the rings. Notice that I keep my hands in close to my body, my arms are in tight, and my false grip is still intact.	Still using my legs to support my weight, I lever forward and pull my elbows back.	I begin to press myself up from the dip position.	To complete the dip, I lock out my arms and then externally rotate my hands.

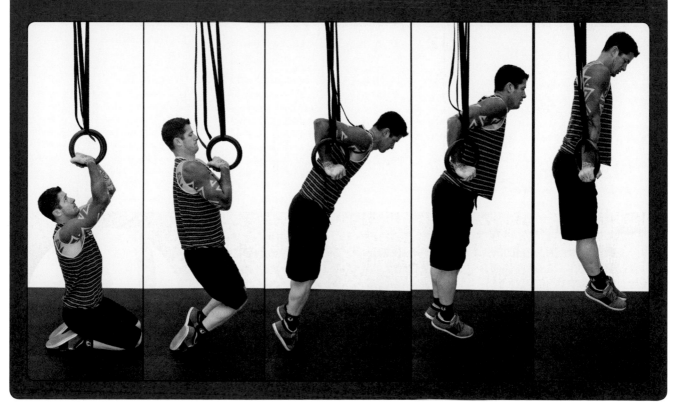

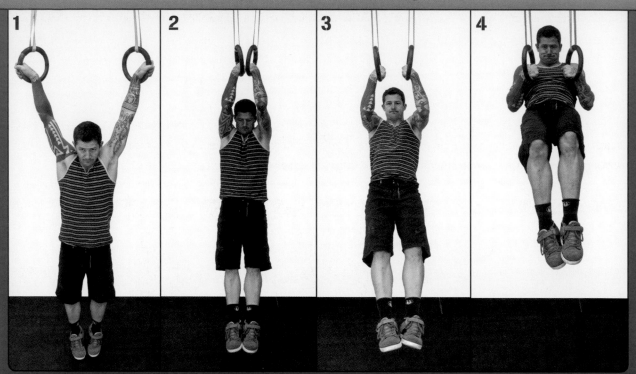

1. I'm hanging from the rings with a false grip.

2. Keeping my false grip intact, I internally rotate my hands and bring the rings together overhead.

3. Keeping my arms in tight, I pull myself up to the rings.

4. I pull my chest up to the rings.

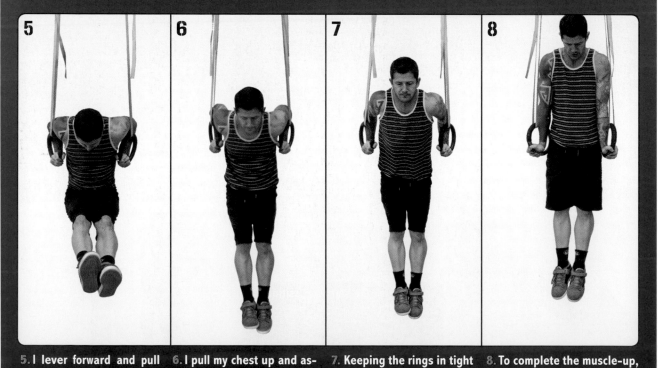

5. I lever forward and pull my elbows back.

6. I pull my chest up and assume the proper dip position.

7. Keeping the rings in tight to my body, I begin to press myself up.

8. To complete the muscle-up, I lock out my arms and then externally rotate my hands.

AIR SQUAT

The air squat is one of the most basic and important functional exercises to incorporate into a conditioning circuit because in addition to building strength, speed, power, and flexibility, it also develops cardiovascular and muscular endurance. In the majority of the prescribed workouts, you'll have to do sets of air squats. If you've never learned how to properly squat, this is where you start.

To perform the air squat, drive your hips and hamstrings back while maintaining a flat back, drive your knees out laterally, keep you weight in your heels, and pull your arms up as you descend into the bottom-squat position to counterbalance your weight. If at any point during a workout you feel your weight shift onto the balls of your feet, your midline collapses, your knees start to track inward or over your feet, or your back rounds, take a quick break and then finish your set with solid technique. The air squat is one of the best exercises you can do as a warm-up because it stimulates all the muscles in the legs and increases mobility in the hip, knee, and ankle joints.

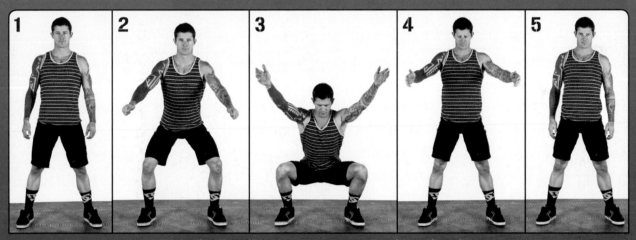

1. I'm standing with my feet slightly wider than shoulder width.

2. I pull my hamstrings back to initiate the squat. As I do this, I raise my arms to counterbalance my weight. It's imperative to initiate the squat with your hamstrings, as if you were reaching back to sit down in a chair. A lot of athletes make the mistake of tracking their knees over their feet to begin the movement. Not only does this put shear force on the knee, but also forces the weight onto the balls of the feet, which shifts the demand onto the quads.

3. Keeping my back flat and my weight driving through my heels, I drop into the bottom-squat position. Notice my arms are still overhead to counterbalance.

4. I extend my hips and knees, lower my arms, and start rising up.

5. As I stand up, I squeeze my glutes and prepare for my next rep.

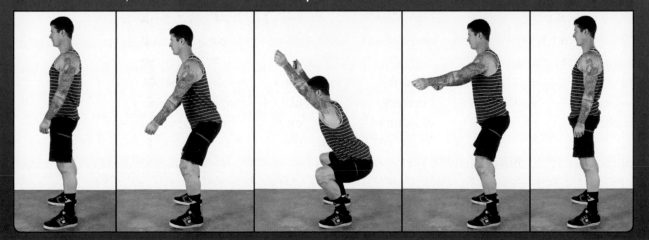

JUMP SQUAT

In this sequence a jump is added to the air squat to develop explosive power and speed. It's important to mention that the jumping technique in this sequence is also used in the broad jump, which requires you to leap forward, as opposed to straight up in the air. The key to doing this exercise correctly—whether you're jumping forward to perform a broad jump or straight up in a jump squat—is to execute an air squat and then explode out of the bottom position by extending your hips, knees, and ankles while simultaneously throwing your arms up. In addition to allowing you to reach triple extension, your arms help accelerate your body off the ground, maximizing the height or distance of your jump. You should land from the jump with your feet parallel and absorb the impact of your weight by dropping into a squat. The former prevents your knees from tracking inward, and the latter cushions your fall and reduces the impact on your hip, knee, and ankle joints.

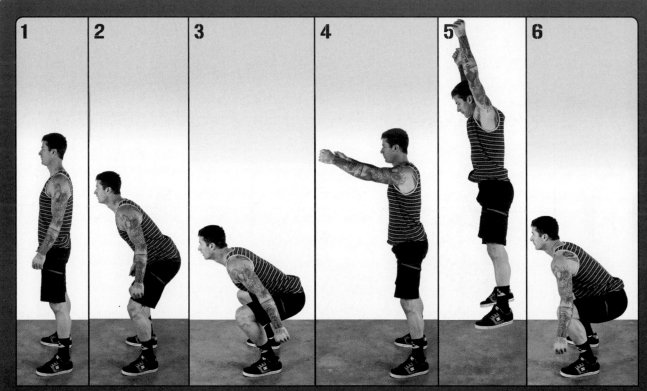

1. I'm standing with my feet slightly wider than my shoulders.

2. I pull my hamstrings back to initiate the squat and start to lower down.

3. I drop into the bottom-squat position. With my arms at my sides, I have to counterbalance my weight by leaning my chest slightly forward.

4. I explode out of the bottom-squat position by extending my knees and hips. To help my acceleration, I raise my arms.

5. Throwing my arms overhead, I jump into the air.

6. As I land, I immediately drop into the bottom-squat position. This not only reduces the impact on my joints, but also allows me to seamlessly transition into my next rep.

PISTOL

The single-leg squat, otherwise referred to as the pistol, is one of the most demanding body weight exercises that you can execute. In addition to making you stronger and more flexible and increasing your coordination and focus, pistols teach you how to exert power through a full range of motion using only one leg. This is incredibly beneficial to runners and cyclist, who have to constantly shift power from one leg to the other.

If you don't have enough range of motion in your hip, knee, or ankle joints to sit down into a full squat, rather than executing the movement as demonstrated, you should sit back on a high box and then stand up on one leg. The single-leg box squat is an excellent way to develop strength, coordination, and proper technique.

Most athletes aren't comfortable dropping deep into a full squat on one leg the first time they try it. To reduce the load on your standing leg, you can do box squats, or you can counterbalance your weight by holding a pole or by standing in a doorway and hanging on to the frame. Grabbing on to a sturdy object not only allows to you to slow down the eccentric progression, which can be difficult to control, but also helps you press out of the bottom position. As you develop strength and coordination, you should momentarily release your grip on your support and practice dropping into the bottom position and pressing out without it. At this stage, it sometimes helps to hold a light weight out in front of your body (Figure A) to counterbalance your weight. Soon you will be ready to execute the freestanding body weight pistol.

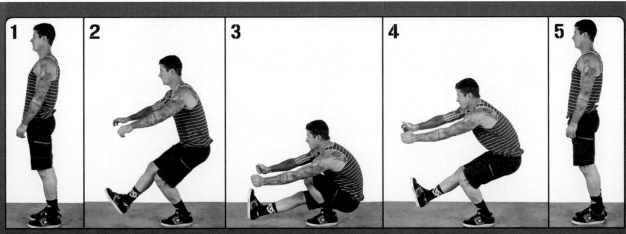

1. I'm standing with my midline stabilized.

2. I shift my weight onto my left leg, extend my right leg in front of me, and drive my hips back. As I lower down, I raise my arms to help counterbalance my weight. It's very important to initiate this movement by driving your hips back as if you were going to sit down in a chair. This not only keeps your weight in your heel, but also keeps your center of mass over your grounded leg.

3. Keeping my right leg straight, I drop into the bottom-squat position.

4. Driving my weight through my left heel, I extend my left hip and knee and begin to stand up. Notice that my arms are still out in front of me to help counterbalance my weight.

5. I stand up, completing the sequence.

Holding a weight out in front of you to counterbalance your own weight can make it easier to press up out of the bottom squat position. You can also use a pole for support, or drop down onto a box if your range of motion or strength are limiting.

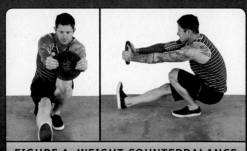

FIGURE A: WEIGHT COUNTERBALANCE

LUNGE

The lunge is another excellent single-leg exercise that develops lower-body strength and endurance. It's important to note that although I demonstrate the basic body-weight forward lunge, there are many other variations. For example, to make this exercise more demanding on your core you can hold a dumbbell in one hand at your side (Figure A), which will develop grip strength and force you to stabilize your midline even more. You can also hold a weight or dumbbell overhead, or wear a weight vest to turn up the volume. Regardless of the variation you execute, you should always lunge forward so that when you touch your rear knee to the ground your lead knee is bent at a 90-degree angle. If you look at the third photo in the sequence below, you'll notice that my lead shin is vertical. This position not only decreases stress on the knee joint, but also recruits the muscles of my posterior chain, which is the whole point of this exercise.

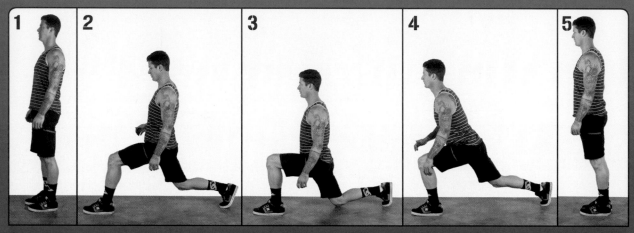

1. I'm standing with my midline stabilized.

2. Keeping my core engaged, I take a giant step forward with my left leg. It's important to take a big enough step forward so that when you touch your opposite knee to the ground your lead shin is perfectly vertical.

3. I touch my right knee to the ground. Notice that my lead shin is vertical. If your lead knee tracks over your foot, you'll place tension and stress on the knee and shift the demand onto your quads, which is less than ideal.

4. Shifting my weight forward onto my left leg, I use my glutes and hamstrings to push off from the bottom position.

5. After driving out of the bottom position, I reset my base and reestablish my starting position. From here, I will lunge forward on the opposite foot. It's important to mention that if you're tired or you lose your balance as you drive out of the bottom, you should reset your base before continuing. In the beginning, you may have to reset every time until you develop the strength and coordination to sequence multiple reps together.

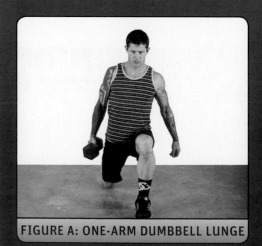

FIGURE A: ONE-ARM DUMBBELL LUNGE

The one-arm dumbbell lunge is just one of countless variations of the lunge. This particular variation increases the challenge on the core and develops coordination and balance. You can hold the weight overhead if you want to get your shoulders involved.

BOX STEP-UPS

Box step-ups are an excellent exercise to implement if you're having trouble with the squat because of a limited range of motion. You can increase the intensity of this exercise by holding weight or by stepping up onto a higher box.

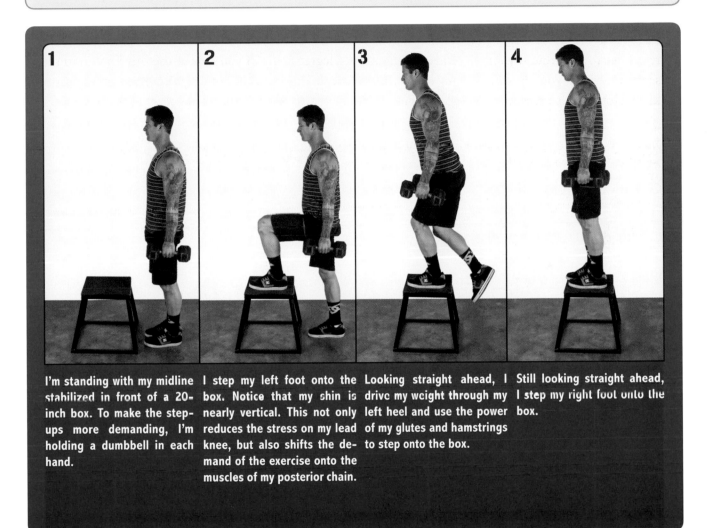

1 I'm standing with my midline stabilized in front of a 20-inch box. To make the step-ups more demanding, I'm holding a dumbbell in each hand.

2 I step my left foot onto the box. Notice that my shin is nearly vertical. This not only reduces the stress on my lead knee, but also shifts the demand of the exercise onto the muscles of my posterior chain.

3 Looking straight ahead, I drive my weight through my left heel and use the power of my glutes and hamstrings to step onto the box.

4 Still looking straight ahead, I step my right foot onto the box.

BOX JUMPS

If you read Chapter 2, you know that running on the balls of your feet is the preferred method. If you're new to this skill, it can be particularly strenuous on your feet and calves. Box jumps are excellent for conditioning your legs for the repeated punishment of running, because in addition to strengthening and building muscle elasticity in your legs, they also develop explosive power. Note: If you're focusing on speed, cardiovascular endurance, and agility, then sequencing multiple reps on an 18-, 20-, or 24-inch box is ideal. If you want to focus on developing explosive power, you should reduce the reps and jump onto a higher box—24 inches or more.

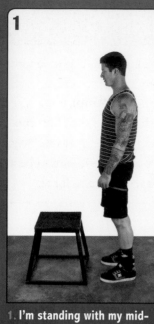

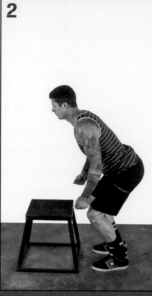

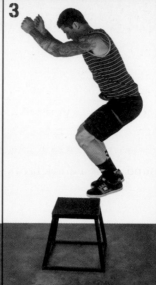

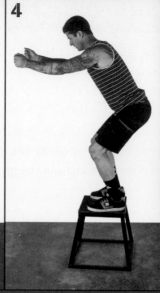

1. I'm standing with my midline stabilized in front of a 20-inch box.

2. To set my body up for the box jump, I lower myself by driving my hips back and bending my knees slightly.

3. Keeping my midline tight, I extend my hips and knees and jump up. Just as in the jump squat, I use my arms to help lift my body off the ground.

4. I land on top of the box.

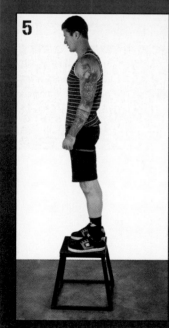

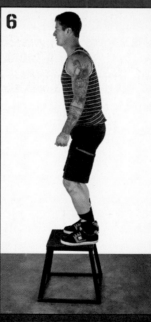

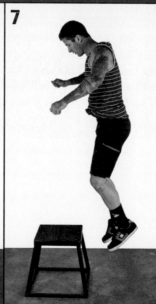

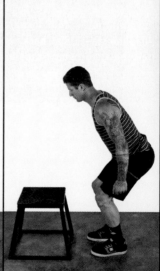

5. I stand up to complete the full range of motion.

6. I dip down slightly by bending my knees.

7. I jump down off the box.

8. I land in a half-squat position. Note that by landing in a half squat, I not only cushion my fall, which reduces the stress on my hip, knee, and ankle joints, but I also position myself to seamlessly transition into my next jump.

BURPEE

The burpee is one the most physically demanding body-weight movements that you can incorporate into your conditioning routine. With each repetition, you strengthen your chest, core, arms, shoulders, and legs. To execute it correctly, assume a plank position, touch your chest to the ground (push-up), jump into a squat, and then drive out of the bottom position into a jump squat. Because the burpee is such a strenuous exercise, it tends to bring on fatigue relatively quickly. If your technique is compromised because, say, you're tired (you start to come up onto the balls of your feet or you're not doing a push-up with your chest and thighs touching the ground), take a quick break and then complete your reps with precise form.

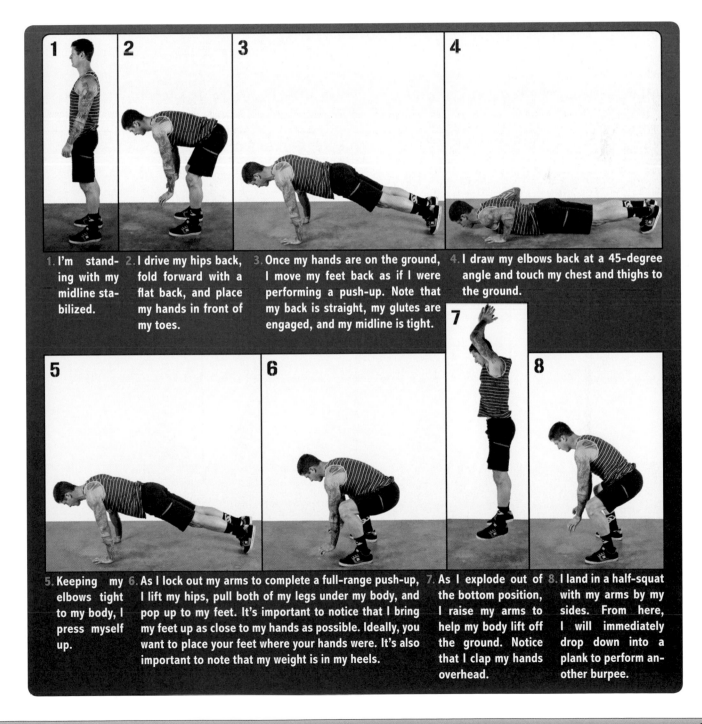

1. I'm standing with my midline stabilized.

2. I drive my hips back, fold forward with a flat back, and place my hands in front of my toes.

3. Once my hands are on the ground, I move my feet back as if I were performing a push-up. Note that my back is straight, my glutes are engaged, and my midline is tight.

4. I draw my elbows back at a 45-degree angle and touch my chest and thighs to the ground.

5. Keeping my elbows tight to my body, I press myself up.

6. As I lock out my arms to complete a full-range push-up, I lift my hips, pull both of my legs under my body, and pop up to my feet. It's important to notice that I bring my feet up as close to my hands as possible. Ideally, you want to place your feet where your hands were. It's also important to note that my weight is in my heels.

7. As I explode out of the bottom position, I raise my arms to help my body lift off the ground. Notice that I clap my hands overhead.

8. I land in a half-squat with my arms by my sides. From here, I will immediately drop down into a plank to perform another burpee.

D-BALL SLAM

The D-ball slam is another full-body exercise that incorporates your legs, arms, shoulders, and core. Like all of the exercises demonstrated in this section, the d-ball slam builds strength and explosive power and develops your cardiovascular system. The key to executing this exercise correctly is to violently throw the ball to the ground as you bend your knees.

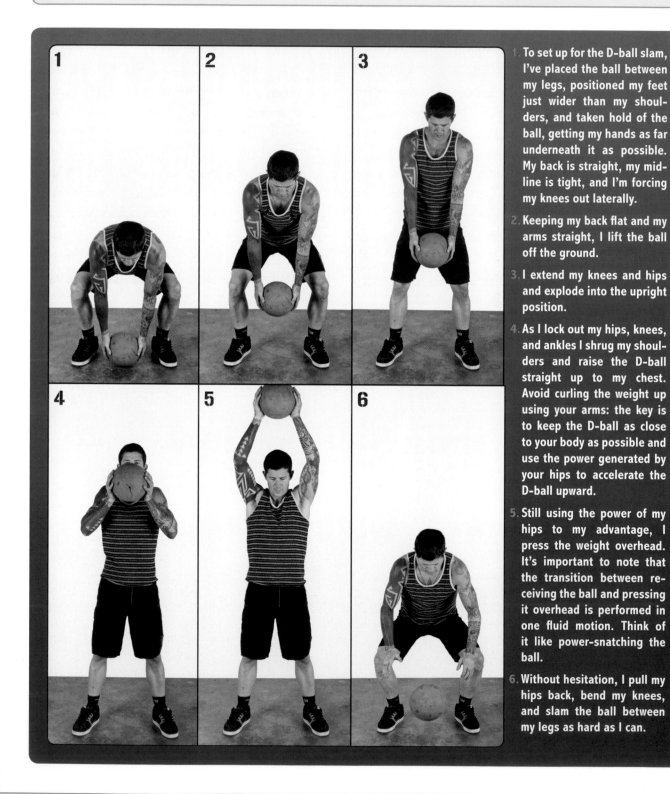

1. To set up for the D-ball slam, I've placed the ball between my legs, positioned my feet just wider than my shoulders, and taken hold of the ball, getting my hands as far underneath it as possible. My back is straight, my midline is tight, and I'm forcing my knees out laterally.

2. Keeping my back flat and my arms straight, I lift the ball off the ground.

3. I extend my knees and hips and explode into the upright position.

4. As I lock out my hips, knees, and ankles I shrug my shoulders and raise the D-ball straight up to my chest. Avoid curling the weight up using your arms: the key is to keep the D-ball as close to your body as possible and use the power generated by your hips to accelerate the D-ball upward.

5. Still using the power of my hips to my advantage, I press the weight overhead. It's important to note that the transition between receiving the ball and pressing it overhead is performed in one fluid motion. Think of it like power-snatching the ball.

6. Without hesitation, I pull my hips back, bend my knees, and slam the ball between my legs as hard as I can.

KETTLEBELL SWING

The kettlebell swing has numerous benefits. It increases aerobic and anaerobic capacity, improves muscular endurance, builds strength, and develops explosive power. It also targets key muscle groups involved in cycling and running, including the glutes, hamstrings, core, lower back, arms, and shoulders. To execute this exercise correctly, you have to let your hips do the work. A common mistake is to pull with the shoulders instead of driving with the hips. You also want to keep your weight in your heels and your back straight. If you break or round forward into flexion, the kettlebell will pull your upper body forward, forcing you to counterbalance by coming onto the balls of your feet. In addition to losing power, this compromise in technique increases your chances of injury.

In the sequence below, I demonstrate an overhead swing, which is standard within the CrossFit community and is commonly referred to as the American swing. By swinging the weight overhead, you open the shoulder joint and increase the range of motion, which not only ups the intensity of this exercise, but also improves shoulder mobility. If you're performing the kettlebell swing with a heavy weight, you can do the Russian version, in which you have to swing the weight only up to chest or eye level. The former (American standard) is good for high-rep conditioning workouts, while the latter (Russian standard) is excellent for developing explosive power in the hips. If you don't have access to a kettlebell, you can use a dumbbell (as demonstrated in Sequence A).

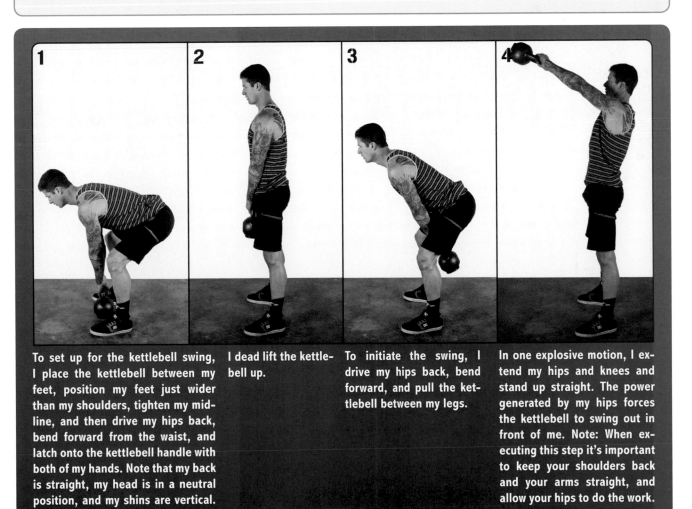

1 To set up for the kettlebell swing, I place the kettlebell between my feet, position my feet just wider than my shoulders, tighten my midline, and then drive my hips back, bend forward from the waist, and latch onto the kettlebell handle with both of my hands. Note that my back is straight, my head is in a neutral position, and my shins are vertical.

2 I dead lift the kettlebell up.

3 To initiate the swing, I drive my hips back, bend forward, and pull the kettlebell between my legs.

4 In one explosive motion, I extend my hips and knees and stand up straight. The power generated by my hips forces the kettlebell to swing out in front of me. Note: When executing this step it's important to keep your shoulders back and your arms straight, and allow your hips to do the work.

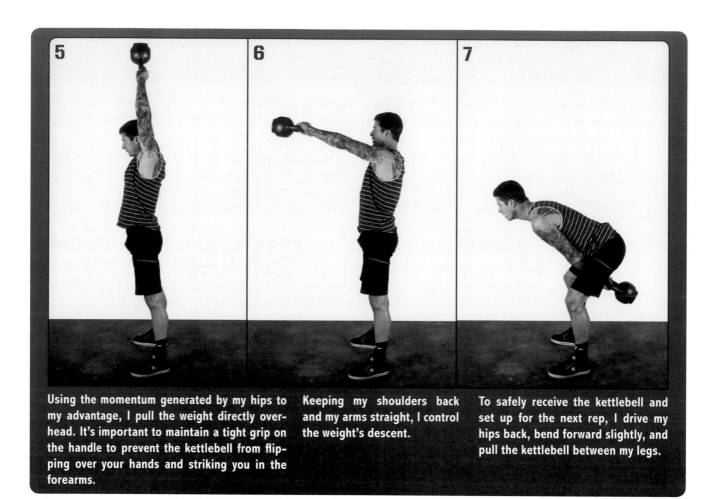

5 Using the momentum generated by my hips to my advantage, I pull the weight directly over-head. It's important to maintain a tight grip on the handle to prevent the kettlebell from flipping over your hands and striking you in the forearms.

6 Keeping my shoulders back and my arms straight, I control the weight's descent.

7 To safely receive the kettlebell and set up for the next rep, I drive my hips back, bend forward slightly, and pull the kettlebell between my legs.

Sequence A: Dumbbell Swing

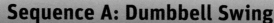

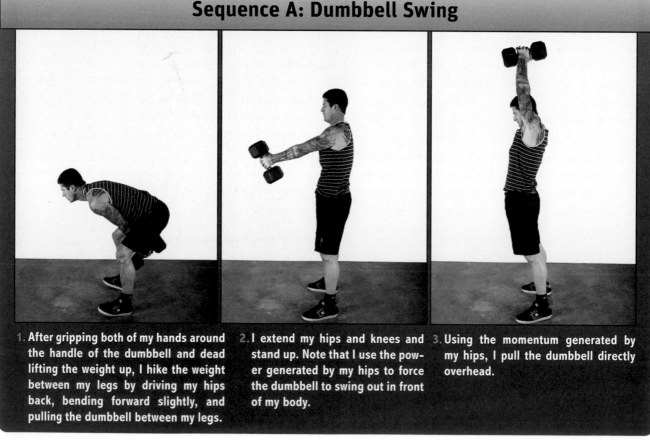

1. After gripping both of my hands around the handle of the dumbbell and dead lifting the weight up, I hike the weight between my legs by driving my hips back, bending forward slightly, and pulling the dumbbell between my legs.

2. I extend my hips and knees and stand up. Note that I use the power generated by my hips to force the dumbbell to swing out in front of my body.

3. Using the momentum generated by my hips, I pull the dumbbell directly overhead.

THRUSTER

The thruster is essentially a combination of the overhead press and the front squat. It is hands down one of the most metabolically demanding full-body movements because you're exerting power through a full range of motion and you have to control the eccentric load after each rep, which requires a ton of energy. In other words, it gets real nasty, real fast. You can perform it using dumbbells (see sequence A), a medicine ball, or a sandbag. Whether you're lifting heavy weight with low reps, or light weight with high reps, you will dramatically improve your cardiovascular endurance and power with this exercise.

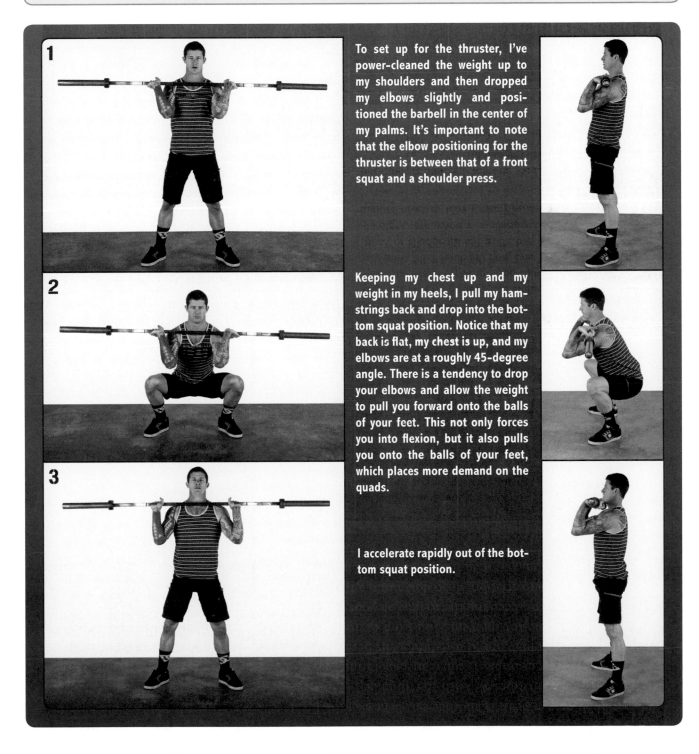

1

To set up for the thruster, I've power-cleaned the weight up to my shoulders and then dropped my elbows slightly and positioned the barbell in the center of my palms. It's important to note that the elbow positioning for the thruster is between that of a front squat and a shoulder press.

2

Keeping my chest up and my weight in my heels, I pull my hamstrings back and drop into the bottom squat position. Notice that my back is flat, my chest is up, and my elbows are at a roughly 45-degree angle. There is a tendency to drop your elbows and allow the weight to pull you forward onto the balls of your feet. This not only forces you into flexion, but it also pulls you onto the balls of your feet, which places more demand on the quads.

3

I accelerate rapidly out of the bottom squat position.

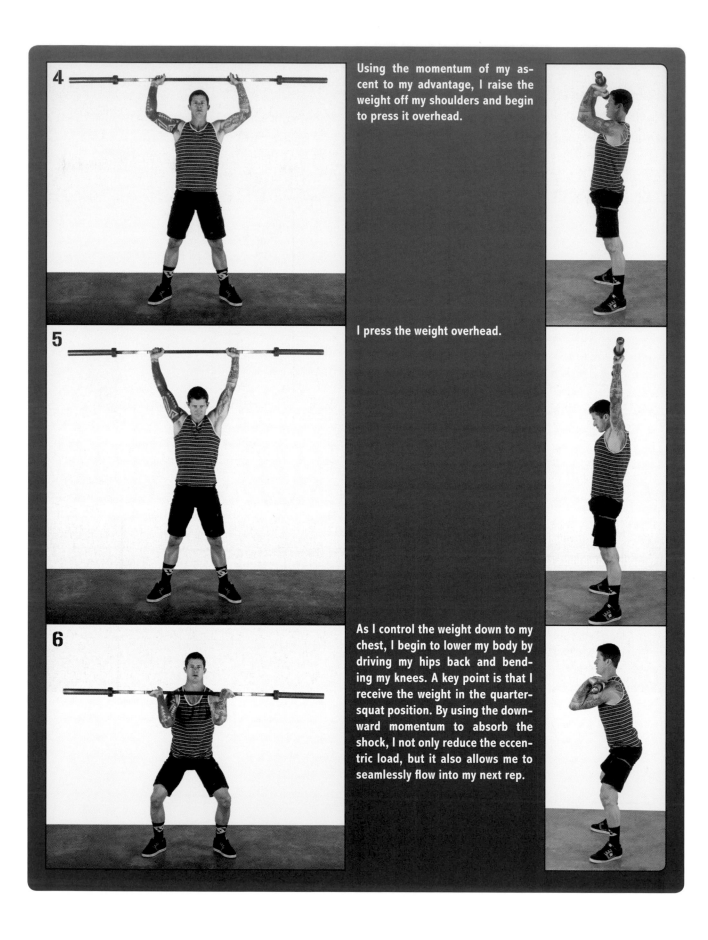

4

Using the momentum of my ascent to my advantage, I raise the weight off my shoulders and begin to press it overhead.

5

I press the weight overhead.

6

As I control the weight down to my chest, I begin to lower my body by driving my hips back and bending my knees. A key point is that I receive the weight in the quarter-squat position. By using the downward momentum to absorb the shock, I not only reduce the eccentric load, but it also allows me to seamlessly flow into my next rep.

Sequence A: Dumbbell Thruster

Performing the thruster using dumbbells improves your balance and coordination because you have to control two weights instead of one. Sometimes the dumbbell thruster is preferred for beginners because it's easier to keep the chest up and it puts less pressure on the lumbar spine. If you're new to this movement, or you're unable to comfortably achieve the front-rack pressing position, this is an excellent variation.

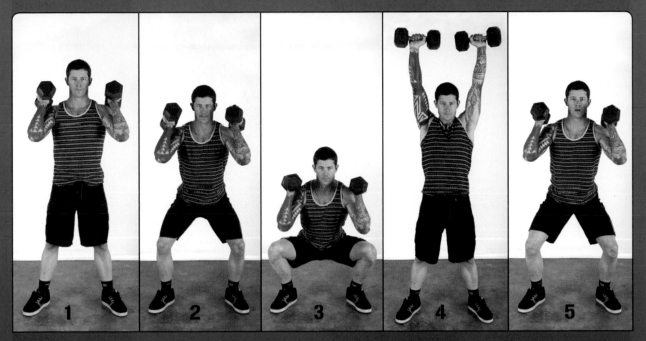

1. I've cleaned the dumbbells up to my shoulders (see next technique).

2. With the dumbbells resting on my shoulders, I pull my hips back and descend into a squat.

3. Keeping my chest up and my weight in my heels, I drop into a bottom squat position.

4. I accelerate rapidly out of the bottom position and press the dumbbells overhead. Note that as I extend my arms overhead, I externally rotate my hands to lock out my shoulders.

5. To effectively receive the weight, I drop into a quarter-squat as I lower the dumbbells to my shoulders. From here, I will seamlessly transition into my next rep.

DUMBBELL POWER CLEAN

The dumbbell power clean is another excellent exercise for developing strength, explosive power, endurance, and coordination. As with the dumbbell thruster, using dumbbells instead of a barbell can minimize faults. For example, if you're incorporating a power clean into a workout that requires a high number of reps, you may opt to use dumbbells because you can receive the weight on your shoulders instead of your chest. This prevents you from caving forward into flexion or rolling onto the balls of your feet as a result of receiving the weight on your chest. You can also perform this exercise as a full clean. To execute that variation, drop down into a full squat and receive the weight on your shoulders in the bottom position, and then front-squat the weight to the standing position.

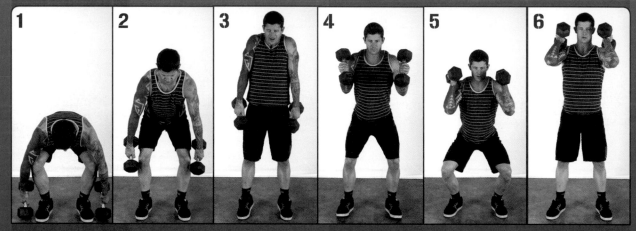

1. After stabilizing my midline and spacing my feet shoulder width apart, I pull my hips back, drive my knees out laterally as I bend forward, and grab the dumbbells. Note that my wrists are relaxed and allow the dumbbells to hang. Fighting to keep the dumbbells at a horizontal angle offers no advantages and will cause your arms to fatigue more quickly.

2. Keeping my arms and back straight, I extend my hips and knees and stand up with the weight.

3. As I reach triple extension, I engage my traps by shrugging my shoulders.

4. The momentum generated by my previous actions causes the dumbbells to accelerate up my body. As this happens, I begin to bend my knees and pull myself under the weight. Note: Avoid using your arms by reverse curling the weight to your chest; instead, rely on the power generated by your hips to accelerate the weight up to your shoulders.

5. As the dumbbells continue to fly upward, I drop into a quarter-squat position, drive my elbows up, and receive the weight on my shoulders.

6. I stand up with the weight.

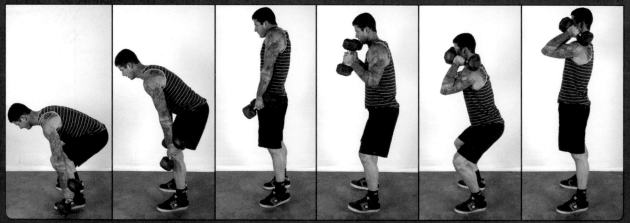

ONE-ARM DUMBBELL SNATCH

The one-arm dumbbell snatch is a tremendous core stabilization exercise that develops total body strength and builds explosive power in the hips. The key to performing this exercise correctly is to keep your arm externally rotated and engage your traps by shrugging your shoulder as you receive the weight overhead: this protects the shoulder from injury and allows you to lock out your arm without restriction.

While it may seem like common sense, I'm going to say it anyway: make sure you perform an equal number of reps with each arm. It's also important to mention that you can perform the one-arm dumbbell snatch as a power variant (Sequence A) or drop into a squat to perform the full snatch (Sequence B). The version depends on the load and your prescribed workout. For example, if you're lifting a lighter weight, you may opt for the power variant to save energy. But if you're tired and you're having trouble getting the weight overhead, you may have to execute the full snatch.

Sequence A: One-Arm Dumbbell Power Snatch

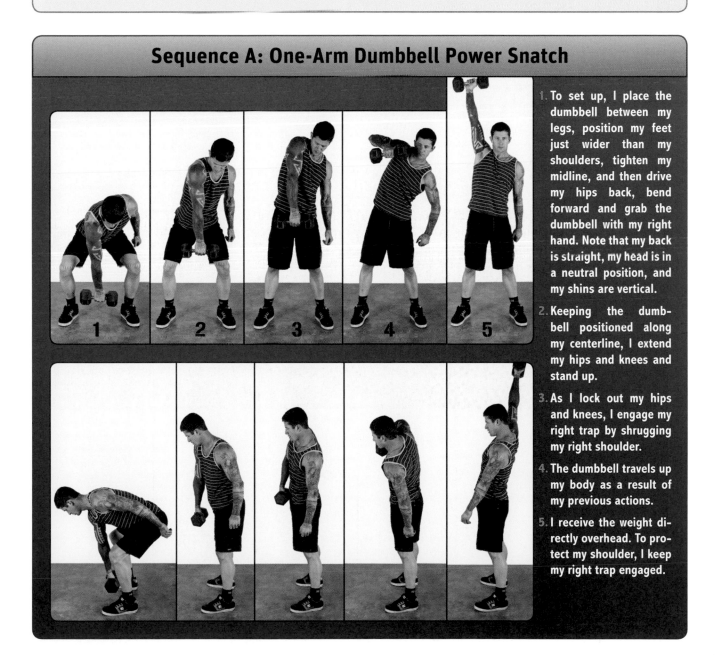

1. To set up, I place the dumbbell between my legs, position my feet just wider than my shoulders, tighten my midline, and then drive my hips back, bend forward and grab the dumbbell with my right hand. Note that my back is straight, my head is in a neutral position, and my shins are vertical.

2. Keeping the dumbbell positioned along my centerline, I extend my hips and knees and stand up.

3. As I lock out my hips and knees, I engage my right trap by shrugging my right shoulder.

4. The dumbbell travels up my body as a result of my previous actions.

5. I receive the weight directly overhead. To protect my shoulder, I keep my right trap engaged.

Sequence B: One-Arm Dumbbell Full Snatch

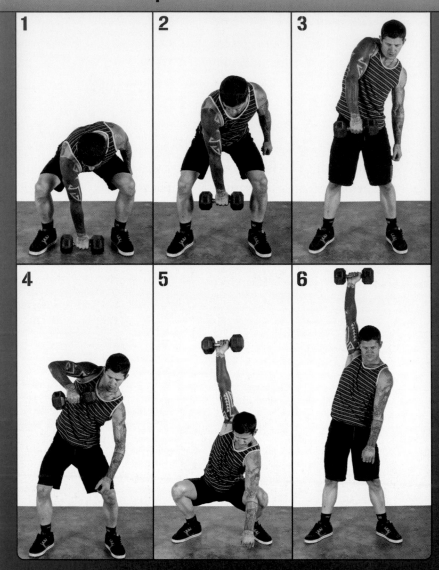

1. I'm set up.

2. Keeping the dumbbell positioned along my centerline, I extend my hips and knees and stand up.

3. As I lock out my hips and knees, I engage my right trap by shrugging my right shoulder.

4. As the dumbbell accelerates up my body as a result of my explosive hip drive, I bend my knees and prepare to receive the weight overhead in the squat position.

5. Keeping my back straight and my weight in my heels, I drop into the squat and receive the weight directly overhead.

6. Still shrugging my right shoulder to stabilize the weight and protect my right arm, I stand up with the dumbbell overhead.

SUMO DEAD LIFT HIGH PULL

The sumo dead lift high pull is a serious posterior-chain and lower-back developer. If you glance at the photos, you'll notice that I assume the same foot positioning as I do when setting up for the sumo dead lift. But instead of taking a flip grip, I establish a narrow double-over grip on the bar with my palms facing toward me. The key to executing this movement correctly is to treat it like an Olympic lift, in that you have to shrug your shoulders as you reach triple extension and use the power generated by your hips to accelerate the weight up your body. A common fault is to pull with your arms as if you were doing a ballistic upright row. This not only diminishes power, but also exhausts your arms and accelerates fatigue. Another common fault is to round the back forward as you control the weight's descent to the ground. As I've continued to stress, it's imperative that you always maintain spinal integrity by keeping your midline tight. If you lose form doing this exercise, you will cause serious low back pain.

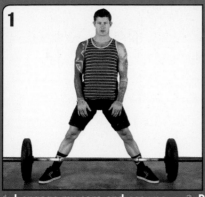

1. I engage my core and assume a sumo dead lift stance.

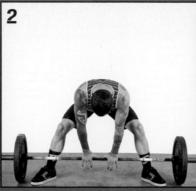

2. Driving my hips back, I fold forward from the hips with a flat back and assume a narrow double-over grip on the bar with my hands positioned a thumb's distance apart.

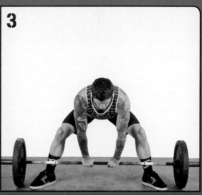

3. I tighten my position by pulling my shins to vertical, slightly elevating my hips, and flattening my back.

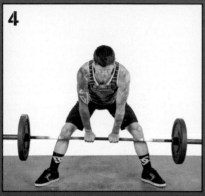

4. Keeping the bar as close to my body as possible, I extend my hips and knees and stand up with the weight.

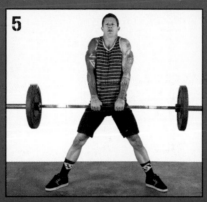

5. As the bar passes my knees, I violently lock out my hips and knees and engage my traps by shrugging my shoulders.

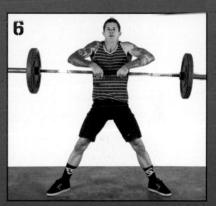

6. The bar flies up my body as a result of my previous actions. It's important to note that I don't pull the weight up using my arms. Instead, I use the momentum generated by my hips to drive the weight up my body.

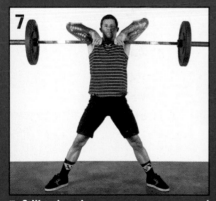

7. Still using the momentum generated by hips to my advantage, I pull the weight up to my collarbones.

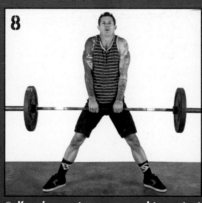

8. Keeping my traps engaged to protect my shoulders, I control the weight's descent to my hips.

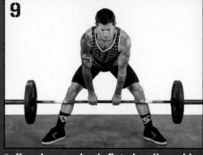

9. Keeping my back flat, I pull my hips back and allow the weight to pass over my knees.

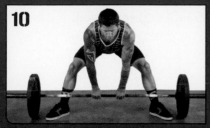

10. Maintaining a tight position, I ease the weight to the ground. Notice that I'm in the same position as when I set up for the lift. From here, I can safely and seamlessly transition into my next rep.

STONE CLEAN

Picking up an awkward object like a stone is something that everybody should do from time to time. It's encoded in our DNA to perform archaic exercises. In addition to developing all of the qualities we've been addressing (but primarily strength and explosive power), the stone clean teaches you how to stabilize under an awkward load. Whether you're picking up a heavy box, moving a log, performing a tire flip (see subsequent technique) or performing the stone clean as demonstrated below, you should always lift the object from under its general center of mass. If the stone is in front of you, you'll never be able to pick it up safely.

To lift up the stone correctly (or whatever you're trying to pick up), you have to get as close as possible and get your hands under it as much as you can. If you look at the photos below, you'll notice that my upper back rounds slightly. While we would usually call this a fault, when lifting an awkward object, like a stone, keeping the upper back completely flat is often impossible. However, that doesn't mean it's dangerous. Just as with all the lifts I demonstrate, to avoid injury you must tighten your core to stabilize your lumbar spine. If your lower back rounds as you set up, stop what you're doing and either set up correctly with a flat lower back or don't do the exercise. It's also important to mention that you should never try to lower the stone back down to the ground. Always drop it in front of your body and make sure to step back to avoid smashing your toes.

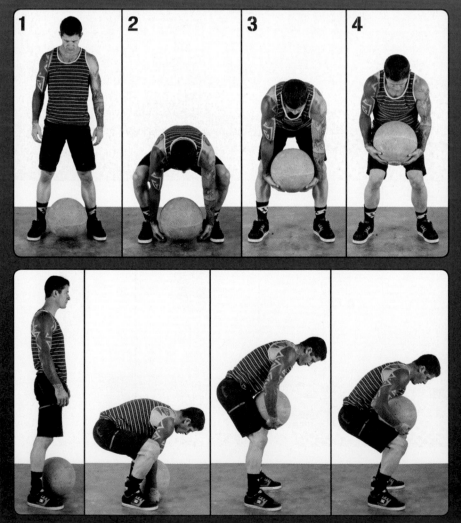

1. To set up for the stone clean, I've placed the stone between my legs, positioned my feet just wider than my shoulders, and stabilized my spine by engaging my core.

2. Driving my hips back, bending my knees, and folding forward from the hips, I grab the stone, getting my hands as far under it as possible. Note that my lower back is flat, my midline is tight, and I'm forcing my knees out laterally.

3. Keeping my lower back and arms straight, I extend my knees and hips, and pick the stone up off the ground.

4. As I lift the stone to hip level, I bend my knees and position both of my legs under the stone. It's important to mention that if you're lifting a lighter load you may be able to clean the weight up to your shoulders without reforming your grip. However, if you're lifting a heavy weight, you'll most likely need to establish a deeper grip around the stone before attempting to lift it up to your shoulders.

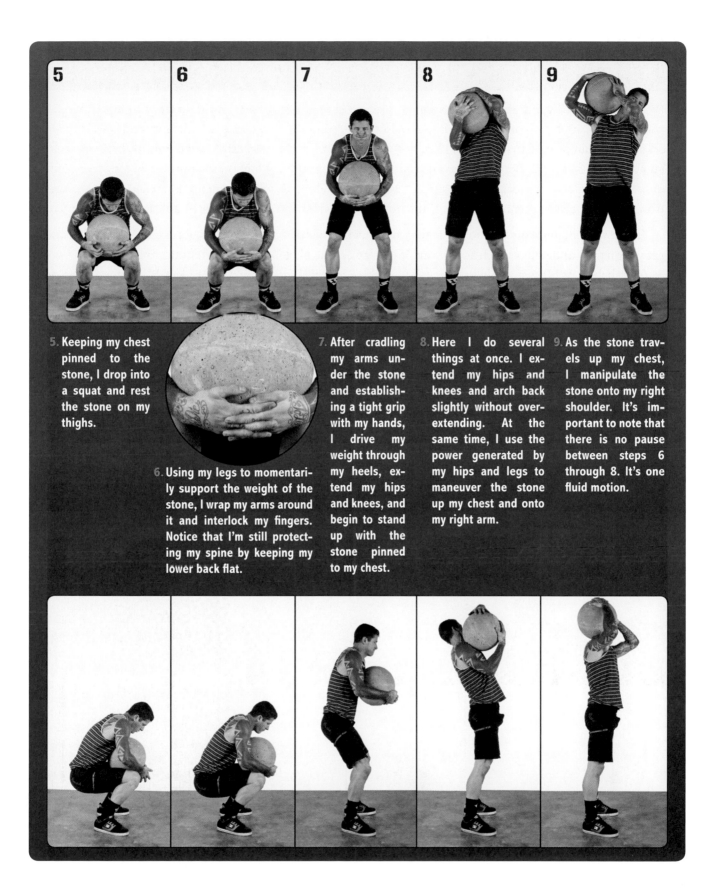

5. Keeping my chest pinned to the stone, I drop into a squat and rest the stone on my thighs.

6. Using my legs to momentarily support the weight of the stone, I wrap my arms around it and interlock my fingers. Notice that I'm still protecting my spine by keeping my lower back flat.

7. After cradling my arms under the stone and establishing a tight grip with my hands, I drive my weight through my heels, extend my hips and knees, and begin to stand up with the stone pinned to my chest.

8. Here I do several things at once. I extend my hips and knees and arch back slightly without over-extending. At the same time, I use the power generated by my hips and legs to maneuver the stone up my chest and onto my right arm.

9. As the stone travels up my chest, I manipulate the stone onto my right shoulder. It's important to note that there is no pause between steps 6 through 8. It's one fluid motion.

TIRE FLIPS

In this sequence, I demonstrate how to correctly perform a tire flip. As you can see from the photos, the set up is very similar to the stone clean in that you want to position yourself as close to the tire as possible and get your hands as far under it as you can. To perform this exercise correctly, it's important that you drive the tire forward at a 45-degree angle as you lift it off the ground. A lot of people mistakenly try to lift the tire straight up as if they were trying to clean it up to their shoulders. This is ineffective because the tire moves away from you as you lift it up, making it an unworkable strategy.

The key is to attach yourself to the tire and remain connected as you lift it up to the vertical position. Ideally, you want to use your explosive hip drive and get the tire lifted in one fluid motion. However, if you're tired, or the tire is too heavy, you may need to slip your knee under the tire as you lift it to hip level. Once accomplished, you can use your knee in conjuncture with your arms and hips to drive the tire over.

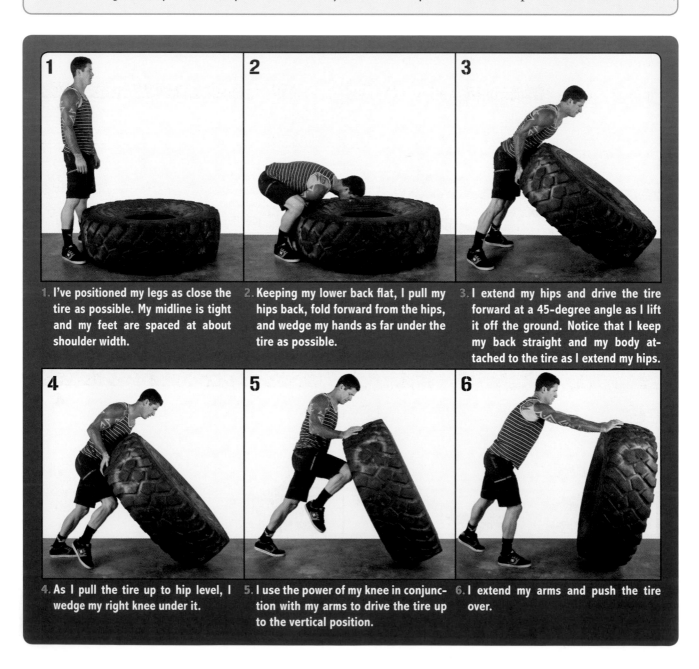

1. I've positioned my legs as close the tire as possible. My midline is tight and my feet are spaced at about shoulder width.

2. Keeping my lower back flat, I pull my hips back, fold forward from the hips, and wedge my hands as far under the tire as possible.

3. I extend my hips and drive the tire forward at a 45-degree angle as I lift it off the ground. Notice that I keep my back straight and my body attached to the tire as I extend my hips.

4. As I pull the tire up to hip level, I wedge my right knee under it.

5. I use the power of my knee in conjunction with my arms to drive the tire up to the vertical position.

6. I extend my arms and push the tire over.

CORRECT ROWING MECHANICS

The row machine is another excellent conditioning tool that can be used in CFE workouts, warm-ups, and cool-downs. If you've got a nagging injury from running or cycling, you can hit the rowing machine and still maintain your endurance fitness. Rowing is also great for a recovery session after a strenuous race or workout.

The key to rowing technique is to chant the same mantra I've been chanting throughout this book: maintain a neutral posture with a flat back. The most common faults in rowing are rounding forward like a hunchback, pulling with the arms before extending the legs, and leaning back to generate more power.

If the ideal rowing technique is too challenging, try setting up without strapping in your feet. This will slow you down and consequently teach you how to time the pull. One of the biggest mistakes you can make is jumping on the rower and pulling with all your might, which ultimately develops dysfunctional movement patterns. That said, it can be helpful in the beginning because it clarifies how important it is not to put too much back into the exercise.

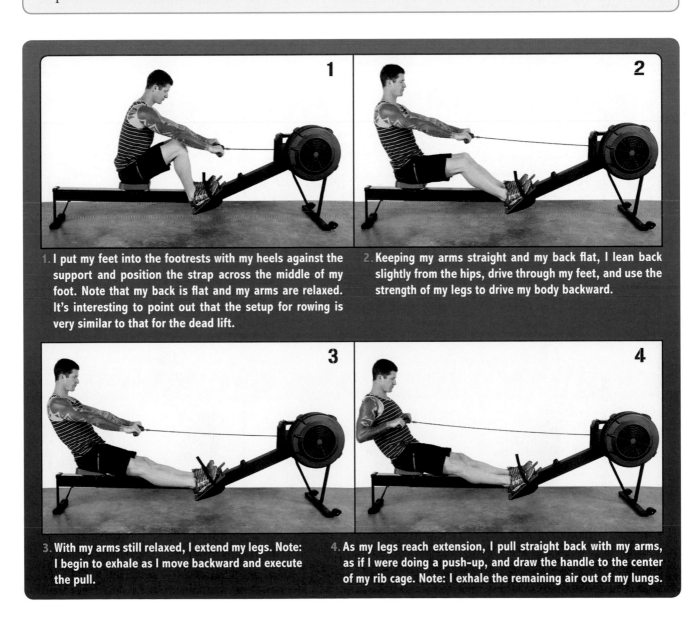

1. I put my feet into the footrests with my heels against the support and position the strap across the middle of my foot. Note that my back is flat and my arms are relaxed. It's interesting to point out that the setup for rowing is very similar to that for the dead lift.

2. Keeping my arms straight and my back flat, I lean back slightly from the hips, drive through my feet, and use the strength of my legs to drive my body backward.

3. With my arms still relaxed, I extend my legs. Note: I begin to exhale as I move backward and execute the pull.

4. As my legs reach extension, I pull straight back with my arms, as if I were doing a push-up, and draw the handle to the center of my rib cage. Note: I exhale the remaining air out of my lungs.

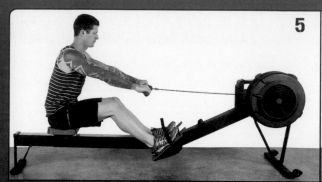

5. As I finish the stroke, I straighten my arms, begin to slide forward, and start to inhale.

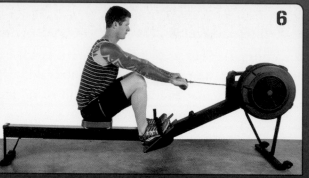

6. As my arms pass my knees, I bend my legs and return to my original position.

Rowing Faults

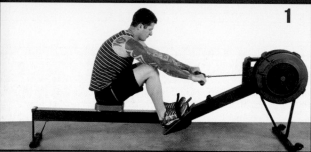

1. I've set up with a rounded back instead of neutral flat back.

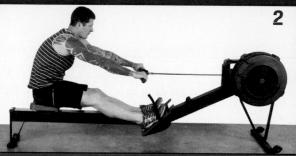

2. I drive through my feet and extend my legs. As you can see, the integrity of my spine is seriously compromised.

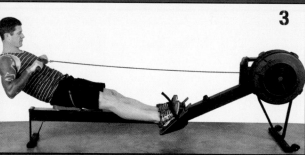

3. I lean too far and complete the pull with my back instead of using the strength of my legs and arms. This is common when athletes try to generate more power at the end of the stroke.

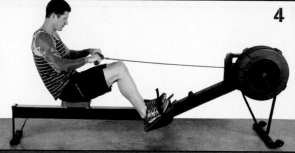

4. I make the mistake of bending my knees before extending my arms, which is another common fault.

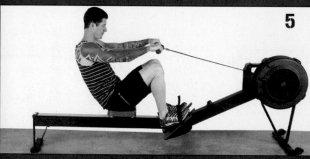

5. I have to move the handle over my knees, seriously compromising the efficiency of the stroke.

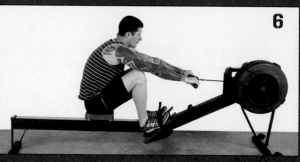

6. I return to my original faulty position.

SLED DRAGS

Dragging a sled has several applications and benefits. You can use it as a recovery tool, to develop weak body parts, to improve and accelerate strength gains, to increase work capacity, and to build cardiovascular and muscular endurance. I usually prescribe sled drags for endurance athletes in a conditioning circuit or as either intervals or a set distance.

Whether as intervals or a set distance, the distance shouldn't be over 50 meters so that the athlete doesn't lose form, which happens at greater distances. Another crucial point is loading. As a rule of thumb, to build explosive power, go shorter distances at max effort with heavier weight. To build muscular and cardiovascular endurance, pull a lighter load over a longer distance.

It's also important to mention that there are countless variations of the sled drag. In the sequences below, I demonstrate two variations of the forward pull and one variation of the backward pull. Although giving other variations a try can be beneficial, the ones demonstrated below are the most basic and important for endurance sports.

Sequence A: Shoulder Grip

The key to executing this variation is to maintain form by keeping your back straight and your hands in front of your body. Rounding or flexing forward will not only cause strain on the shoulders, but it will also shift the demand onto your quads, which defeats the purpose of this exercise. Note: You can walk or run depending on your goals in the workout.

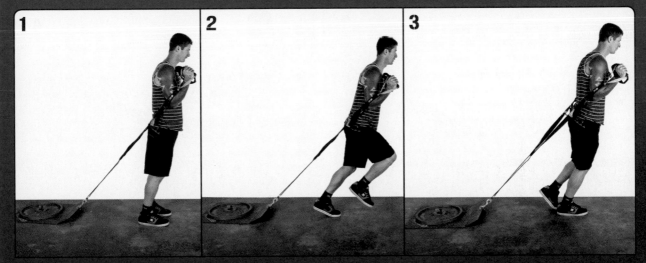

1 I've established the shoulder-grip forward pull position. My arms are tight to my body, my head is in a neutral position, and my core is engaged.

2 Keeping my body straight, I lean forward slightly and step forward with my right foot.

3 I shift support onto my right leg as I continue to pull the sled forward.

Sequence B: Low Grip

The low-grip forward pull puts more demand on your core, arms, and legs All the same principles as the shoulder-grip forward pull apply: keep your core engaged, your back straight, and your arms in front of your body. And just like the previous variation, you can run or walk, depending on your workout agenda.

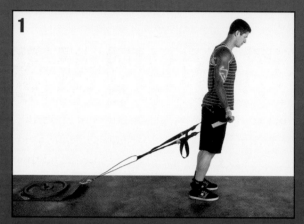

I've secured the low-grip forward pull position. My arms are tight to my body, my palms are facing away from me, my core is engaged, and my head is in a neutral position.

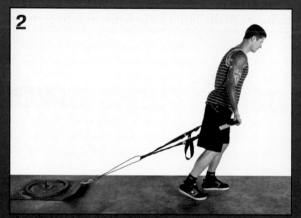

Keeping my body straight, I lean forward and take a small step with my left foot to generate forward momentum.

Sequence C: Reverse Sled Drags

The reverse sled drags targets your quads, VMOs, and lower back, all of which play a crucial role in running and cycling. Just like the forward pulls, keep your back straight and lean slightly in the direction you're heading.

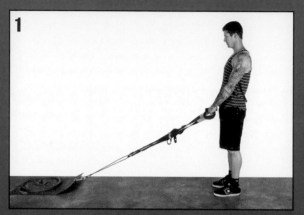

I've secured the reverse sled drag position.

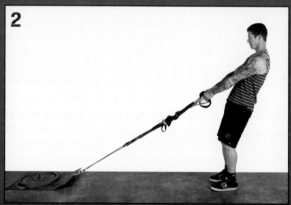

Keeping my shoulders back and my body straight, I lean back slightly.

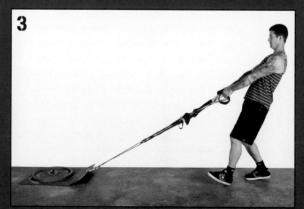

Driving off my left heel, I step back with my right leg. Notice that my right foot is directly under my hips as I shift supports. From here, I will continue to pull the sled backward until I reach my set distance.

HOLLOW ROCK

If you read Chapter 2, you know how to establish the hollow rock position to find midline stabilization. In this sequence, I demonstrate the same drill but as an exercise. If you look at the photos below, you'll notice that once I achieve the hollow rock position, I lift my rib cage as if I were doing a crunch, and then, keeping my body tight, rock back and forth. If your goal is a set number of repetitions, then an up plus a down equals one rep. However, I normally prescribe hollow rocks for time. For example, you can do Tabata hollow rocks (20 seconds of work, 10 seconds of rest) for four minutes.

If you break in the rib cage or you can't maintain a solid position while rocking back and forth, simply do the hollow rock as a hold. If achieving the hollow rock position proves difficult, you can bend your legs and place your arms at your sides or incorporate plank holds (sequence follows) to build stabilization strength. It's important to start wherever you are and work to gradually build up to being able to perform the real-deal exercise correctly.

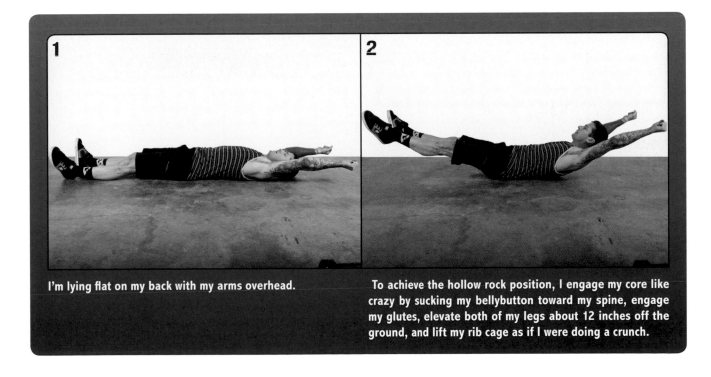

1 I'm lying flat on my back with my arms overhead.

2 To achieve the hollow rock position, I engage my core like crazy by sucking my bellybutton toward my spine, engage my glutes, elevate both of my legs about 12 inches off the ground, and lift my rib cage as if I were doing a crunch.

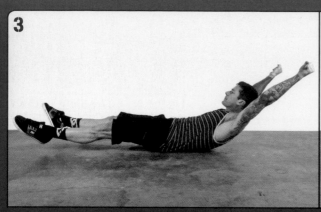

3

Staying tight and keeping my legs straight, I kick my feet toward the ground and rock onto my lower back.

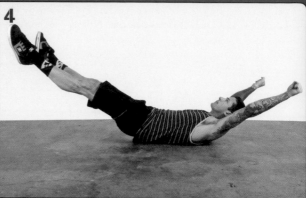

4

Having created some momentum with my previous action, I drive my arms back slightly and roll onto my upper back. The hollow rock exercise is like a rocking chair: once you generate some momentum, you have to move only slightly to keep it going.

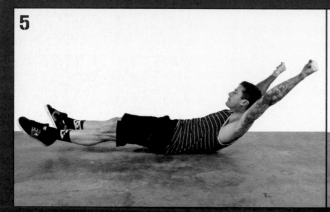

5

Keeping my rib cage and legs locked in place, I rock forward onto my lower back.

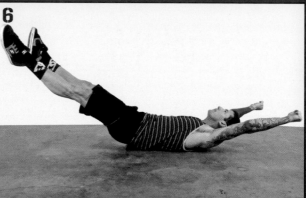

6

Because my midline is tight and my body is in a rounded, fixed position, I roll onto my upper back.

PLANK

Unlike the hollow rock, which requires you to support the weight of your limbs, the plank uses your arms and toes to support the weight of your body, helping to develop a baseline of core strength and stability. The key to this exercise is to achieve a hollow-tight position and maintain it. Once fatigue sets in, you'll want to lift into a pike position or drop into a cobra stretch to give your abs a break. Fight these tendencies at all costs: if your back is not flat, you're probably not doing the exercise correctly.

This is another exercise that you do for a set time, which means it's an awesome way to build total body-strength endurance. If you're new to this exercise, you can start with the push-up plank (Figure A), and then progress to the bent-arm version (Figure B). If you already have a good base level of core strength, you can increase the intensity by adding a weight or a sandbag to your back (Figure C). If there's no one around to assist you by adding weight to your back, you can lift one leg off the ground or extend an arm out in front of you.

Figure A: Push-up Plank

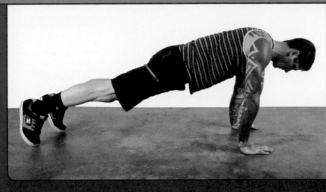

I've achieved the push-up plank position. To maintain a tight position, I've engaged my glutes, erectors, and core. My back is flat, my arms are locked out, my shoulders are externally rotated, and my hands are shoulder width apart.

Figure B: Bent-Arm Plank

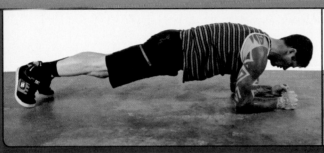

I've achieved the bent-arm plank position. To maintain a tight position, I've engaged my glutes, erectors, and core. My back is flat, my elbows are bent at a 90-degree angle, and they are right under my shoulders. My forearms are parallel and my arms are straight. This is the stable position of the shoulder. If you put your hands together, which is common, your shoulders will roll forward into a compensated position.

Figure C: Weighted Plank

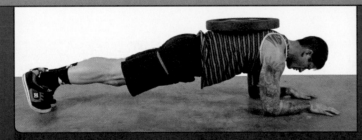

To make the bent-arm plank more challenging, I've added a weight to my midback.

PLANK PUSH-UPS

Plank push-ups add a challenge to the classic plank hold by mixing movement and a static hold. In addition to strengthening the core and forcing you to find stability while in motion, plank push-ups also develop strength in the shoulders and arms. A common fault is to wiggle back and forth like a snake as you lift and lower your body: keep your body straight and your core engaged as if your life depended on it as you perform this exercise.

1 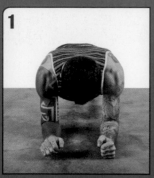 I've achieved the bent-arm plank position.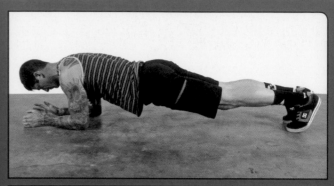

2 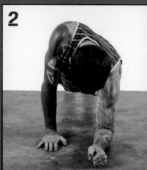 Keeping my body straight, I shift my weight onto my left arm and press my right palm down.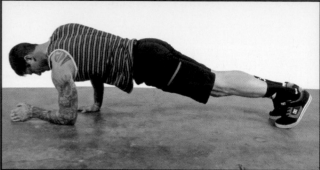

3 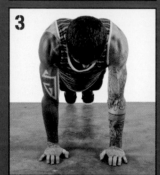 I press my left palm down and achieve the push-up plank position.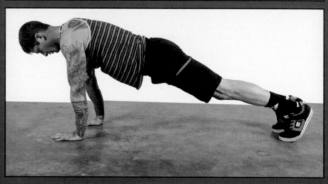

4 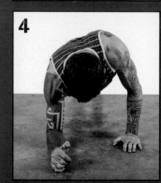 I come down onto my right elbow, initiating the transition back into the bent-arm plank with the same arm that initiated the transition into a push-up plank.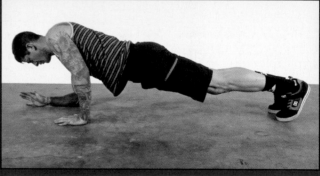

5 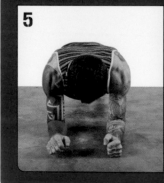 I come down onto my left elbow and reestablish the bent-arm plank position. From here, I will initiate the next repetition using my opposite arm, which in this case happens to be my left.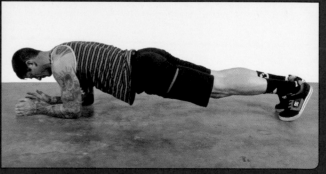

L-SIT

The L-sit strengthens and increases endurance in the core stabilizers and hip flexors. Whether you're performing it on the ground or using parallettes, as demonstrated below, make sure your hands are directly at your sides. If you're using parallettes, you can establish their correct distance apart by measuring the length of your lower arm. Once you've got your hands in place, bring your knees up to your chest and then straighten your legs. If you're unable to straighten your legs, you can hold the first step until you build up enough strength to progress to the full L-sit. Just as with the other stabilization exercises, this one should be held for a specific amount of time.

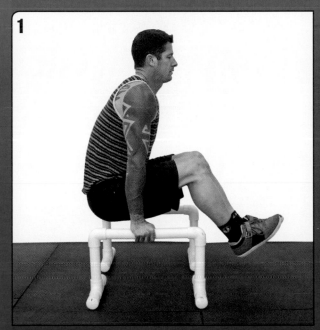

1

I've spaced the parallettes approximately shoulder width apart (i.e., the length of my lower arm). I position myself in the middle of the parallettes, assume my grip, and then lift my knees to my chest. The more bend you have in your knees, the easier it is to hold the position. Initially, you may have to keep your knees bent at a 90-degree angle. But as you get stronger, you can start to straighten you legs until you reach the full L-sit.

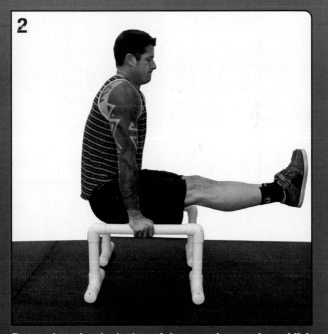

2

From a bent-leg L-sit, I straighten my legs and establish the full L-sit position. Notice that I've created a 90-degree angle between my upper and lower body. The goal is to maintain this angle for the prescribed time. You can increase the intensity of this exercise by lifting your legs higher in the air, decreasing the angle between your upper and lower body. This not only tasks your core to work harder, but also fires your triceps and shoulders.

DRAGON FLAGS

Dragon flags are a core-stabilization exercise requiring tremendous strength. To perform them, keep your erectors off the bench, maintain a straight body, and slowly lower yourself, ideally to a 45-degree angle (see last photo). It's important to mention that this is an advanced stabilization exercise. If you're unable to perform this movement without losing form, work on midline stabilization by doing the plank, hollow rock, and L-sit progressions.

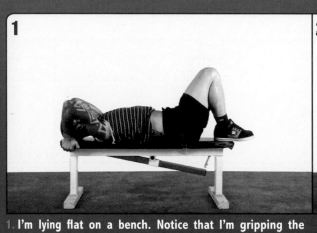

1. I'm lying flat on a bench. Notice that I'm gripping the bench near my ears. I will use this grip in conjunction with my erectors and abs to support the weight of my body as I go through the sequence.

2. Using my handgrips to keep my upper back pinned to the bench, I draw my knees to my chest and roll onto my shoulders.

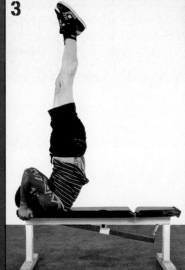

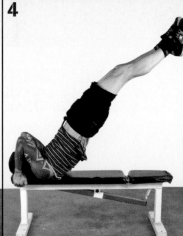

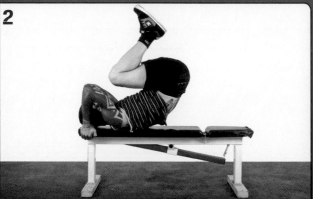

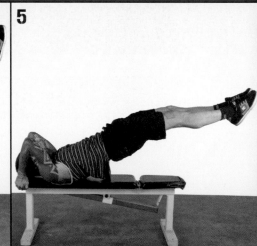

3. I lift my legs toward the ceiling. To keep my body straight, I keep my glutes and core engaged.

4. Keeping my body straight, I slowly lower my legs. This may be as far as you can go without breaking. If so, pull yourself back into the vertical position and repeat, lowering your legs only as far as you can without losing form, until you've completed your set number of reps. As you get stronger, work to lower your legs until you can bring them to a 45-degree angle, as illustrated in the next step.

5. I lower my legs until they reach a 45-degree angle. This is the ideal angle and is obviously the most difficult to achieve. From here, I will lift my legs back to vertical with perfect form and repeat, until I've done my reps.

SIT-UP

The sit-up is a classic exercise for building a base level of core strength. As with all the exercises I demonstrate, you should always perform it through its end range. With this particular exercise, that means becoming completely upright. To get the best results, use your arms to help accelerate your back off the floor and kick up into the seated position ballistically. There are two versions for you to choose from: the classic sit-up (Sequence A) and the butterfly sit-up (Sequence B). The former engages your hip flexors, which makes it easier to explode into the upright position, while the latter takes your hip flexors out of the equation, shifting more demand to your core.

Sequence A: Classic Sit-Up

1
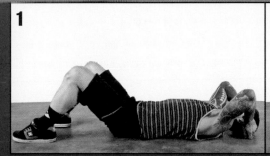

I'm lying on my back with my arms overhead. Notice that my feet are flat on the ground and that my knees are bent at a 45-degree angle. If you want to make doing multiple reps easier, you can anchor your feet to the ground by having someone hold your feet or by wedging your toes under a couple of heavy dumbbells.

2
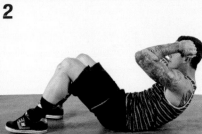

I engage my hip flexors and core, drive my elbows toward my knees, and lift my rib cage as if I were doing a crunch.

3
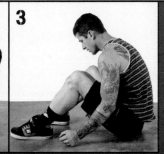

To complete the movement, I throw my arms down to help accelerate my upper body into the upright position. Notice that I sit all the way up so that my chest is nearly touching my thighs.

Sequence B: Butterfly Sit-Up

1
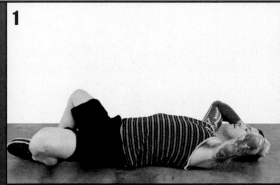

I'm lying on my back with my arms overhead. Notice that my feet are together and that my legs are bowed out to the side as if I were performing a butterfly stretch.

2
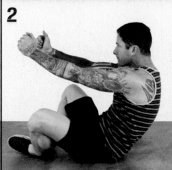

I throw my arms toward my legs and use the power of my core to sit up.

3
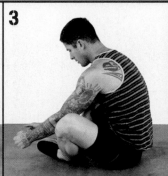

I sit all the way up to complete a full range of motion.

V-UP

The v-up will also strengthen the core and hip flexors. Unlike the classic sit-up, which allows you to temporarily disengage your abs, the v-up requires that you to stay in a hollow-tight position for the duration. If you can't sit up and touch your toes, as demonstrated below, ditch this exercise and stick with the hollow rock and classic sit-up.

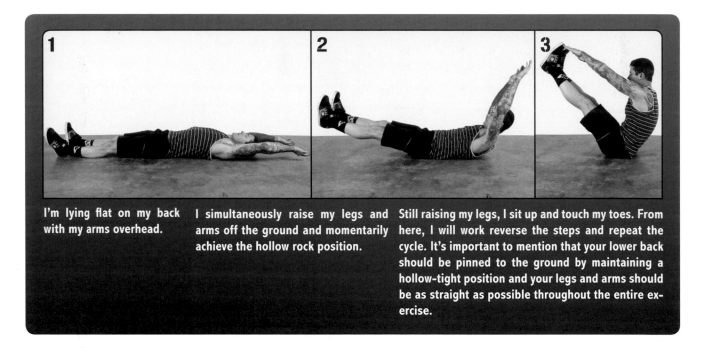

1 I'm lying flat on my back with my arms overhead.

2 I simultaneously raise my legs and arms off the ground and momentarily achieve the hollow rock position.

3 Still raising my legs, I sit up and touch my toes. From here, I will work reverse the steps and repeat the cycle. It's important to mention that your lower back should be pinned to the ground by maintaining a hollow-tight position and your legs and arms should be as straight as possible throughout the entire exercise.

GLUTE-HAMSTRING SIT-UP

Although glute-hamstring sit-ups build tremendous strength and explosive power in the core, you have to be extremely careful about progressing with this exercise. Not only is back injury possible, but there is also a high risk of developing rhabdomyolysis, or rhabdo, which in simple terms is the break down of muscle tissue as a result of overexertion. To avoid these unfortunate outcomes, first make sure that you're set up correctly on the glute-hamstring machine, and then progress slowly by doing moderate sets and reps. If you experience any pain or discomfort in your back, stop immediately. If you're new to this exercise it's imperative that you start off slowly.

The glute-hamstring sit-up is deceptive: you can perform several reps without discomfort, and it isn't until you unhook your feet and get off the machine that you realize how much demand you've put on your core. For that reason, I suggest that you start out doing something like three sets of about three to five reps. As you build up, you can steadily increase the number of reps in each set until you can do fifteen reps.

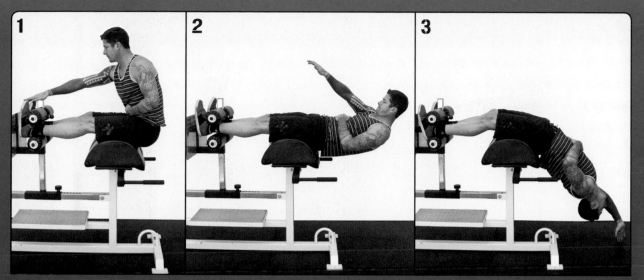

1. To set up for the glute-hamstring sit-up, I adjust the machine so that my butt hangs slightly off the pad and my knees are bent slightly. A common mistake is to set up too low on the machine with your butt square on the bench. This not only places a ton of pressure on your spine as you roll backward, but also takes your legs out of the equation, which restricts your ability to explode up into the seated position. It's also important to notice where my arms are. My right arm is extended while my left arm is positioned across my belly. By throwing only one arm overhead, I can control my descent and use my arm to accelerate my body into the seated position without placing too much pressure on my back. Two arms overhead not only makes the movement harder to control, but also places a ton of stress on your lower back.

2. Keeping my knees bent slightly and my core engaged to control my descent, I slowly lower my upper body toward the ground.

3. I maneuver my right arm overhead as I roll back to my end range.

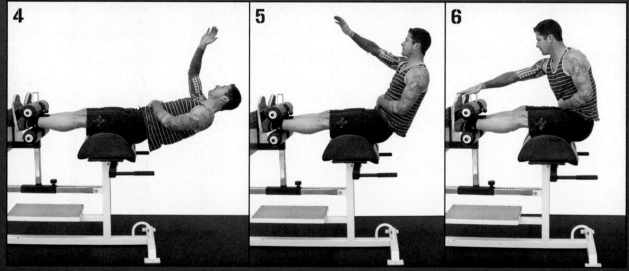

4. In one fluid motion, I throw my right arm forward to help accelerate my upper body into the seated position while simultaneously extending my knees. It's very important that you extend your knees as you explode into the seated position. This not only helps you sit up, but it also takes pressure off your lower back as you sit up.

5. I continue to sit up.

6. I touch the foot harness with my right hand to complete the movement. From here, I will switch my arms, placing my right arm across my belly and extending my left arm, and repeat the sequence.

BACK EXTENSION

You don't want to focus solely on the core without developing the extensor and stabilizer muscles in your back. In this sequence, I demonstrate the back extension, which is one of the best exercises to accomplish this goal. When studying the photos below, you'll notice that I snake my back up and then straighten out as I reach the end range of the movement. A lot of people have the tendency to pull with their hips and hamstrings, taking tension off the back. As you will see shortly, this is a totally different exercise with a slightly different focus. To get the best result from the back extensions, perform each rep as illustrated in the photos below.

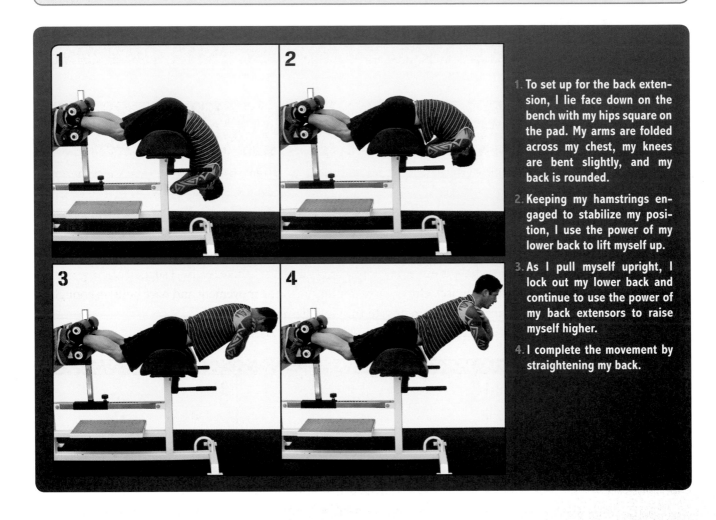

1. To set up for the back extension, I lie face down on the bench with my hips square on the pad. My arms are folded across my chest, my knees are bent slightly, and my back is rounded.

2. Keeping my hamstrings engaged to stabilize my position, I use the power of my lower back to lift myself up.

3. As I pull myself upright, I lock out my lower back and continue to use the power of my back extensors to raise myself higher.

4. I complete the movement by straightening my back.

HIP EXTENSION

Hip extensions are very similar to back extensions, but instead of rounding your back and then flattening out at the top, you maintain a straight back throughout the duration of the movement. This shifts a portion of the focus to your hamstrings and glutes, while still engaging the back extensors. It's important to mention that the hip extension is an excellent progression for the glute-hamstring raise (see next sequence). If you've never performed a glute-hamstring raise, I recommend that you start out with the hip extension until you've built up your posterior chain.

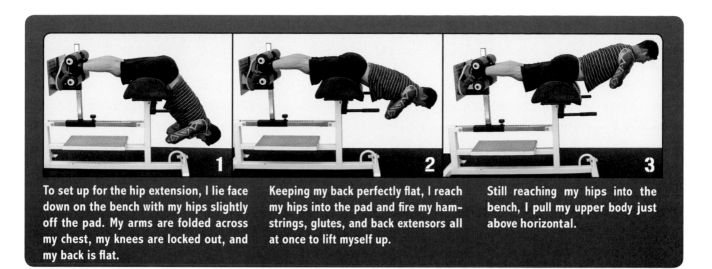

To set up for the hip extension, I lie face down on the bench with my hips slightly off the pad. My arms are folded across my chest, my knees are locked out, and my back is flat.

Keeping my back perfectly flat, I reach my hips into the pad and fire my hamstrings, glutes, and back extensors all at once to lift myself up.

Still reaching my hips into the bench, I pull my upper body just above horizontal.

GLUTE-HAMSTRING RAISE

The glute-hamstring raise is one of the best exercises for developing strength and endurance in the posterior chain. In fact, the glute-hamstring raise is one of the only exercises that trains the hamstrings through their full range. If you glance at the photos, you'll notice that I flex at the hip and then at the knee as I pull myself upright. Unlike the majority of the posterior-chain leg developers previously demonstrated, which targets either the lower or upper half of the hamstrings, glute-hamstring raises fire both the lower and upper hamstrings equally. If your posterior chain is underdeveloped or you're new to this exercise, I suggest starting with the hip extensions (see previous exercise). Once you're familiar with the movement and have built up enough strength in your posterior chain, you can progress to the glute-hamstring raise.

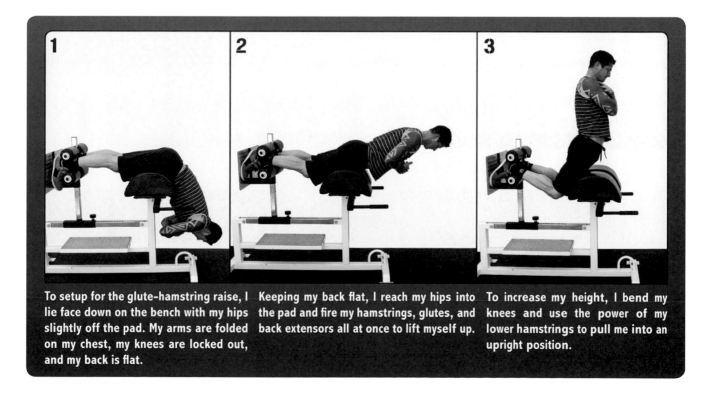

To setup for the glute-hamstring raise, I lie face down on the bench with my hips slightly off the pad. My arms are folded on my chest, my knees are locked out, and my back is flat.

Keeping my back flat, I reach my hips into the pad and fire my hamstrings, glutes, and back extensors all at once to lift myself up.

To increase my height, I bend my knees and use the power of my lower hamstrings to pull me into an upright position.

MOBILITY AS A SKILL

BY KELLY STARRETT

"ASIDE FROM BECOMING A BETTER ATHLETE, CFE HAS MADE ME A STRONGER, MORE CAPABLE HUMAN BEING WITH A MORE ENJOYABLE LIFESTYLE. I PLAN ON BEING ON THIS EARTH FOR A WHILE AND I PLAN ON CONQUERING A LOT MORE THAN A FEW RACES. CROSSFIT ENDURANCE HAS GIVEN ME STRENGTH AND SKILLS THAT TRANSCEND THE BOUNDARIES OF A SPECIFIC SPORT. I CARE ABOUT BEING FIT TO WIN, BUT I CARE MORE ABOUT BEING FIT FOR LIFE. CFE GAVE ME BOTH."

SARAH WILSON

I f you have participated in endurance sports for a long enough time, there's a good chance that you have suffered some sort of injury. As discussed in earlier chapters, injuries that are common to endurance athletes— plantar fasciitis, a pulled hamstring, IT band syndrome, lower-back pain, etc.—generally occur because a) the athlete's movements are dysfunctional and mechanically poor, or b) the athlete doesn't have the range of motion to get into the correct positions for efficient movement.

The former is a motor-control issue, while the latter is a mobility issue. For example, if you never learned proper running technique and you always run in shoes, then suddenly start running barefoot, you are unlikely to have the skill or strength to go very far. You may not understand how to use gravity to your advantage, maintain a neutral foot position, pull using the strength of your hamstrings, or the importance of landing on the ball of your foot. You can assume, based on your lack of technical running experience, that you exhibit one or more of the following faults when you go out for a run:

☐   Poor body posture (rounded forward, overextended back)

☐   Landing in front of the body (braking)

☐   Heel striking (no elasticity)

☐   Landing on a straight leg (stress on the knee joint)

☐   Pushing off from the back foot

☐   Foot on the ground too long (prolonged contraction)

These faults can and will cause performance-inhibiting injuries. However, if you learn how to work with gravity instead of against it, as well as ingrain the correct mechanics, you can increase your efficiency and reduce your chances of these faults.

But what if you physically can't get into the correct position required for efficient movement? For example, say you don't have full range of motion in your ankles when you run, so that you can't maintain a neutral foot position when you land. Every time you strike the ground with an open foot, your ankle collapses, which compromises the stability of your transition from one support to the other. Over time, the compromised landing position causes a ripple effect up and down the athletic chain, causing foot, ankle, knee, hip, and low back problems. Put simply, your limited range of motion prevents you from setting up, transitioning, or completing a movement in an ideal position. As a result, your body has no choice but to find stability elsewhere— knee, hip, etc.—and that elsewhere wasn't designed to handle the responsibility, which is how injuries occur.

Let's use another simple example to illustrate this point. Imagine an athlete who sits at a desk all day. He is stuck in a flexed position, and he doesn't take the time to mobilize between long sitting sessions. How do you think this will impact his ability to achieve a neutral posture in his sport?

Remember, the positions you spend your days in and the activities you perform impact your range of motion. In other words, if you have to endure a closed-hip position for prolonged periods of time, it's no surprise that your hip flexors will become adaptively short and stiff. To help you understand how this affects your entire body, perform this simple test:

Skin-Pinch Test

Bend forward, grab a chunk of skin on the front of your hips, and then try to stand up. What happens? I would suspect that your knees remain bent and your back is overextended to compensate for your limited range. This is exactly what happens when you sit or ride for extended periods of time. The hip flexors adapt and start to reflect your habits, becoming short and stiff. It's as if you stapled those tissues together and then tried to establish a neutral posture in full extension. It's just not going to happen. Overextending and bending your knees is your body's way of buffering the problem.

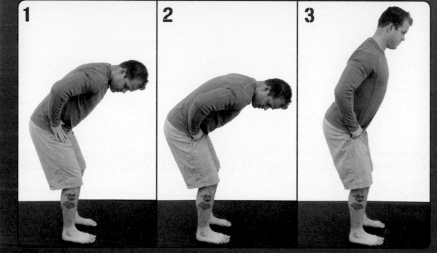

1. I bend forward at the hips and place my hands over my front hip creases.

2. Having created slack in the front of my hips, I close my hands and grab a chunk of skin.

3. Still pinching the skin, I attempt to stand up. With my skin essentially stapled together, I'm unable to fully extend. To compensate, I overextend my back and default into a broken position. The skin pinch is a reflection of the underlying tissue, which becomes shortened after long periods of flexion.

Now imagine trying to sprint or squat a heavy load when you can't reach full extension. It doesn't matter if you know how to establish a neutral posture with a stabilized midline (or understand how to perform the movement correctly!). If you're missing range of motion—regardless of whether it's in your ankles, hips, or shoulders—establishing the ideal position for efficient movement is impossible. Perform the movement with enough intensity, load, and volume, and injury is inevitable. To fix your position, you have to address muscle stiffness and restore normal range to your tissues.

Think of mobility exercises as a tool to improve position. A lot of coaches and athletes mistakenly think that they have to treat specific areas of the body with specific exercises rather than focus on improving the position they need to be in. For example, the first thing that comes to mind when you say "shoulder injury" is torn rotator cuff. The most popular protocol—whether to recover from the injury or prevent it in the future—is to spend a lot of time strengthening the rotator cuff. The logic is that by strengthening the rotator cuff you can prevent it from tearing, or rehabilitate the area to keep it from happening again. While this is a legitimate tactic, it addresses only a small piece of the problem. What is missing from this conversation is the housing of the rotator cuff, or the scapula. If the scapula is in a good position, a lot of the problems that would otherwise signify a weak rotator cuff spontaneously resolve themselves. Here's why:

Say you can't put your arms overhead because of limited range of motion, but you're an athlete, and athletes train, so you train anyway. You lift heavy weight overhead and swim laps in the pool despite your handicap. In the beginning everything is fine, but over time you notice a slight pinch in your shoulder. You continue to follow your same training protocol because you're tough and "real" athletes train through pain.

After a heavy day of pressing, your shoulder lights up, and "out of nowhere" you can't even lift your arm. You go to the doctor and he delivers the bad news: "You have a torn rotator cuff." Now, let's consider the potential causes. Did it tear because you had a weak rotator cuff or because you did countless movement repetitions from a bad position and stressed your joint into submission? I would suspect the latter.

In short, your body adapts to the stimulus you throw at it. If you never learn how to correctly perform the movement or task you're attempting, you will break mechanical laws, which will result in wasted energy and injury. However, if you rule out motor control as the root cause of your movement faults, you have to address the mobility issue that is preventing you from achieving a good position. Not only that, you have to perform maintenance on your body using mobilization exercises to prevent muscles from becoming adaptively short from training and toxic habits like sitting.

Remember, mobility is the only attribute that can improve position. The better your position, the more efficiently you move, and the less likely you are to sustain injury.

Having already demonstrated the proper positions of stability as well as having outlined several skill-based drills aimed at teaching the proper mechanics of running, swimming, cycling, and functional exercise, this chapter focuses solely on mobilization techniques that can be used to rehabilitate injuries and restore normal range of motion to your joints and muscles. Unlike conventional stretching and recovery protocol, Starrett's Movement and Mobility Method, presented in this chapter, will equip you with all the tools needed to perform basic body maintenance.

MECHANICAL LAW:
TWO RULES THAT CAUSE INJURY

There are two ways you can get injured when you perform a movement incorrectly: by stopping the movement or by creating leverage.

- Stopping a movement refers to faults that impede motion and is otherwise referred to as an overtension injury. For example, landing out in front of the body when you run, otherwise known as putting on the brakes, would fall into this category. This could also refer to stopping abruptly while performing a squat or dead lift.

- Creating leverage occurs when you put too much force/stress on a given joint or tissue and is otherwise referred to as an overuse injury. Think of performing a push-press out in front of your body instead of straight overhead. The leverage created on the tissue places shearing stress on the joint, inevitably causing injury. Add volume, intensity, and load to the equation, and you accelerate the process.

If you don't understand how to perform a movement correctly, or you're lacking range of motion, which prevents you from establishing the ideal positions, you break mechanical law and join the ranks of "the injured."

Mobility Checklist

As mentioned in the introduction to this book, if you don't attach purpose to your actions as it relates to performance, it's difficult if not impossible to improve as an athlete. Mobility is no different. In order to reduce your chances of injury, improve positions of stability, or accelerate recovery following an injury, you have to take a systematic approach to your warm-up, cool-down, and daily maintenance. It should come as no surprise that this ritual should be structured around the movement/exercise being performed. For example, if you know that you're going to back squat, it makes sense to implement mobility exercises that will improve the start and finishing position of the squat. Conversely, if you're going for a run, warming up with skill-based exercises will not only prepare your body for the movement by activating key muscle groups, but also help ingrain proper running technique.

Along these same lines, you should cool off or end your workout by lengthening the tissues that have been exhausted or shortened (i.e., contracted) during the training session. So if you went out for a hard ride, the front of your hips and your upper back are going to need your attention the moment you finish your ride. Similarly, if there are areas that you know need extra work, taking the time to mobilize these problem spots is the best way to elicit lasting change.

To help you piece together your mobility puzzle, I've provided a mobility checklist, which will elucidate universal guidelines for implementing the forthcoming techniques. Just as in the previous skills chapters, this is a systems approach to training aimed at improving the overall efficiency of your movement. And the checklist ensures that you get the most out of the techniques demonstrated.

MOBILITY CHECKLIST

- ☑ **Mobilize the Movement**
- ☑ **Identify the Problem (What Is Your Position of Restriction?)**
- ☑ **Mobilize Upstream/Downstream of the Problem**
- ☑ **Test/Retest**

Mobilize the Movement

When you approach the concept of mobility, it's important to always think along the lines of how a particular mobilization technique will improve your position for an upcoming task. Unless you have an incredible amount of time on your hands, you can't treat every single mobility issue in one session. A much better approach is to attack the areas that will improve the positions of your next workout. For example, if you are dead lifting, focusing on mobilization techniques that will improve the start and finishing position of the dead lift is your best bet.

Here's a sample mobility prescription:

Mobility Rx for Dead Lift

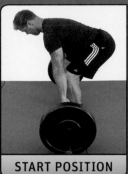

START POSITION

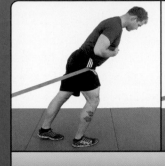 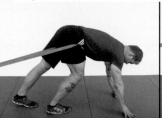 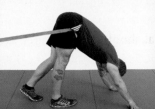

HAMSTRING FLOSS: Relieves muscle stiffness and improves range in the posterior chain, allowing for an easier setup.

HAMSTRING FLOSS

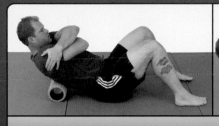 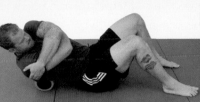 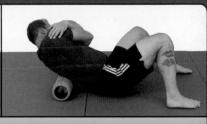

T-SPINE SMASH

T-SPINE SMASH: Allows you to pull your shoulders back and achieve a flat back, which is critical for power and stability.

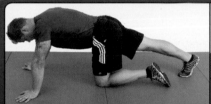 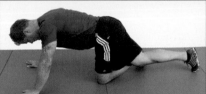 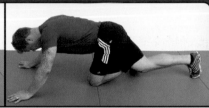

HIP CAPSULE

HIP CAPSULE: Increases external-rotation torque from the hips, which improves stability and power as you pull.

FINISH POSITION

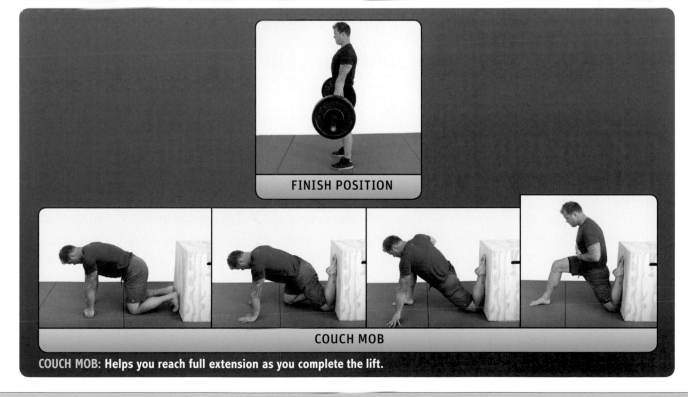

COUCH MOB

COUCH MOB: Helps you reach full extension as you complete the lift.

Identify the Problem (What Is Your Position of Restriction?)

While understanding the biomechanics of a common fault can be extremely complex and difficult to comprehend, fixing the problem is usually not very complicated. First, you identify the fault. Second, you narrow the limiting factors. Is it a motor-control issue, or a lack of the mobility required to achieve the position? If it's a motor-control issue, you have to isolate the movement and work to correct your mechanics. If it's lack of mobility, you need to restore normal range of motion to the area of restriction so that you can achieve the ideal position and perform the movement correctly.

Here's a simple example: Say your foot spins out to the side at the end of each stride. By externally rotating your leg in extension, you land with an open foot, which not only compromises the efficiency of your stride, but also invites injury. The first step is to isolate the movement by performing simple drills that focus on pulling mechanics to see if it's a motor-control issue. Having read all about running mechanics (Chapter 2), you know that the correct technique for pulling and landing is to maintain a neutral foot position, meaning that your foot, knee, and hip are pointed straight ahead and are in line. If you can't correct the movement fault because you lack the capacity to achieve the position, you automatically know that you're missing a normal range of motion. In such a situation, you have to work to restore internal rotation in the position of restriction by biasing the movement.

Mobility Rx for Internal Rotation of the Foot, Knee, and Hip

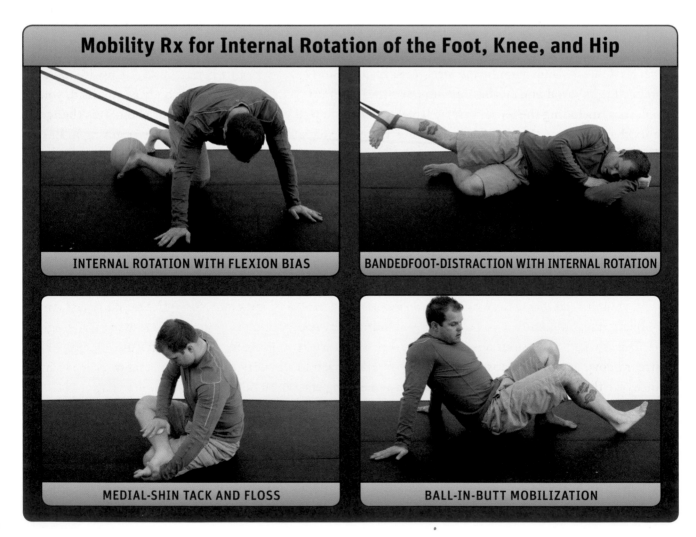

INTERNAL ROTATION WITH FLEXION BIAS

BANDEDFOOT-DISTRACTION WITH INTERNAL ROTATION

MEDIAL-SHIN TACK AND FLOSS

BALL-IN-BUTT MOBILIZATION

Mobilize Upstream/Downstream of the Problem

Identifying where you are feeling resistance and then working to restore/improve range of motion in that area will help bring you into good form. However, this is not the only way to approach mobility. For example, say you have knee pain. Every time you finish a hard run, your knee lights up and hurts for days. By now you know that your knee pain is more than likely a result of poor movement mechanics. To avoid further issues, you have to make sure that you or your coach diagnoses the problem and make the necessary adjustments. In the meantime, you have knee pain and you need to know what to do about it.

The first step is to ask yourself this simple question: What tissues/muscles above and below the knee affect that joint? You don't need a lesson in anatomy to figure this out. What are the big players? Below the knee is your calf (i.e., gastroc and soleus), and below that is your Achilles tendon. Above your knee is your thigh (quadriceps and hamstrings), and above that is your hip and butt (glutes, etc.). If any of these muscles/tendons are tight, the functioning of the knee joint will be affected, which can lead to pain/injury.

This is how it works: You are encased in a web of connective tissue (fascia), which transmits movement throughout your body. If a muscle above or below a joint is tight, it's going to have a domino effect on whatever is nearby. So if a muscle in proximity to your knee (say your quad) is stiff, the fascia surrounding it, which in turn will also be tight, will tug on the knee joint. By bringing mobility to the musculature upstream and downstream of the issue, in this case the knee (by stretching your calf muscles, flossing your hamstrings, doing sliding-surface mobilization techniques on your quad, etc.), you will restore normal function to the muscles that are compromising the unrestricted functioning of the knee.

Here's a specific example: Say your quads and hip flexors are inflamed. With the fascia tugging on your knee, it can be difficult to pull your heel toward your butt (knee flexion) when running. To avoid leaving your trail leg behind you as you shift supports and position your foot under your body as you land, your hip flexors (including the tensor fasciae latae) take over to pull your knee toward your chest. This changes the mechanics of your pull and compromises the efficiency of your movement, usually resulting in knee pain. If you look upstream of the problem (i.e., knee pain), you'll realize that your quads and hip flexors are the culprits. By using some of the mobilization techniques shown in this chapter, you can completely resolve the issue. It's that simple.

Test/Retest

Did the mobility prescription work? Can you get into position? Are you more efficient? Are you faster? Any mobilization techniques that you apply should have observable, repeatable, measurable results every single time. This is what the test/retest is for. It doesn't matter if you're mobilizing areas of restriction or using the upstream/downstream diagnostic, the test/retest allows you to quantify change. If no change is apparent, chances are that you didn't implement the techniques long enough or perhaps targeted the wrong area.

Think of the test/retest as your diagnostic tool for measuring progress. For example, if you're trying to improve your dead lift, you can assess your area(s) of restriction by setting up for the pull. Once you've identified where you are being held back from achieving optimal form, perform some mobility therapeutics on those tissues, and then do a retest. Do you feel a difference in your pull? Is it easier to get into the setup position? If you followed the correct mobility protocol, I suspect that the answer will be a resounding yes.

THE TUNNEL

By now it goes without saying that if you start a movement from a bad position, you will end the movement in a bad position. The setup is what I refer to as entering the tunnel.

The goal is to always enter the tunnel in a position of impeccable form so that you can maximize the efficiency and power of the movement that follows. However, just because you enter the tunnel in a good position doesn't necessarily mean you will exit the tunnel in a good position. You may, for example, establish a perfect running stance, but that doesn't mean that as you take off you won't fall into old patterns and start to roll your shoulders forward to compensate for your lack of shoulder mobility, that is, because you don't have enough internal rotation (pulling the arm behind the body). It's your job to be mindful of your body positioning at all times until flawless technique become unconscious action.

Let me give you an example to help imagine transitioning from the propulsive phase of the swimming stroke to the recovery phase. At this particular step, you need to vault over your supporting hand, which is extended in front of you, shift forces by rotating sides while pulling your opposite arm out of the water. Now, if you've got limited range of motion in your shoulder, you're going to have to roll your shoulder forward to compensate for the lack of internal rotation. You entered the tunnel (started the movement) from an ideal position but because you don't have full range of motion at the midway point, you exit in a bad position.

In summary, you have to address the starting position as well as the finishing position to determine whether or not you have the range needed to perform the movement correctly.

TOOLS OF MOBILITY

Equipment:

- Resistant/Stretch Band
- Voodoo Band
- Roller
- Lacrosse Ball
- Barbell

Techniques:

- Sliding Surfaces: Sliding surfaces are a component of the human mechanical system, which include motor control, joint capsule, and muscle dynamics. Put simply, the term "sliding surfaces" refers to how tissues slide over one another. This can be skin over tendons, intramuscular over intra-muscular surfaces, nerves gliding in nerve beds, muscles sliding under fascia, etc. Sliding-surface issues are largely dealt with using lacrosse balls, rollers, smashing, pressure waving, and voodoo flossing. Note that hydration and other factors also play a role.

Sliding Surface Test

To ensure ideal ranges of motion in your joints and muscles, your skin should slide smoothly over the underlying tissue. To give you an idea of how this works, take your left index finger, press down on the top of your right hand (making sure to keep your right hand open), and move your finger back and forth. Your skin slides back and forth without struggle, right? This is what a sliding surface ought to feel like. Now, to test something more telling: Flex your foot, and try to pinch or slide your skin over the back of your Achilles tendon. Does it move? Can you pinch the skin? If not, that's going to present huge problems down the road and no amount of stretching is going to help. To restore suppleness you have to unadhere that skin to the underlying tissue using sliding-surface mobilization technique (e.g., ball whack, barbell smash, smash and floss, etc.).

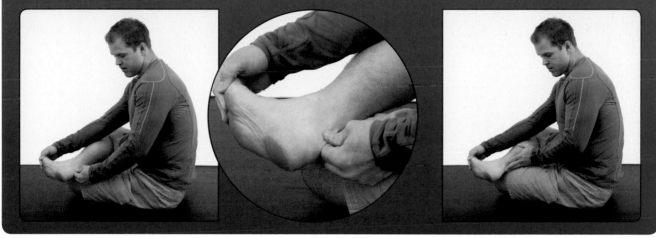

- **Pressure Waving:** A technique used to work through deeper sliding surfaces. This is accomplished by applying as much pressure as possible over the area in question while remaining completely relaxed, usually by distributing your weight over a lacrosse ball or roller. Once a tight area is identified, create a pressure wave by slowly rolling the tissue over the ball using the full weight of your body. This is high pressure, acute self-myofascial sliding-surface treatment.

- **Distracted Mobilization:** Incorporates the use of a band to restore normal intra-articular-joint motion. The joint capsule is often the most restricted motion component in the system and the least addressed. By idealizing joint position using a stretch band, you bias joint-capsule restriction. For most mobilizations, if you are not using a band, you are wasting your time.

- **Flossing:** A technique that deals with muscle stiffness. With the joint held in an optimal position by a stretch band, you move that joint in a full range of motion, thereby "flossing" the tissue in the newly challenged range. This technique addresses both joint-capsule restriction and sliding-surface dysfunction in that working range.

- **Smash and Floss:** A technique in which tissue is pinned (tacked) or pressured by a barbell, roller, or mob ball. Once a "tack" has been applied to an area of resistance, the limb is moved through as much range of motion as possible, thereby "flossing" the tissues being compressed (pinned, or tacked, down).

- **Contract-Relax:** Neuromuscular mobilization technique used to restore normal muscle dynamics (reset overlapping contractile muscular features). It can be used to increase range while stretching or to get deeper compression during sliding-surface mobilization. To execute this technique, create a strong co-contracted tension around the position of restriction by engaging that muscle for no less than 5 seconds. After the desired movement has been resisted for 5 seconds, immediately release tension and move into the new, desired range for 10 seconds. This tension-relax sequence is repeated for 5 or 6 cycles for no less than 2 minutes, or until you stop experiencing improvement. Note that this is a technique focused on position, not tissue.

WARM UP! COOL DOWN!

Warming up and cooling down are paramount to staying injury-free and promoting performance gains in training and events. A common mistake athletes make is to rush through a warm-up, charge directly into a hard workout, and then skip the cool-down.

Here's the formula: The shorter and more intense the effort (like 800-meter repeats), the longer your warm-up; the longer the effort (like an ultra marathon), the shorter your warm-up.

Here is an example of how you should warm up for a short-distance maximum-effort run. Depending on the intensity of your effort, your warm-up and cool-down should constitute 40 to 50 minutes of your workout.

WARM UP

5-10 minutes: Increasing Pace

• Start off easy and steadily increase the intensity of your effort. This could be in the form of a very light 400-meter jog, skill-based exercises, and dynamic stretching (leg swings, arm circles), etc.

*NOTE: 5 minutes if you're doing a 5K; 10 minutes for 800-meter repeats.

5-10 minutes: Mobility

• As already discussed, you should approach your mobility in terms of the activity or movement being performed. For example, if you're going for a run, you want to address the ankles, knees, and hips, focusing on the areas that need the most work. Remember, this is different for everybody, so use the checklist to identify your problem areas.

5-10 minutes: Skills and Pace Increase

• After doing some mobility work, implement skills in the form of a drill as demonstrated in Chapter 2. Just like your mobility work, the drills should address your areas of weakness.

• In addition, you need to do some higher-intensity intervals—like 5 to 8 100-meter sprints at 50 to 70 percent intensity. The key is to work some skills while incorporating some light sprints as you continue to pick up the pace of your warm-up.

• You can also throw in some dynamic stretching to help loosen up areas that are still tight.

5 minutes: Rest Before Workout

• This gives you some time to recover before you segue into your training.

5 minutes: Skill Work

- 5 minutes max of skill work to stimulate the central nervous system and help ingrain proper motor patterns while you are in recovery mode.

10-20 minutes: Movement and Mobility

- To complete the cool-down you want to continue to move at a slow pace, maybe by just walking or doing some body-weight squats or lunges to stretch out your body. In addition, you should target the muscles used, as well as your problem areas, by spending an ample amount of time on mobility techniques.

POSITION IS POWER EVEN WITH MOBILITY

You never want to mobilize with bad form (back rounded forward, overextended, etc.). As with all of the movements in this book, you never want to breach neutral posture or compromise your form for the sake of range.

NEVER TAKE A DAY OFF

You should always find time for mobility exercises: 15 minutes is plenty of time to deal with your business. Whether you are sore, stiff, or lacking range, make time everyday to aggregate change.

SKILL TRAINING

Think of the techniques presented in this chapter as an arsenal of tools that can be used not only to treat injuries, but also to bring efficient movement to areas where you are feeling resistance. To make navigating through this section easier, the techniques are organized into three main sections: 1) Feet, Ankles, and Calves; 2) Upper Legs (quads, hamstrings, adductors) Hips, and Trunk; and 3) Thoracic Spine, Shoulders, and Neck. Use the checklist as your guide to determine which areas need to be addressed—like a "choose your own adventure" for your body—and go from there. Remember, to avoid injury and improve efficiency, you have to make mobility practice a daily ritual and deal with the issues in your tissues before they become a problem.

MINIMUM EFFECTIVE DOSE IS TWO MINUTES

To instigate change, you have to spend at least two minutes with target mobilization exercises. For example, if you're doing the couch mobilization, you have to spend at least two minutes mobilizing each hip to restore normal motion. Ideally, you want to start working up to four to six minutes on each leg.

IF IT FEELS SKETCHY, IT'S SKETCHY

It's really simple: Never mobilize into hot, nervy pain. The numbness and tingling sensation you feel when you go past your comfort zone are signals from damage to come. Don't do it.

STAY HYDRATED

Being dehydrated impedes performance, affects mobility, and increases your susceptibility to injury big time. Stay hydrated at all times. For more information on hydration protocol, flip to page 352.

SORT OUT YOUR IMBALANCES

For most of us, one side will be tighter than the other. To be an efficient and well-balanced athlete both sides of you should have the same degree of range. If, say, your left hip has less mobility than your right one, it can compromise your movement pattern, which leads to other areas trying to compensate for the imbalance, which potentially leads to problems.

MOBILIZE YOUR STIFF AREAS

You have to remember that your tissues and musculature are not self-equalizing, meaning that soreness and stiffness isn't distributed equally throughout your entire body. Some areas will be sore, some not. Give some tender, loving care to the sensitive and hot spots and ignore anything that doesn't make you uncomfortable.

EXPLORE YOUR BUSINESS (INFORMED FREESTYLE)

It's important to mention that although the exercises in this chapter illustrate proper technique, you're not limited to performing them exactly as the photos indicate. Every individual has his own corners that need to be hit. As long as you maintain good form, explore your business by freestyling into some crazy positions. This idea of hunting for your stiffness is call informed freestyle.

IF POSSIBLE, ALWAYS USE A BAND

Using a resistant band allows you to pull the joint into a good position and mobilize into ideal ranges. Remember, your posture reflects the realities of your mobility. For example, if you sit all day long with you hips locked at a 90 degree angle, the head of your femur will adapt to the position by moving to the front of your hip socket. In order to have full faculty of your hip in motion, you need the head of your femur centered in the hip capsule (sac surrounding the head of the femur). If it moves to the front of the socket, it not only limits range of motion, but also creates an impingement in the front of your hip, which is your femur running into your acetabulum (housing for the head of the femur). By hooking your leg through a band and creating a distraction (tension in the band) you draw the head of the femur into the center of the hip capsule, allowing you to safely and comfortably stretch into ideal ranges. Not only that, you address hip capsule stiffness as well as muscular stiffness, making it a two for one mobilization.

One of the basic rules of distracted mobility is that if you want to improve extension, you mobilize to the front of the socket. If you want to improve flexion, you mobilize to the back of the socket. This allows you to get to the end range of the joint and articulate mobility from these positions. These positions tend to be the places where we have the most problems, which is why it is so effective.

Foot, Ankle, and Calf Mobilization

Foot, ankle, and calf mobilization is at the core of the supple-leopard program and one of the most important ingredients for endurance athletes to add to their daily routine. The bottom line is that the heel cords (Achilles tendons) do a ton of work, and they don't get enough attention. Think about it: A cyclist puts in thousands, if not tens of thousands, of contractions on a ride. Do you think your Achilles tendon can do that amount of volume without getting stiff? Absolutely not!

If you have tight heel cords or calves, your issues won't end there. For example, if you're following a CFE program that calls for a hard-interval ride one day, and then a strength session that includes squats the next, how do you think your squats will look/feel if you don't spend some time mobilizing your feet, ankles, and calves between workouts? Are you missing range of motion in your ankles? Are your knees tracking forward in the bottom of the squat? Do you have knee pain? These are all symptoms of tight heel cords and poor ankle and calf mobility. Here's the deal: If you're an endurance athlete, you need to be obsessed with increasing the range of motion in your feet, ankles, and calves. You need to spend as much time as possible on the mobilization exercises that follow or suffer the consequences.

Dorsiflexion

In this sequence, I'm demonstrating a normal range of motion for the foot in dorsiflexion, which should be about 20 to 30 degrees. To perform this test, sit down with your legs extended and flex your foot as far as you can. Can you pull your foot past 90 degrees? No? Then that's going to pose a serious problem. If you're training on a foot that has zero range of motion, you're at risk of an overtension injury, which is the case for the majority of endurance athletes. To avoid/fix such a problem, you have to unglue those tissues from the bone using the subsequent sliding-surface techniques (downstream foot mobilization, barbell calf smash).

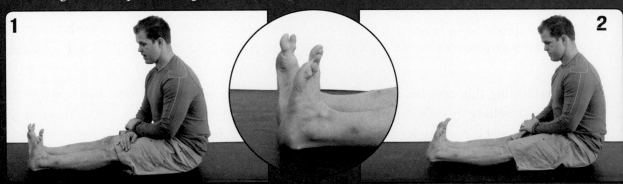

1 I'm demonstrating a normal range of motion with my left foot, which is about 20 to 30 degrees, and a poor range of motion with my right foot, which is about 90 degrees.

2 In order to move as efficiently as possible and avoid injuries, you must be able to flex both of your feet past 90 degrees, as demonstrated here.

Plantarflexion

In the photos below, I'm demonstrating a normal range of motion in plantarflexion, which is about 40 degrees, when measured from the bottom of the foot. Just like the dorsiflexion test, this should give you a little information about the stiffness of your lower leg. If the front of your shin (anterior tibialis) is tight, your range is going to be less than what's considered normal, and that will explain why you get shin splints every time you run.

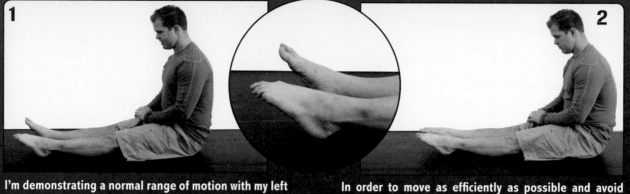

1 I'm demonstrating a normal range of motion with my left foot, which is about 40 degrees, and a short range of motion with my right foot.

2 In order to move as efficiently as possible and avoid overtension injuries, you must be able to point your toes at least to 40 degrees.

THE DOWNSTREAM FOOT

Most runners are familiar with the term, or have experienced, plantar fasciitis. It is caused when the connective tissue on the sole of the foot (plantar fascia) becomes inflamed, often as a result of poor running mechanics. To prevent/treat this injury, you have to not only address your running mechanics, but also go through the entire arsenal of mobility tools. If you're looking downstream of the ankle, the first thing to check is whether or not your skin is sliding over the underlying tissues. Think of the bottom of the plantar surface like the Achilles tendon for the bottom of the foot. In order for the foot to function as it was designed to, it needs to be supple, flexible, and elastic.

The foot is highly dynamic and sensitive. In addition to being part of the body's shock-absorbing system, the foot provides a lot of feedback about how you are moving. If its skin is matted to the underlying tissues, which is the case for most runners, then the Achilles is going to feel like a steel cable. In such a situation, your main priority should be to restore suppleness to the foot. One of the best ways to accomplish that is through the sliding-surface mobilization technique demonstrated below (see Plantar Surface).

When performing this exercise, it's important to take it slow. A lot of athletes rush through the process by hastily rolling their foot up and down the ball without any intention or focus. This will get you nowhere. The goal is nothing less than quality tissue mobilization. For example, if you're pressure-waving, it should take you up to 40 seconds to traverse from the back to the front of the foot. It's also important to note that you're not limited to just going up and down the foot, as demonstrated below. You can make circles, rolling the ball from side to side over a particularly nasty area. You can also "tack" the tissue down and move your toes around. Regardless of the method you choose, the key is to really take your time with the ball so that you can affect the tissues you're rolling over.

Plantar Surface

I'm showing you the plantar fascia area, which is where you want to roll the ball. As you can see, you want to cover not only the muscular insertion point, which is where I'm holding the ball, but also all of the salient structures along the foot.

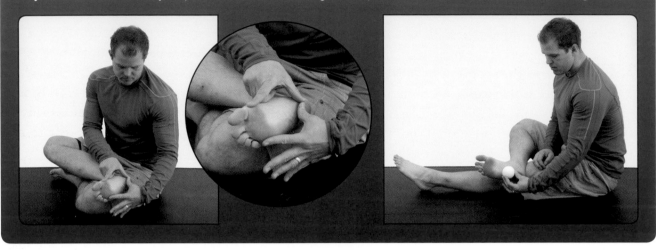

Downstream Foot Mobilization

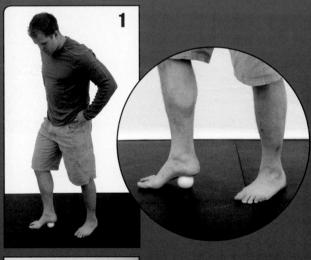

1. I've positioned my foot over the ball right at the insertion point for the posterior tibialis—which is the muscle that gives your foot arch support. This is your starting point. Be sure to take your time, as this area gets rather nasty.

2. Moving slowly, I pressure-wave the tissue by moving my foot backward, allowing the ball to roll under my foot.

3. I continue to slowly move my foot backward until the ball rolls under the length of my foot.

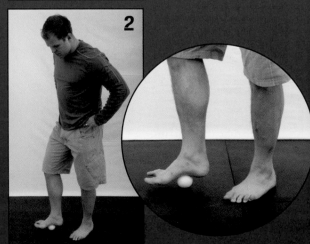

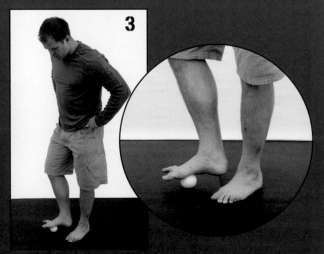

THE UPSTREAM FOOT
(RESTORING ANKLE MOBILITY)

To assess how your skin slides, perform the sliding-surface test (see page 301) by flexing your foot and pinching the skin behind your Achilles tendon. If you fail the test, work on ungluing the skin that is matted to the fascia by using the subsequent techniques. It's important to note that there are three areas you should investigate when performing the test: the Achilles tendon, the inside of the ankle, and the outside of the ankle. In treating each area, position the lacrosse ball against the skin with one hand, applying as much pressure as possible, and then use your other hand to whack the ball into the skin. You can also just move the ball back and forth, but if you can position yourself correctly and maintain enough pressure, a firm whack seems to yield the best results.

Achilles Tendon

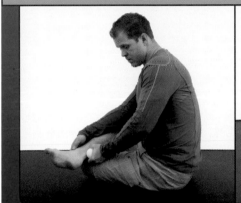
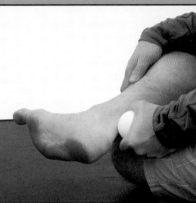

I've placed the lacrosse ball on my Achilles tendon. I can maneuver the ball up and down while applying as much pressure as possible or keep it pinned in place while striking the ball with my other hand.

Inside Ankle

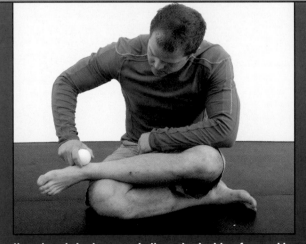

I've placed the lacrosse ball on the inside of my ankle. From here, I can maneuver the ball up and down while applying as much pressure as possible or keep it pinned in place while striking the ball with my other hand.

Outside Ankle

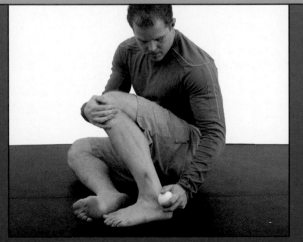

I've placed the lacrosse ball on the outside of my ankle. I can either maneuver the ball up and down while applying as much pressure as possible or keep it pinned in place while striking the ball with my other hand.

Barbell Calf Smash

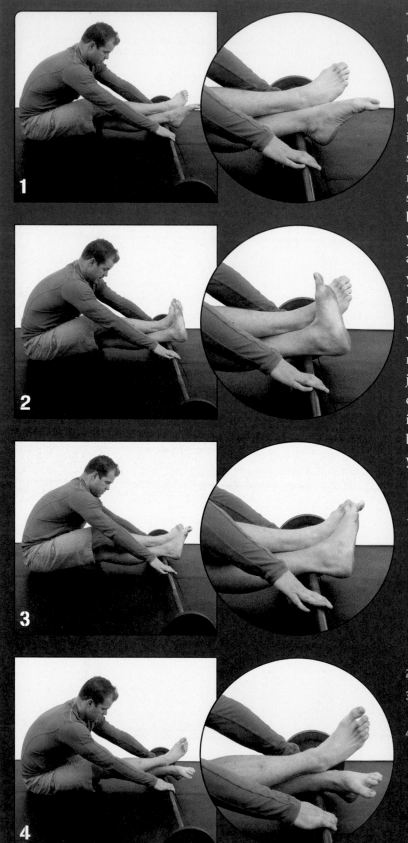

This is another highly effective way to release tension in the Achilles tendon, restore sliding surfaces, and treat a very stiff calf. With your heel cord anchored to the barbell, you can tack and stretch by pulling and pointing your foot, as well as rotating from side to side. Just as when doing a quad mobilization, the idea is to explore all sides of the tissue by rolling the barbell up and down the ankle/calf until you encounter a tight or matted-down area. As I already mentioned, when you start working through various ranges, you're going to find some areas that aren't tight while other areas are very tight: focus on the tight areas and move past the areas that are feeling juicy. It's important to note that if you don't have a barbell at hand, you can improvise using a rolling pin, lacrosse ball, or anything that you can anchor your heel cord on.

1. I've crossed my right foot over my left foot, anchoring my left Achilles tendon to the barbell. Having tacked down the tissue, I begin to explore my range by pointing my foot. It's important to note that if the pressure is too great, you can just do one foot. Applying additional pressure using this method is for my running ninjas.

2. I flex my foot.

3. To ensure that I find all my problem areas, I rotate my foot to the left.

4. I rotate my foot to the right. From here, I'll roll the barbell up my leg and continue to tack and stretch the tissue while rotating my foot.

Equipment Options

Although a barbell is ideal, you can improvise with other equipment, such as a rolling pin or lacrosse ball.

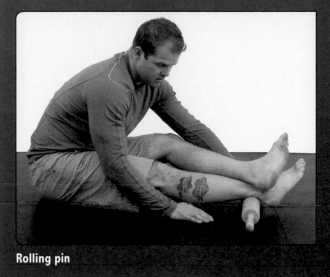

Rolling pin

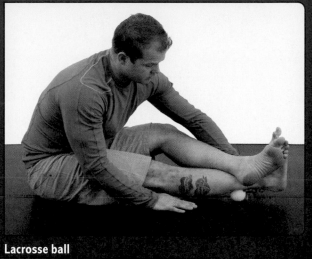

Lacrosse ball

Super-Friend Variation

If you have a super-friend on hand, you can do the same exercise by having him or her tack your leg to a foam roller, while you pull, point, and rotate your foot from side to side.

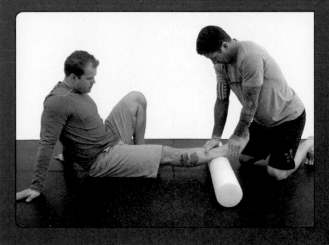

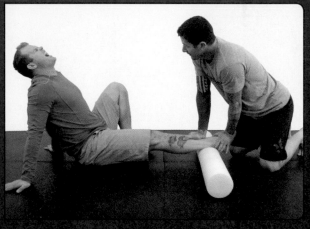

MEDIAL-SHIN TACK AND FLOSS

Whenever you correct a movement fault, you're going to get really sore and stiff because you're turning on muscles that haven't been used for a long time. For example, if you run with your feet angled out to the side as you reach the end of your stride, your foot is going to collapse every time you strike the ground. This fault overstretches the muscle (posterior tibialis) and tissue that give your foot arch support. The moment you put your ankle into good position and start landing with a neutral foot, that musculature turns on. Having been dormant for way too long, your shin is going to become extremely tender as you begin running with proper technique. To ease that discomfort, press a lacrosse ball to the medial side of your shinbone. Just as with all of the sliding-surface mobilizations, traverse the entire length of the muscle, working from the top to the bottom. When you find a hot area, hang out for a little bit and spend some quality time there before moving on.

There are a couple of ways you can execute this mobilization technique. You can pin the ball down using both of your hands while moving your foot around in circles (option 1) or pin the ball in place with one hand and use your other hand to move your foot around (Option 2). The former allows you to apply more downward pressure to stiff areas, while the latter forces your foot into ideal ranges. If you don't have a lacrosse ball, you can sit in a chair, cross your foot over your knee, and drive your elbow into the inside of your shin. As long as you're mobilizing in a good position and targeting your tender areas, you can get creative in exploring options.

Option 1

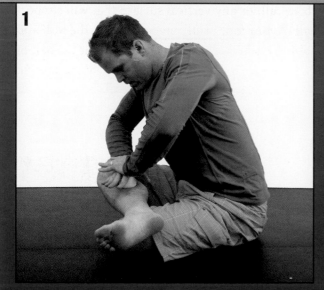

1 Starting high on my calf, I place the lacrosse ball on the medial side of my shinbone, and then press down on it with both hands. With my skin and tissues tacked down, I will move my foot in a circular fashion.

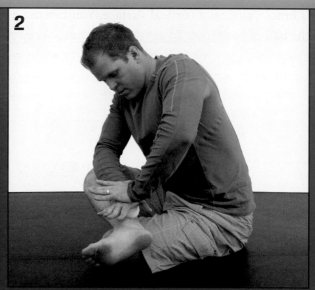

2 I work my way down my leg—tack and stretching and contracting and relaxing—until I reach my ankle.

Option 2

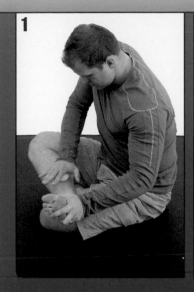
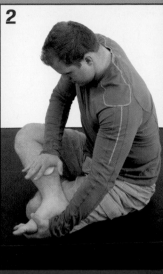

1. I've pinned the lacrosse ball on the medial side of my right shinbone with my right hand and latched on to the bottom of my right foot with my left hand. To begin, I press down on the lacrosse ball, and then pull my foot upward using my left hand. From here, I may hold the position or rotate my foot in search of tender areas.

2. Still applying downward pressure on the lacrosse ball, I push my foot toward the ground. It's important to note that you're not limited only to pulling and pushing your foot up and down. You can move it laterally, diagonally, and in circles. The key is to work the length of your shin—from your knee to your ankle—spending lots of time on stiff and tender spots and working your foot into all the ideal ranges.

CALF MOBILIZATION

The wall stretch has two variations. The first, done with a straight leg, focuses on the upper calf and the back of the knee (high-gastroc area). The second, done with a slight bend in the knee, focuses on the heel cord, isolating the soleus-related tissues. If you look at the photos, you'll notice that the ball of my foot is braced against a vertical surface. You can use a curb, a wall, or any vertical surface that will support the ball of your foot. To get the best results, keep the ball of your foot firmly braced against the wall and avoid bending your toes. With this particular mobilization, it's helpful to wear shoes so that the ball of your foot doesn't slide down the vertical surface as you drive your weight forward to initiate the stretch.

Option 1: Straight Leg

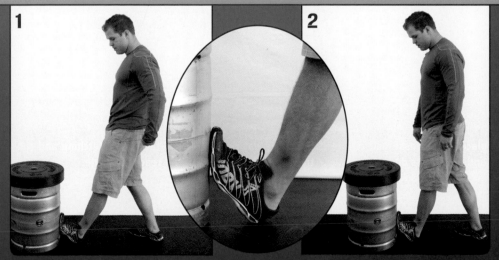

1. To begin, I brace the ball of my left foot against the keg, extend my leg, and squeeze my left glute.

2. Keeping my leg straight and my glute engaged, I shift my weight forward and drive my hips toward the wall.

Option 2: Knee Bend

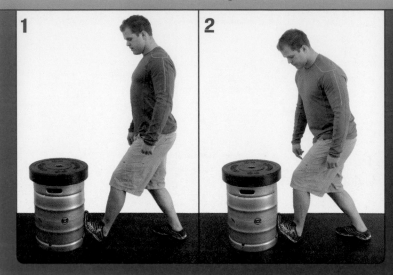

1. After spending some time in the previous position (2 minutes minimum), I bend my knee. It's important to note that by bending my knee I take tension off my gastrocsso so that I can focus on my Achilles.

2. To increase the intensity of the stretch, I shift my weight forward, lower my body, and rotate my torso in a counterclockwise direction.

Calf Mobilization with Distraction

As I mentioned in the introduction to this chapter, if your joint capsules are tight, it's difficult to achieve a full range of motion with a stretch because you are starting from a compromised position. For instance, many people experience a pinch in the joint capsule when they mobilize their ankles using the techniques previously demonstrated. In such a situation, you need to prioritize the positioning of your joint by wrapping a band around your instep and creating tension. In addition to pulling the joint into an ideal position, you focus on the tissues surrounding the joint, allowing you to stretch to your end range. You can use the distraction of bracing your foot against a vertical surface, as in the previous exercise, or a foam roller, as demonstrated in the photos below.

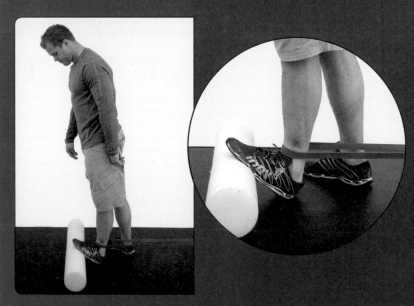

To make sure that my ankle joint is locked in a good position, I've wrapped a resistance band around my instep and created tension. Then I brace the ball of my foot against a foam roller, engage my glutes, and drive my hips forward.

Ankle Flossing

You can't expect to change the joint or tissues in question unless you understand how to achieve an ideal position. In this sequence, I demonstrate another highly effective ankle/calf mobilization that can be used to open up and lengthen the tissues of your lower posterior chain. To correctly execute this technique, start with your foot flat on the ground, shift the majority of your weight over the ankle you're mobilizing, and then drive your knee over your foot. The key is to externally rotate at the hip and drive your knee out laterally as you shift your weight forward. This not only allows you to reach your end range, but also prevents your ankle from collapsing inward, which would compromise the integrity of the joint. It's important to note that unlike the previous techniques, you don't want to hang out at end range. To get the best results, floss the tissues around that ideal joint position by oscillating back and forth as if you were trying to snap a credit card. This will free up those tissues and open up the joint capsule so that you can reach your end range.

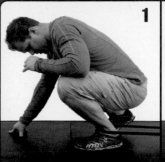 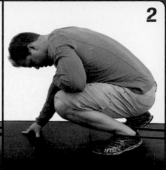

To ensure that my ankle joint is locked in a good position, I've wrapped a resistance band around my instep and created tension. To initiate the stretch, I shift my weight onto my left leg—keeping my left heel planted on the ground—and lean forward. It's important to note that I'm driving my left knee forward and out laterally. This prevents my ankle from collapsing and allows me to reach my end range.

I continue to drive my left knee out and over my left foot until I reach my end range. After touching end range, I will momentarily return to the starting position before returning to end range. Remember, the goal is to target those tissues around that ideal joint position by flossing back and forth.

SHIN MOBILIZATION

There are three engines used to power the human machine. The shoulders and hips are the primary engine, the knees are the secondary engine, and the calves and feet are the third engine. If you were to physiologically break down the calf and foot, you would realize that they're not designed to generate a lot of force; they're designed to generate a lot of low-level power for repeated and extended efforts. Think of a swimmer constantly kicking with her feet extended, a runner landing on the ball of his foot, or a cyclist driving through the pedal stroke. In each case, the calf and foot are in a state of constant resistance. No wonder your calves and feet are stiff after every workout. Although we do regularly mobilize our calves to alleviate stiffness, we almost never address the other giant muscle that bears a lot of the load, which is the front of the shin. In fact, ask any endurance athlete when was the last time he stretched the front of his shin and he probably couldn't tell you.

Remember, you have to look at the system as a whole. If your calf is tight, you not only have to mobilize the bottom of your foot, heel cords, and calf, but also the front of your shin. Think about it. Your calf is responsible for pushing your toes away. So if the front of your shin is tight, your calf doesn't have slack to pull because the muscle on the other side of the leg is stiff. It's a classic situation in which you are playing gaso-brako: you have one foot pressing on the gas and controlling the speed of the vehicle with your other foot on the brake. In other words, you're accelerating the wear and tear on your third engine.

Option 1: Double-Leg Mobilization

1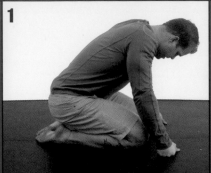

To begin, I kneel down, position my knees roughly shoulder width apart, and cross my right big toe over my left big toe.

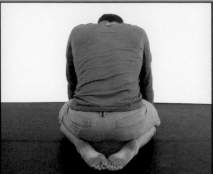

2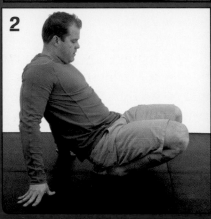

Keeping my core engaged, I lean back, placing my hands behind me for support, and pull both my knees off the ground. The nice part about this technique is that you can treat both of your legs at the same time. However, it doesn't offer the same freedom or maneuverability as the single-leg mobilization.

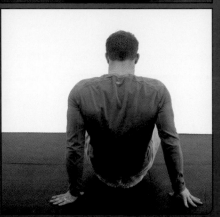

Option 2: Single-Leg Mobilization

1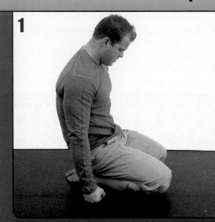

2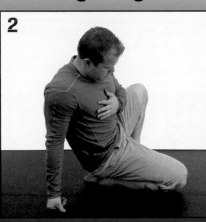

3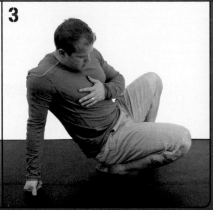

I start from the kneeling position.

I post up on my left foot and shift my weight toward my right side. Notice that I use my right hand to support the weight of my body.

Just as in the double-leg mobilization, I keep my midline engaged to maintain a neutral posture, lean my upper body back, and pull my right knee off the ground. An important point worth noting, which separates this mob from the double leg mobilization, is the ability to maneuver your knee from side to side to treat extra-stiff areas.

Upper Leg, Hip, and Trunk Mobilization

Modern humans do a lot of sitting. We sit when we drive, when we eat, when we work—we sit to do pretty much everything. As a result, the main engine that powers athletic performance (the hips) shuts down. The tissues of the posterior chain, especially the glutes, get matted down and extremely stiff. We hang on our psoas, causing the muscles that contribute to flexion and external rotation of the hips (the elements that give you power and stability) to get ropy. In addition, being in a closed-hip position for prolonged periods of time causes the muscles in the front of your hips and upper legs to shorten, which limits extension (see Skin-Pinch Test, page 294). Even if you sit with your core engaged and in a neutral posture, you can't prevent these repercussions if you sit in a chair all day.

To keep your primary engine running smoothly, stay away from the chair as much as possible (unless it's being used as a mobilization tool) and spend some serious time mobilizing the front of your hips, upper legs, psoas, and posterior chain. Unfortunately, the world we live in makes sitting unavoidable and as endurance athletes we have to work within limited ranges, which slowly kills our athletic performance. However, if you use the mobility tools in this section and take the time to deal with your issues before you experience pain, you can restore suppleness to the areas that are directly responsible for powering the human machine and defy the death of your athletic performance.

PATELLAR-POUCH AND DISTAL-QUAD SMASH AND FLOSS

Endurance athletics, especially running and cycling, causes a lot of overuse issues. Think of a cyclist repeatedly powering through the pedal stroke. The leg and hip reach extension with each stroke, but not to the end range. This can cause a lot of stiffness in the lower quad, right above the knee, which puts a lot of strain on the knee joint. When the tissues above the knee are matted down, it takes up an enormous amount of slack, creating tension on the kneecap. To restore slack to those angry tissues, you have to open up the suprapatellar pouch, right above the knee, and work the area of stiffness at the VMO—the teardrop-shaped muscle just above the inside of your knee. This is the upstream/downstream concept in action. If you're having knee pain, the first thing you should do is get some slack in the joint by opening up the calf as well as the quads and hamstrings.

Target Area

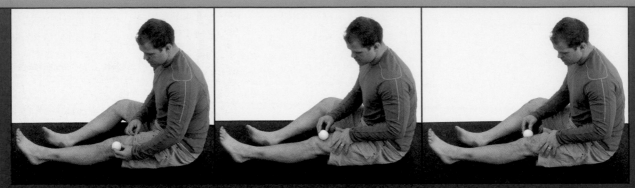

When performing this sliding-surface mobilization, focus on the patellar pouch, right above the knee. Here I show you where to position the ball as you rotate your leg from side to side. As you can see, I go from the outside of the leg, just above the knee, which is the insertion point for the IT band, toward the inside of the leg, where the VMO is located.

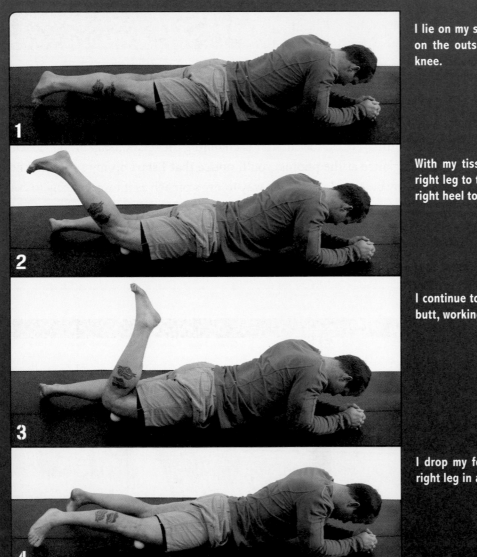

1 I lie on my stomach, with the lacrosse ball on the outside of my leg, just above my knee.

2 With my tissue tacked down, I rotate my right leg to the right and begin pulling my right heel toward my butt.

3 I continue to pull my right heel toward my butt, working my leg through its full range.

4 I drop my foot to the mat and rotate my right leg in a counterclockwise direction.

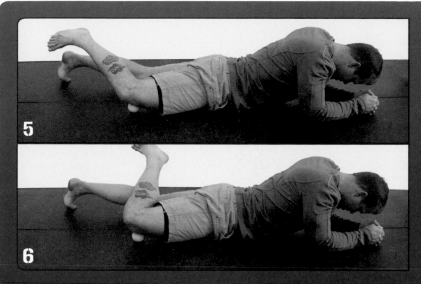

I tack down the tissue around my VMO and start pulling my heel toward my butt. Notice that I keep my leg at an angle to ensure that the tissue remains immobilized.

I slowly pull my heel toward my butt. Just as I did before, I make sure to work my leg through its full range.

QUAD/HIP SMASH

The most common mistake people make when using a foam roller is to hastily roll back and forth without intention. Remember, a warrior leopard thinks along the lines of quality, not quantity. You're not going to restore suppleness and range of motion by rushing through the mobility process. If you're rolling out your quads, the best approach is to pressure wave from side to side as opposed to rolling front to back. It doesn't matter that the muscle fibers are longitudinal; what does matter is changing the relationship of the muscle bundle to the tissues around it. If you glance at the photos, you'll notice that I start on my side with the roller positioned high on my hip near my butt, and roll all the way to my stomach as if I were trying to cut off my leg. By chopping the leg up into sections and taking your time to roll through the area, you become acutely aware of stiff, angry, painful spots that are dying for some extra attention. Roll across the leg until you encounter an ugly spot. When you do, stop, tack, and stretch and pressure-wave back and forth until you experience change.

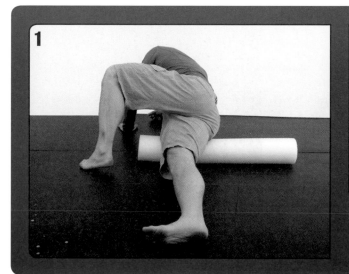

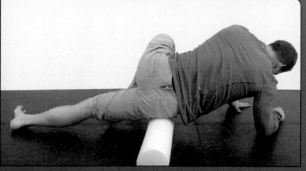

I've positioned the foam roller directly under my right hip. To keep my weight distributed over my leg, I've planted my left foot down and I'm supporting the weight of my upper body with my arms.

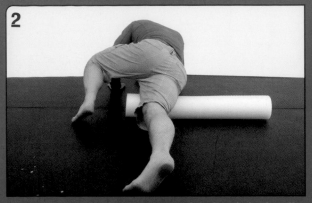

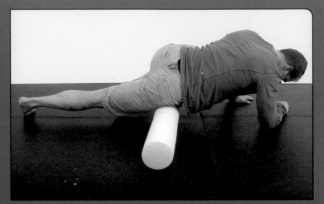

With my weight distributed over my right leg, I slowly roll to the left.

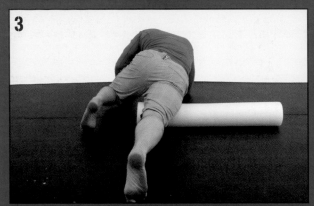

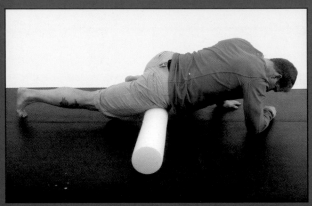

I continue to roll toward my belly, mashing the tissue laterally.

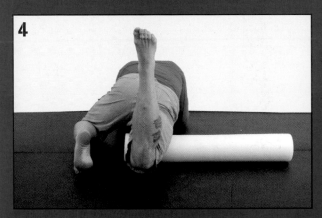

As I roll onto my stomach, I encounter a really stiff area. Instead of rolling past it, I tack the tissue down, and then curl my heel toward my butt. You're not limited to just one pull. Move your leg around as many times as it takes to find some relief in the underlying tissue.

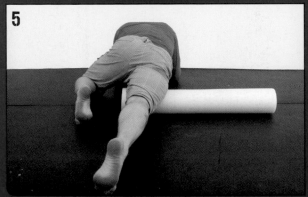

I straighten my leg.

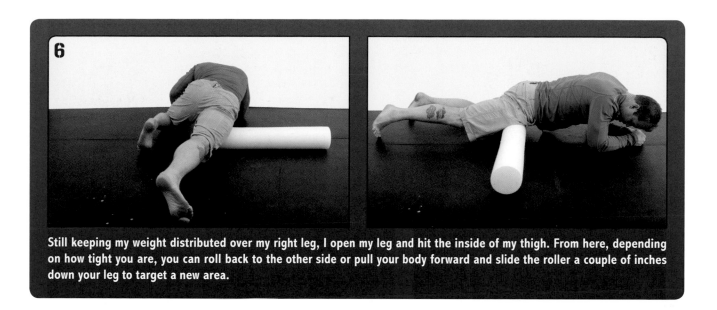

6

Still keeping my weight distributed over my right leg, I open my leg and hit the inside of my thigh. From here, depending on how tight you are, you can roll back to the other side or pull your body forward and slide the roller a couple of inches down your leg to target a new area.

ANTERIOR- AND MEDIAL-HIP SMASH

To write your own mobility prescription, you have to not only examine the positions you spend your day in, but also when you exercise. For example, if you go for a hard ride, you know that you're going to be stuck in a flexed position for an extended period of time. For starters, you can assume that, based on your position on the bike, the front of your hips are going to get tight. Rather than wait for the problem to become worse and affect other parts of your body, you should repair the damage immediately after your ride. There are a couple of methods you can employ in such a situation. The couch stretch is an excellent option, but it's not an end-all cure. To restore suppleness and open up the front of your hips, you need to mash a ball into the gnarled tissue. Don't wait for your body to seize up to formulate a mobility program. If you're performing an activity that causes stiffness (and let's face it, if you're an athlete, there's no escaping that reality), plan ahead and target the hotspot before it becomes a problem.

Target Area

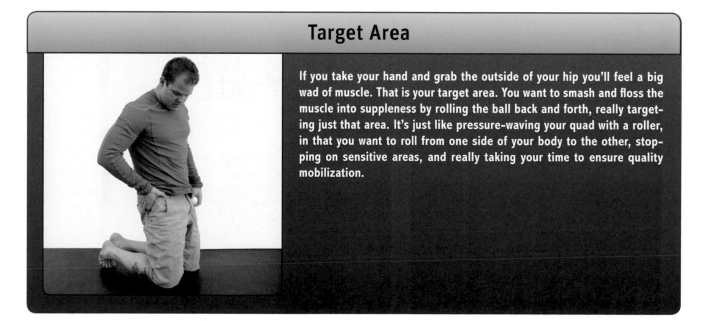

If you take your hand and grab the outside of your hip you'll feel a big wad of muscle. That is your target area. You want to smash and floss the muscle into suppleness by rolling the ball back and forth, really targeting just that area. It's just like pressure-waving your quad with a roller, in that you want to roll from one side of your body to the other, stopping on sensitive areas, and really taking your time to ensure quality mobilization.

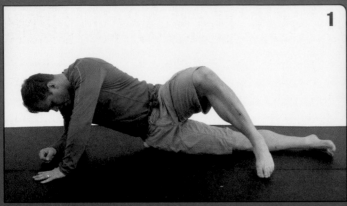

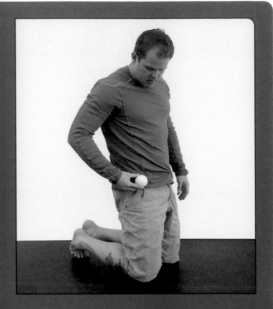

1

I've positioned the lacrosse ball on the outside of my right hip. In order to get the best results from this mobilization, I must distribute all of my weight over the lacrosse ball. To accomplish this, I plant my left foot in front of my right leg, reach my right leg back, and use my right elbow and left hand for support.

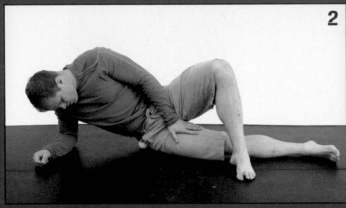

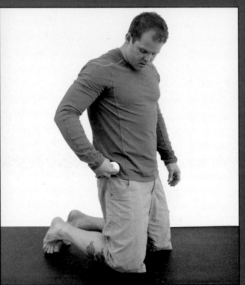

2

With all of my weight distributed over the lacrosse ball, I slowly roll toward my back, mashing the ball into the bound-up tissue.

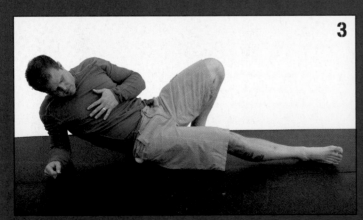

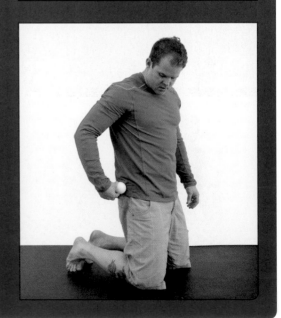

3

I slowly work my way toward my butt. From here, I'll reverse the sequence and work my way back to the starting position.

BALL-IN-HIP MOBILIZATION

In the sequence below, I demonstrate a simple sliding-service technique that will restore normal range of motion to the areas that get matted down after a long time sitting. This is one of the most popular sliding-surface mobilizations because it provides instant relief and automatic mobility; it's like receiving a free super power. You reduce discomfort and pain, decrease your susceptibility to injury, improve movement efficiency, and increase power. And the best part is that it can be done anywhere. Yes, you can work on becoming a faster runner while answering e-mails at work. It's not complicated. Just stick a ball in the side of your butt and you're good to go.

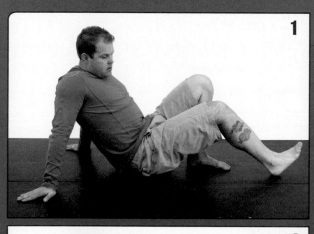

1 I'm sitting on a lacrosse ball, which is in the side of my butt. Notice that I support myself on my hands, lean back slightly, and keep my legs curled. This helps distribute the majority of my body weight over the lacrosse ball to ensure optimal pressure.

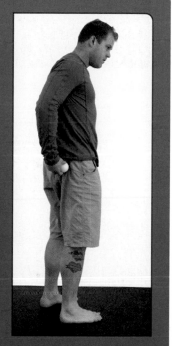

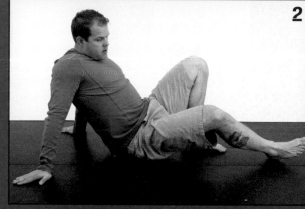

2 I move my body over the ball until I find some ugliness.

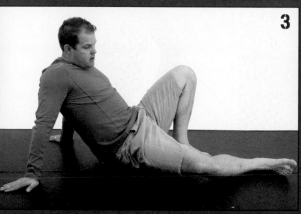

3 Having found a stiff area, I stop, tack the underlying tissue down, and move my leg to the side. It's important to note that you're not limited to the movements shown below. For example, you can cross your right leg over your left leg and then squirm around. Straighten your leg and mash over the tissue. Sit in a chair. There are many variations. It's not complicated. Just pressure that ball into the side of your butt and go hunting for sensitive areas.

CLASSIC POSTERIOR-CHAIN MOBILIZATION

You can use the following two mobilization options to increase hamstring flexibility. But these are just two of many variations. Whether you're lying on your back and pulling your leg up (Option 1), propping your foot on a box and leaning forward (Option 2), or keeping both of your feet on the ground and leaning forward from the hip (see page 297), always wrap a resistance band around your hip crease, create tension, and pull the joint back into the hip capsule. As in all mobilization stretches, if you don't distract the joint into an ideal position, you're going to get jammed. You can still mobilize the surrounding tissue, but you'll never be able to take the limb through a full range of motion. With the distraction of the hip capsule, you bias the leg into assuming an ideal position and restore its normal range of motion, which allows you to pull your leg to its end range.

Option 1

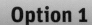

1 With my leg distracted into an ideal position, I sit up and grab my ankle.

2 Keeping my leg locked out and my arms straight, I roll onto my back. Note: You should be able to lie down with your back flat on the ground and your leg straight as your base range. If this isn't possible, you can bias your leg into a normal range by wrapping your hands around the back of your knee. Don't try to grab your ankle or high on your leg if you lack range. In most cases, this will force your lumbar spine into overextension as you roll toward your back. Remember, always mobilize in a good position by maintaining a neutral posture.

Option 2

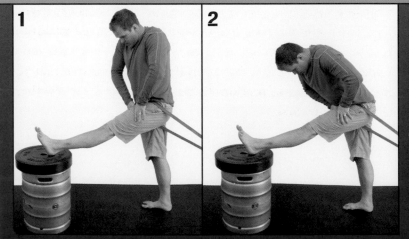

1. I've wrapped a band around my hip crease, created tension, and then placed my foot against a keg. To prevent my knee from flexing, I'm pressing down on my thigh with both hands.

2. Keeping my spine in a neutral position, I hinge at the hips and lean forward, forcing my hamstrings to lengthen to their end range.

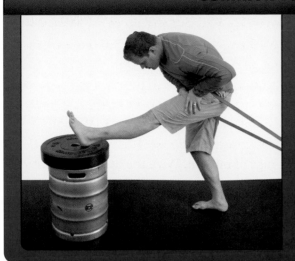

Here I'm demonstrating one of the most common faults with this stretch. The key with this particular technique is to make sure you don't sacrifice an ideal spinal position to stretch your posterior leg and hip. If your hamstrings are tight, the tendency is to compensate with a rounded lumbar spine. This not only reinforces a poor movement pattern, but also puts stress on the tissues of the back. Keep your spine in a neutral position, stabilize your core, and hinge forward from the hip, as demonstrated here.

HIP-CAPSULE MOBILIZATION

Unless you were born with a debilitating condition or suffered a catastrophic accident, you should be able to do a full squat—humans are designed to. However, most endurance athletes can't get their thighs below parallel without rounding forward or overextending. Most chalk this up to tight hamstrings and other posterior-chain issues, but that is only partly true. Another, often overlooked, limiting factor is the hip capsule. The hip capsule and glutes get extremely tight after hard runs and rides. If you don't work to reverse that situation, you'll lose flexion in the hip and wind up with an overtension injury.

In this sequence, I demonstrate a very important mobilization exercise that should be practiced on a daily basis to ensure proper hip function. What you'll find is that by driving the head of your femur into the back of the hip capsule, where it belongs, you can restore the normal position of the femur head in the socket, which improves the joint capsule's range of motion, increases flexion of the hip, lengthens the hamstrings, and improves external rotation. Consequently, you'll have more depth and power in the bottom of your squat, be able to generate more power in the pedal stroke, and run more efficiently.

Although you can mobilize the hip capsule without a resistance band, many athletes experience an impingement in the front of their hips. That is because the femur is positioned at the front of the hip capsule, which causes a slight pinch of the tissue. In such a situation, you should stop what you're doing and start over using a band. The idea is to distract the hip laterally or posteriorly so that you can account for that tight joint and increase your range of motion. If you continue to stretch with an impinged hip, you're just going to make that pinch worse.

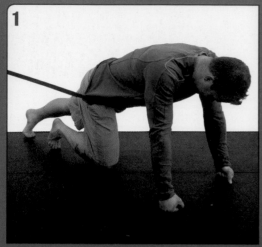
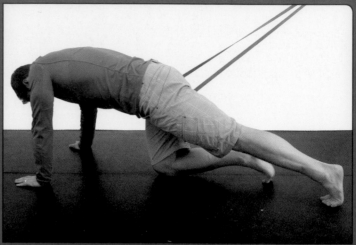

I've wrapped a resistance band around my hip crease and created tension with a lateral distraction. To load my hip, I've distributed the majority of my weight over my right knee. For the best results, drive your knee into the ground and let your weight drop until your femur feels like it's going to pop out the side of your hip.

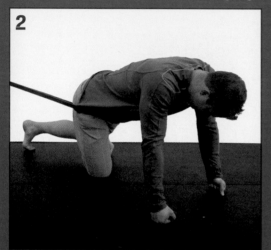
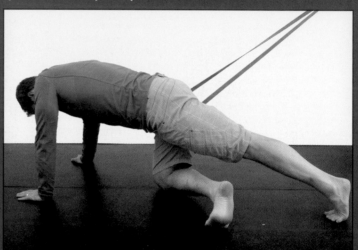

With my line of force directly over my right femur, I kick my leg across my body into external rotation.

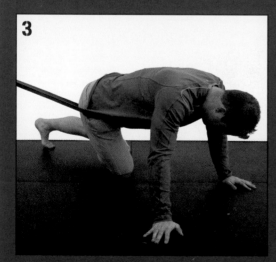
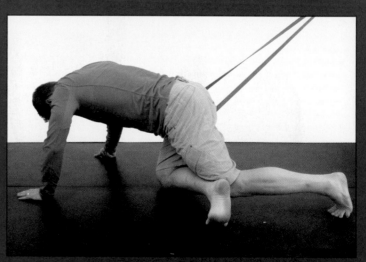

With my leg external rotated, thanks to the band, I bring my left knee up to my right calf, pinning my leg in place. From here, I'll spend a minimum of 2 minutes oscillating in and out of end-range tension. The goal is to hit an area of resistance, retreat, touch resistance, come out, and repeat, until you feel significant improvement.

FLEXION WITH EXTERNAL ROTATION OF THE HIP: OPTION 1

The key with this technique is to make sure you block the foot and the knee so that you can fold your upper body forward from a stable position. After bending your upper body over your leg, start hunting for stiff areas by rotating your bellybutton over your knee—which I like to call the pigeon sweep—and then over your foot. If you experience outside knee pain or you're unable to get into this position because you're too tight in the hips, throw your leg up on a box, chair, or table, as demonstrated in the following sequence.

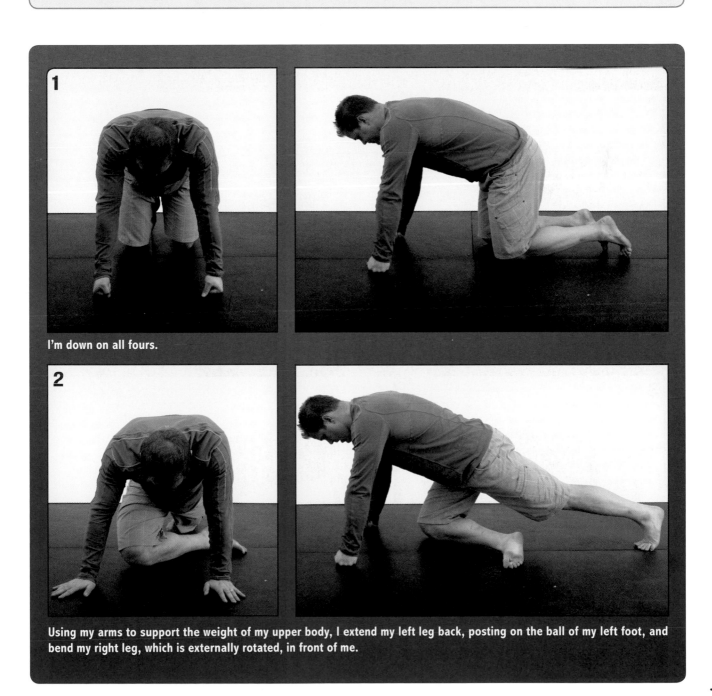

1 I'm down on all fours.

2 Using my arms to support the weight of my upper body, I extend my left leg back, posting on the ball of my left foot, and bend my right leg, which is externally rotated, in front of me.

1

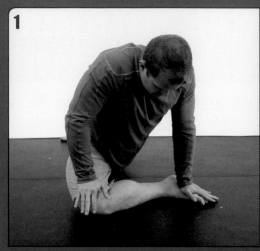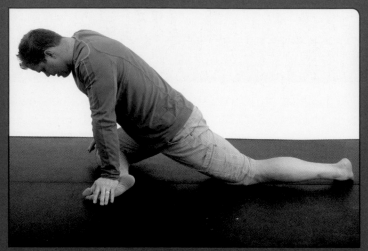

As I lower my hips, I point my left foot so that the top of it is on the mat, and shift my weight back slightly. To keep my right leg from moving, I place my left hand over my foot, and my right hand on my right knee. Next, I fold forward to initiate the stretch.

2

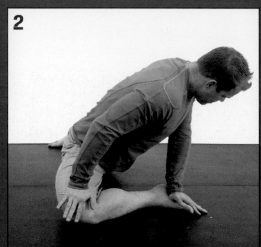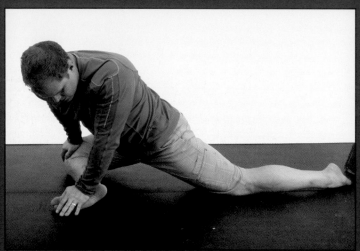

Pressing my right hand into my right knee, I begin hunting for stiff areas by twisting toward my left side. Notice that I maintain neutral spinal alignment despite the rotation in my torso.

3

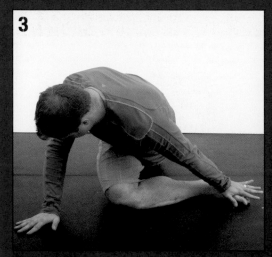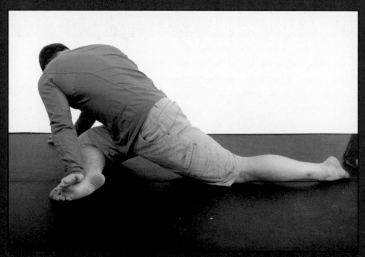

I continue to search for tightness by sweeping my upper body toward to the right, trying to get my bellybutton over my knee.

FLEXION WITH EXTERNAL ROTATION OF THE HIP: OPTION 2 (CHAIR/BOX/TABLE)

If tight hip flexors prevent you from getting your knee and hip flush with the ground, elevating your leg on a box, chair, or table is an excellent option. With less tension in the pelvis, you can place your leg in a neutral position, achieve more flexion in the hip, and keep your torso straight. The key is to load the hip first by driving your hips back, just as you would when setting up for a dead lift. You can then fold forward and begin hunting from side to side for stiff areas. If you're extremely tight in the posterior and anterior hips, you may have some knee discomfort when you attempt to bring your leg into a perpendicular position. To alleviate the pressure on your knee, drop your foot off the side of the chair, box, table, or whatever you're using to prop your leg up. This is a lot less aggressive, but still allows you to open up the hip in flexion and external rotation, which is the goal of this mobilization. Just as in the previous technique, you want to hinge forward from the hip and hunt for tight areas by rotating your torso from side to side.

Sequence A

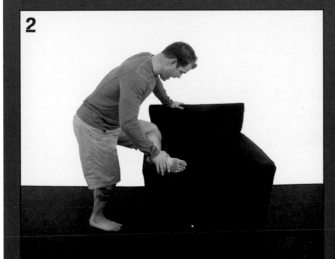

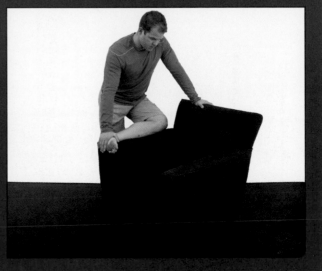

1. My left leg is perpendicular to my body on the side of the armchair. To keep my leg fixed in position, I place my right hand over my left foot.

2. I load my hip by driving my butt back.

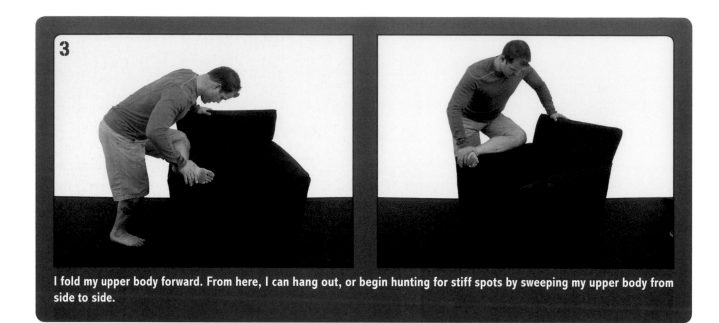

3

I fold my upper body forward. From here, I can hang out, or begin hunting for stiff spots by sweeping my upper body from side to side.

Sequence B

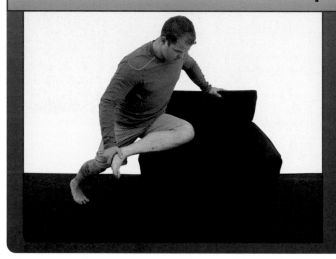

To alleviate some of the pressure on my knee, I let my left foot fall off the arm of the chair and lean forward. I can still sweep from side to side in search of hot spots.

FLEXION WITH EXTERNAL-ROTATION BIAS: OPTION 1

In the previous mobilization pieces, I focused on external rotation first, then added tension with flexion. In this sequence, I do the exact opposite. I place my foot flat on the ground and bias the leg into hip flexion, then add external rotation to the load to increase the stretch. Both variations are important because flexion and external rotation go hand in hand. Think about dropping down into a squat. You need flexion to drop below parallel, and you need external rotation to generate power and sustain an ideal body position. However, you may need to focus on one instead of the other depending on where you're weak and what exercise you're doing. For instance, cycling is a more flexion-based exercise and requires very little external rotation, making the following mobility piece mandatory after hard rides.

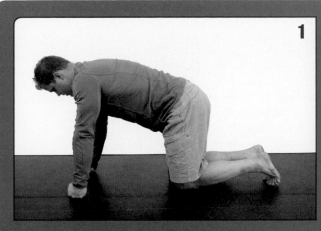

1 I'm down on all fours.

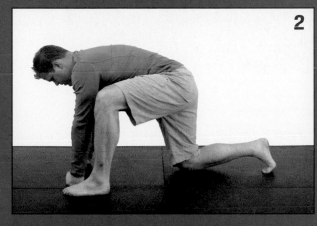

2 I plant my left foot down.

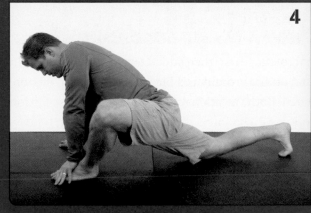

3 Keeping my left shin vertical, I extend my right leg back and drop into deep flexion. It's important to notice that my left hand is on top of my left foot. This prevents my big toe from leaving the ground as I externally rotate that leg.

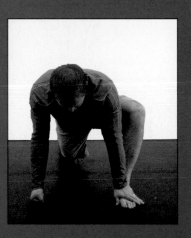

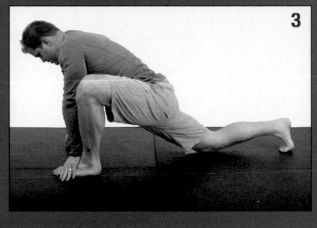

4 I drive my left knee out laterally into external rotation.

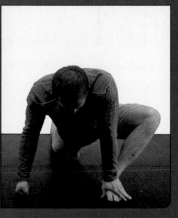

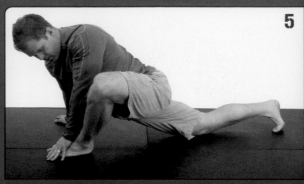

5 Keeping my back flat, I begin searching for tight areas by rotating my upper body in a counterclockwise direction.

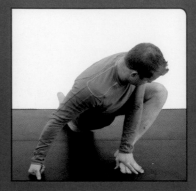

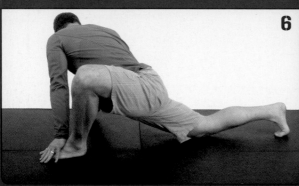

6 Still searching for tightness, I sweep my upper body toward my right side.

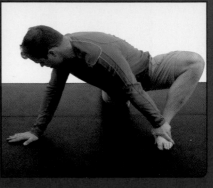

Distraction Option

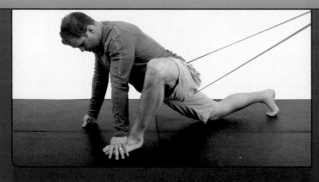

Whenever possible you should mobilize with a resistance band. Here I demonstrate the same stretch but with a distraction. Notice that the band is wrapped around my hip crease and pulling the head of my femur into the back of my hip socket, which is the ideal joint position.

FLEXION WITH EXTERNAL-ROTATION BIAS: OPTION 2

This is very similar to the previous mobilization exercise, in that it combines flexion with an external rotation bias. But instead of working from the ground, as demonstrated in the previous sequence, you prop your foot up on a box, chair, or table. Although this is an excellent variation that all endurance athletes should implement, it's particularly effective for really stiff athletes who struggle getting into these random ranges from the floor. By propping your foot up on a box, you can force that leg into deep flexion and really work the end ranges. The key with this technique is to wind the tissue up by driving your hips back and then exaggerate the flexion by leaning forward and bringing your knee toward your chest.

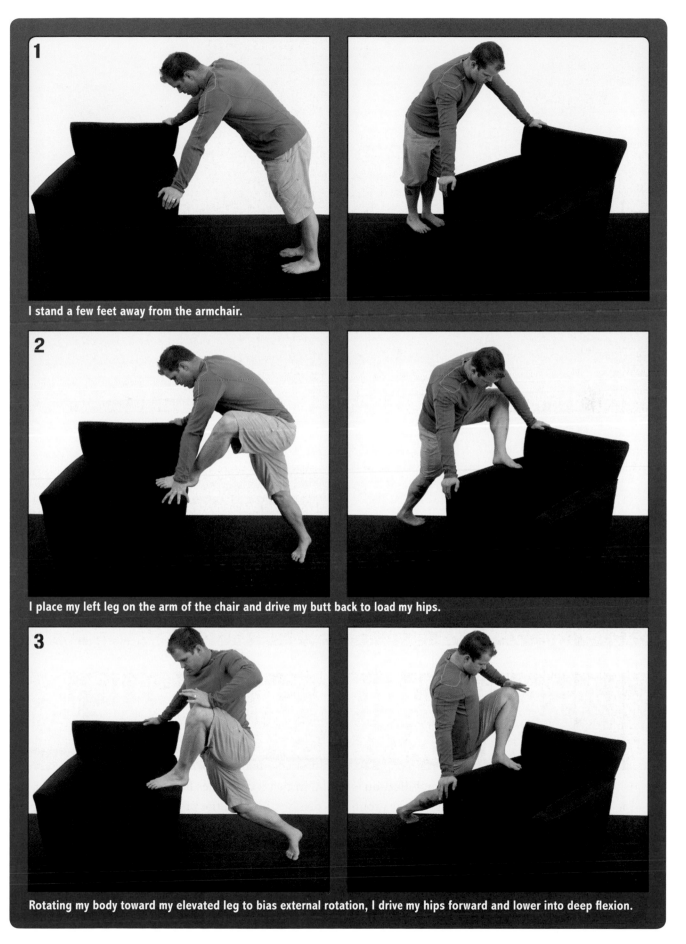

1

I stand a few feet away from the armchair.

2

I place my left leg on the arm of the chair and drive my butt back to load my hips.

3

Rotating my body toward my elevated leg to bias external rotation, I drive my hips forward and lower into deep flexion.

INTERNAL ROTATION WITH FLEXION BIAS

When you think about internal rotation, the first thing that should come to mind is extension. Think of a split jerk, a running stride, or proper kicking mechanics for swimming. In each of these movements, your leg is in extension, which means that in order to create the most stable and powerful position possible you need to internally rotate your leg. If you're missing a normal internal rotation range of motion, you're going to externally rotate in these positions, which as you already know is a mechanism for injury and power loss. In addition, missing internal rotation also limits your ability to drive your knees out laterally (externally rotate) when your leg is in flexion (squat). Allow me to explain.

As you already know, for your hip to function correctly you have to be able to lift your leg straight up to your chest with ease. Previously, I discussed the potential limiting factors, which include having tight hip flexors and hamstrings. However, what I didn't discuss is the role internal rotation plays in flexion. Let's assume that you don't have any limiting factors, and the only thing you're missing is internal rotation. In such a situation, bringing your leg straight up to your chest is difficult because there's no capsular slack. So even though you're not necessarily working on internal rotation when you pull your leg into flexion, you need a certain degree of freedom in the joint. Otherwise, you have to compensate for that lack of capsular range by externally rotating your leg. This is why people turn their feet out when they squat; otherwise, they couldn't reach deep flexion and squat below parallel.

Think of a cyclist who kicks his leg out to the side every time he enters the recovery phase of the pedal stroke (brings his knee up to his chest). If he lacks capsular slack, he can't keep his knee pointed forward, which is necessary for generating power and maintaining rhythm in the pedal stroke. In addition to losing power and compromising stability, this creates an open-circuit fault that will inevitably lead to injury.

One of the first things taken off the table when you're missing internal rotation is the capacity to get into flexion while in an internally rotated position. In the sequence below, I demonstrate a similar mobilization technique to the hip-capsule stretch. But instead of crossing my leg under my body, I kick my leg out and pin my foot in front of a medicine ball, kettlebell, or friend's foot so that I can get my leg into an internally rotated position. Just as in the hip-capsule stretch, the key is to distract your hip laterally using a resistance band, shift all your weight over your knee, and drive your femur through the side of your hip. Once accomplished, you want to worry those tissues around by shoving your hip out laterally, bringing your knee under your body, and flossing around tender areas. It's important to note that if you don't account for the joint capsule you're going to feel an impingement in the front of the hip, which reduces the effectiveness of the stretch. For more information on how to improve internal rotation with a flexion bias, check out mobilitywod.com.

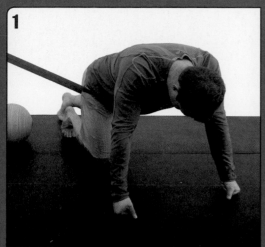
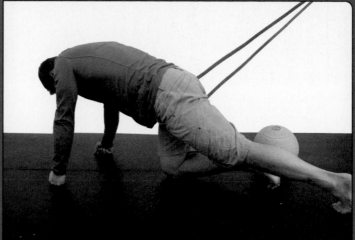

1

I've wrapped a resistance band around my hip crease and created tension with a lateral distraction. To load my hip, I've distributed the majority of my weight over my right knee.

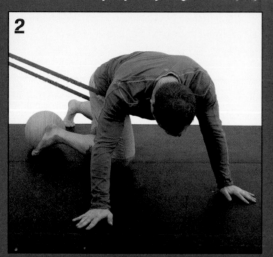
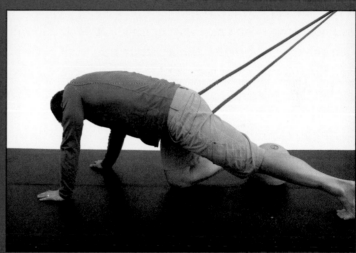

2

I kick my right leg out laterally and pin my foot behind a heavy medicine ball.

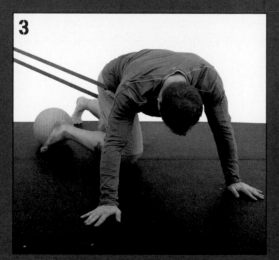
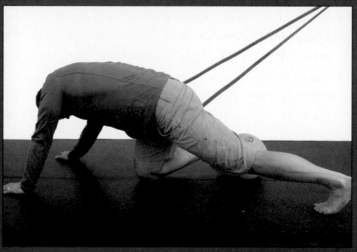

3

With my leg eased into an internally rotated position, I work on shoving my femur out the side of my hip—just as I would if I were doing the hip-capsule mobilization. From here, I'll spend at least 2 minutes oscillating in and out of end-range tension. The goal is to hit an area of resistance, come out, touch resistance, come out, and repeat, until you feel you get some release.

BANDED-FOOT DISTRACTION WITH INTERNAL ROTATION

When runners can't internally rotate their leg in extension, they end up spinning it out to the side as they reach the end of their stride. In other words, they start running like a duck, with their feet, knees, and hips turned out. If you externally rotate your leg at the end of your stride, your foot and knee collapse, causing you to enter the tunnel of movement from a bad position. Reinforce this motor pattern enough, and you're going to end up with an injury that is hard to fix. To prevent that from happening, you need to restore internal rotation so that your feet, ankles, knees, and hips can function as they're designed to.

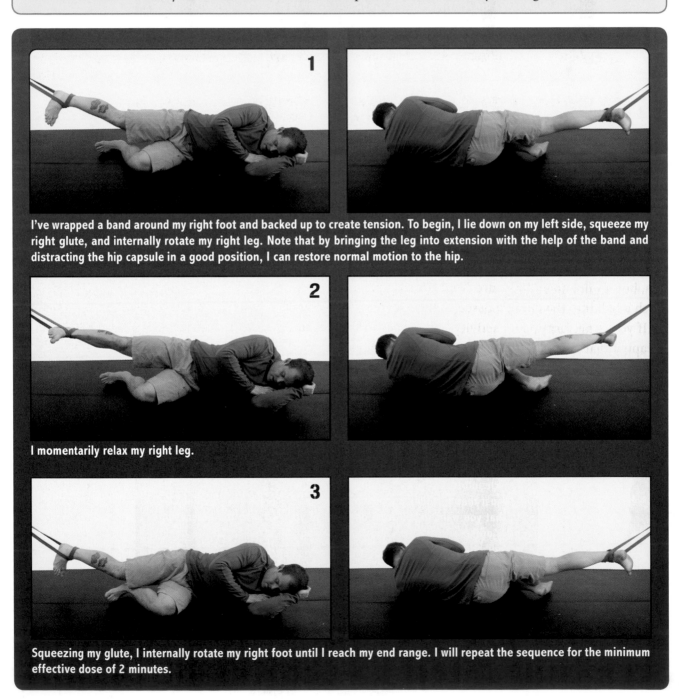

1

I've wrapped a band around my right foot and backed up to create tension. To begin, I lie down on my left side, squeeze my right glute, and internally rotate my right leg. Note that by bringing the leg into extension with the help of the band and distracting the hip capsule in a good position, I can restore normal motion to the hip.

2

I momentarily relax my right leg.

3

Squeezing my glute, I internally rotate my right foot until I reach my end range. I will repeat the sequence for the minimum effective dose of 2 minutes.

BANDED HIP

One more time: If you're an athlete who spends a lot of time seated—whether it's in a chair, in a car, or on a bicycle—you've got to spend your time mobilizing the front of your hip. Although I always opt for the couch stretch to lengthening the tissues, this is another simple yet effective mobilization technique that you can implement if you have access to a band. Just as in the couch stretch, the key is to maintain a neutral posture as you drive your hips forward. Most athletes have a very hard time keeping a neutral posture, causing them to lose form and overextend as they try to open up their hips. To prevent this from happening, your upper body and pelvis need to feel as if they are fused into solidarity and you need to engage your glutes with as much force as possible. Another important aspect of this technique is distracting the hip into a good position before you shift forward to initiate the stretch. If you glance at the photos, you'll notice that I start by loading back, squeezing my glutes, and then slowly pressing forward with a stable trunk. With the band pulling the head of the femur into the front of the socket I can ease in and out of tension, open the hip into full extension, and floss all of the tissue that is limiting the front of my leg.

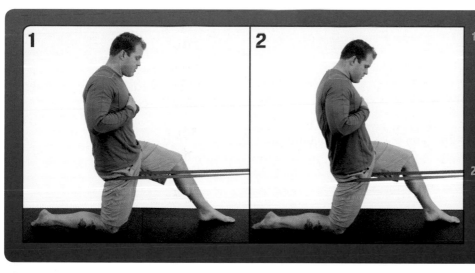

1. I've created a distraction of the hip by wrapping a band around the back of my right leg. With my hip in a good position, I load my weight back and squeeze my right glute to establish proper lumbar positioning.

2. Keeping my glute and my core engaged to maintain a neutral posture, I shift my weight forward and open my hips.

Common Fault: Overextension

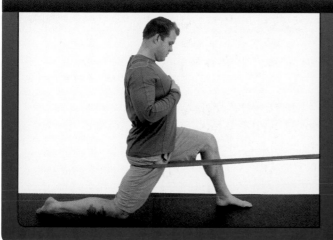

If you don't address your lumbar spine by engaging your glutes, opening your hips with a stable trunk is difficult. The tendency in such a situation is to overextend, which reduces the effectiveness of the technique. To perform this stretch correctly, you need to maintain a neutral posture and open your hips with a stable trunk by keeping your core and glutes engaged.

COUCH MOBILIZATION

One of the central themes of the Movement and Mobility Method is to pinpoint your biggest area of weakness and work on restoring suppleness to it with daily maintenance. For the majority of endurance athletes, and athletes in general, the anterior hip usually demands the most attention. Endurance athletes spend a lot of time in slightly flexed positions, causing the front of their hips to get extremely short. It takes a lot of time to restore suppleness to compromised areas, and to get the job done you have to be consistent. The challenge is to fit daily mobility into your already hectic training and work schedule. You have to find opportunities to sneak it in. Whether you're hanging out watching TV, waiting for a flight at an airport, or just drinking your morning coffee, don't waste your time sitting down. Throw your leg against the back of the chair or wall and start mobilizing the front of your hip. This is how the couch mobilization originated. It's one of the nastiest and most aggressive mobilization stretches you can implement and lies at the core of the supple leopard program. If there is one thing that you should do every day, it's the couch mobilization.

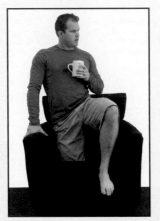

Although you're never restricted to the movements illustrated in the photos, there are two main positions you want to hit. First, set up by putting your knee in the corner with your foot flush against the wall (or back of the couch) and then posting up on your opposite leg. With your arms supporting your upper body, engage your glutes and press your hip into extension. At this point, most of you will feel a big mobilization stretch. From here, you can start hunting for stiff areas by moving laterally or driving forward into some crazy positions. The key is to keep your lumbar protected and your midline stabilized with a tightly squeezed core and butt. After you've spent some time hanging out in the first position, lift your torso into an upright position. This will increase the tension of the stretch by forcing your leg into deep flexion and driving your hip into full extension. Remember: Keep your butt squeezed as you lift your torso upright to avoid losing form. If you relax or give into the pain, you'll immediately overextend, which is never o.k.

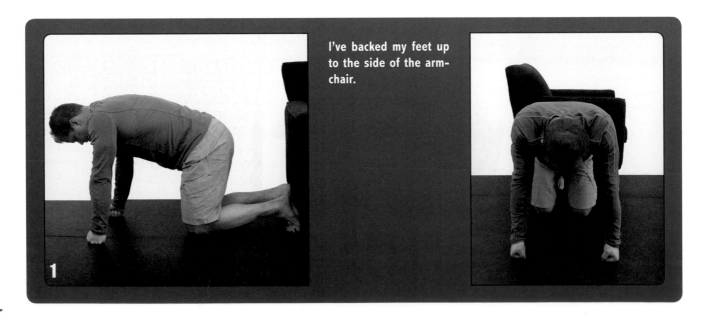

I've backed my feet up to the side of the arm-chair.

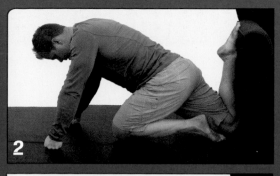

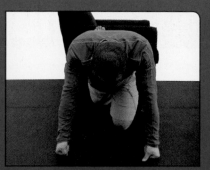

I slide my right leg back and position my right shin and foot flush with the side of the chair.

2

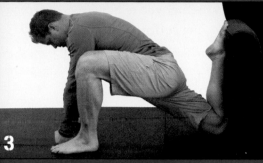

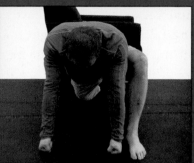

Squeezing my butt to stabilize my lower back, I post up on my left foot, keeping my shin vertical, and drive my hips forward.

3

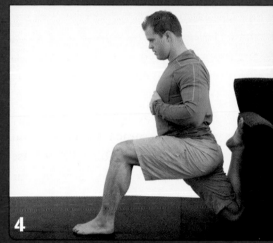

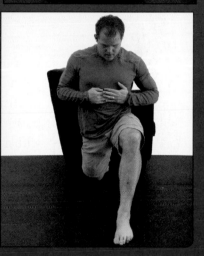

After hanging out in the previous position for a minute or two, I lift my torso into the upright position. It's important to mention that sometimes it's difficult to support the weight of your upper body from the upright position. If that happens, position a chair, box, or bench in front of you for extra stability.

4

Common Fault: Overextension

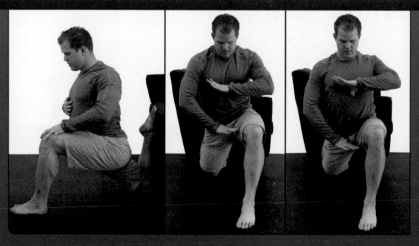

If you don't squeeze your butt to stabilize your lumbar spine, you're going to naturally overextend. Because the stretch can be pretty painful, sometimes it can be difficult to feel yourself overextend. In such a situation, implement the two-hand test to ensure a neutral posture: Place one hand on your sternum and the other on the top of your pelvis. Keeping your hands flat and as straight as possible, lift your torso into the second position. If your hands remain parallel to each other, you're in a neutral posture. If your hands separate and open, you're overextended.

PSOAS SMASH AND FLOSS

Before I discuss the upstream repercussions of compromised hip flexion, it's important to note that hip flexion is a function of your hip flexors working in conjunction with your psoas—which is responsible for stabilizing and flexing the base of the spine, as well as rotating the hips. So imagine that you're trying to pedal a bike, squat, or set up for an Olympic lift with a hip that won't let you to bring your knee above hip level. To make up for the lack of range, you have to feed slack to the system. In this particular scenario, the only way you can reach deep flexion is to yank on your psoas and pull yourself into overextension.

Need proof? Lie flat on your back and bring your knee to your chest. Unless you have a full range of motion, the moment you pass your end range—which for most of you is probably around 90 degrees—you'll notice that you immediately arch your back (i.e., overextend). This is your psoas overcompensating for your lack of hip flexion. Overextend repeatedly, and you're going to end up with a chronically tight psoas, which can cause a plethora of issues, including low back pain. The antidote is to not only lengthen and loosen the adhesions in the front of your hip, but to also release tension on your psoas.

Having already demonstrated several ways to restore suppleness to the front of your hips, I will now show you how to manage a tight psoas. The first option is to lie face down on a lacrosse ball, positioning the ball alongside your bellybutton and creating a pressure wave through that abdominal tissue by mashing back and forth. You can also smash and floss on a stiff area by curling your heel toward your butt and swinging your foot from side to side. To create additional pressure, simply take a big breath in through your belly as you roll over stiff areas. Another option is to lie on your back and use a kettlebell to drive the lacrosse ball deep into your psoas. From here, you can really tack the tissue down and move your leg in all kinds of directions. Remember, we live off our hip flexors and psoas all day long, so they're going to get tight. Don't wait for back pain to rear its ugly head—get in there and address your business.

Target Area

Here I'm demonstrating the target area. For the best results, you want to start just below your ribcage a couple of centimeters from your sternum and work your way down to your pelvis.

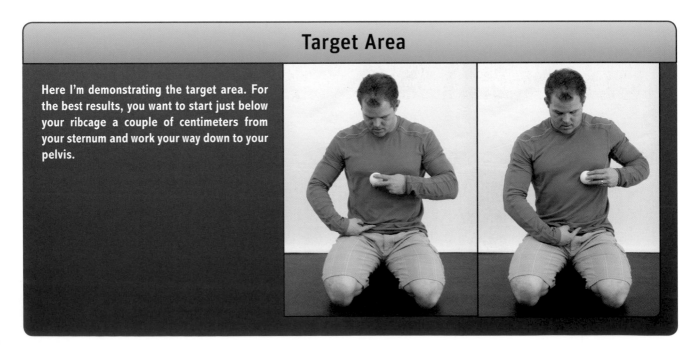

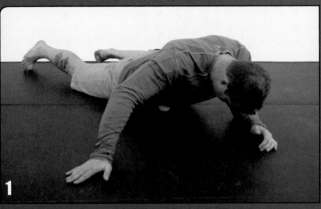

I'm lying face down on the lacrosse ball, positioning it just to the side of my bellybutton. To create maximum pressure, I keep my hips pressed to the ground and use my arms to support my upper body.

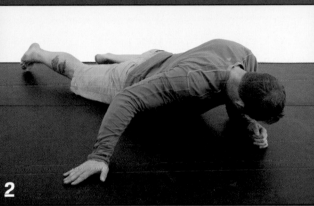

I mash the ball into my psoas and start rolling back and forth across the muscle.

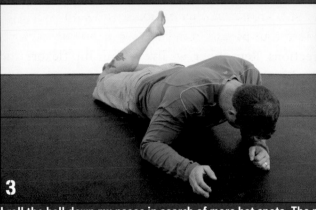
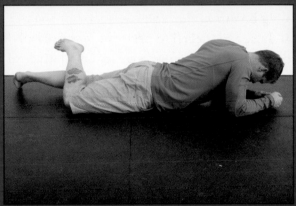

I roll the ball down my psoas in search of more hot spots. The moment I find a stiff area, I pin the ball in place, curl my right heel toward my butt, and rotate my leg toward my left side.

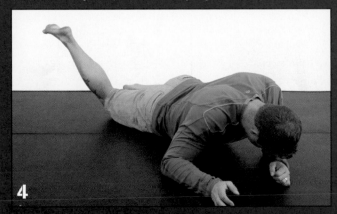
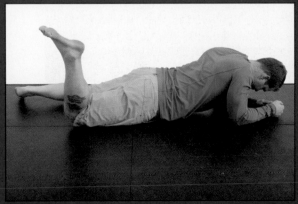

I continue to tack and stretch by moving my right leg toward my right side.

T-Spine and Shoulder Mobilization

It doesn't matter if you're running, cycling, swimming, or lifting—a neutral posture is critical to moving safely and efficiently. In order to achieve that goal, you not only have to activate your abdominal muscles and glutes, but also address your thoracic spine. If you're tight in the upper back, aligning your head over your spine and pulling your shoulders into a strong externally rotated position is difficult to manage. As a result, your posture will be compromised and you therefore won't be able to assume optimal form and perform with utmost efficiency.

T-SPINE SMASH

In order to improve the mechanical efficiency of your hips and set your shoulders and head in the proper position, you have to make sure your thoracic spine is in the game. If your upper back rounds, it's going to have a domino effect up and down the kinetic chain. For example, a tight thoracic spine puts a lot of stress on the lumbar spine, which can cause lower-back pain and reduce proper hip function. If you're looking upstream, a stiff upper back can cause a number of movement faults in the head and shoulders: it can, for example, make your head jut out, leading to serious neck pain. It will also limit your ability to raise your arms overhead, affecting your ability to swim or press.

Fortunately there is an easy way to mobilize those tissues and restore a normal range of motion to your back. By taping two lacrosse balls together, as demonstrated below, you can create a very low tech and inexpensive mobility tool that can be used to restore normal range to the thoracic spine. It's important to note that the single lacrosse ball can be used effectively on the ribs, shoulder blades, and other areas of the back, but not to mobilize the spine. To restore suppleness to your thoracic spine, you need to block the facet joints—which are the weight-bearing stabilizing structures located behind and between the adjacent vertebrae—using two lacrosse balls. In the sequence below, I demonstrate the proper placement of the balls when you start and finish the mobilization. The key is to not roll hastily up and down the back without purpose. Instead, you need to block the motion segment of the vertebrae using the double balls, extend over that segment, hang out for as long as it takes to feel a difference in the tissues—which in this case would be 1 to 2 minutes—and then move on to the next segment. Just as with all the mobilization exercises, hang out where it hurts, roll on past the areas that don't.

Peanut LAX Ball

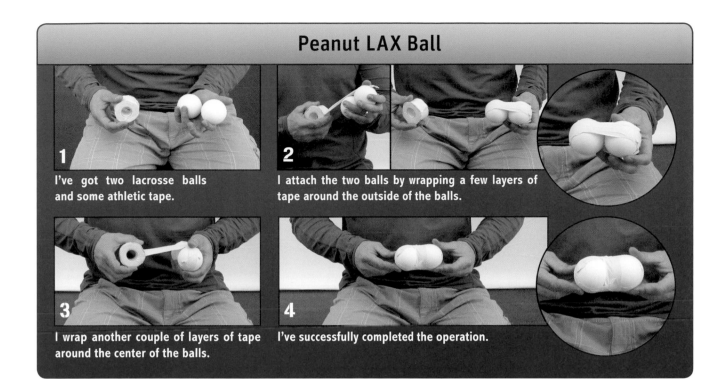

1 I've got two lacrosse balls and some athletic tape.

2 I attach the two balls by wrapping a few layers of tape around the outside of the balls.

3 I wrap another couple of layers of tape around the center of the balls.

4 I've successfully completed the operation.

Target Area

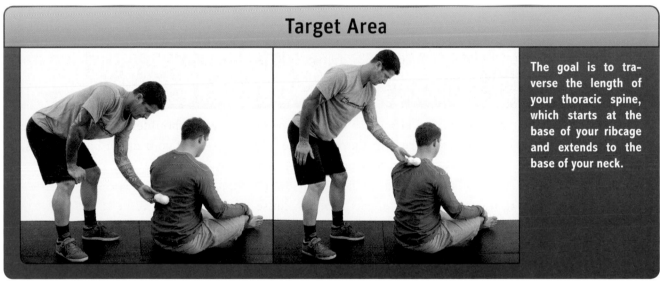

The goal is to traverse the length of your thoracic spine, which starts at the base of your ribcage and extends to the base of your neck.

Option 1: Body Hug

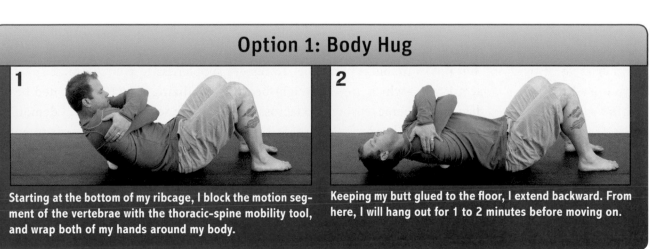

1 Starting at the bottom of my ribcage, I block the motion segment of the vertebrae with the thoracic-spine mobility tool, and wrap both of my hands around my body.

2 Keeping my butt glued to the floor, I extend backward. From here, I will hang out for 1 to 2 minutes before moving on.

OVERHEAD T-SPINE MOBILIZATION

Another add-on to the body hug is to raise your arms overhead as you extend over the blocked segment. There are two things going on here: we're trying to mobilize the upper back, and we're trying to get the arms into a good position. As I've repeatedly stated, you always want to mobilize within the context of movements. Simply hugging your arms across your chest will definitely mobilize the back, but you're not really mobilizing all of the tissues in the context of the movement. For example, if you're swimming or pressing anything overhead with a stiff upper back, chances are you're going to overextend and lose form. The only way to express that ideal position is to mobilize in the positions that you're going to find yourself in. For the best results, I recommend combining the two exercises. First, hug your body and extend over that blocked segment. Then, after your back is loosened up, return to the starting position and extend back while slowly raising your arms overhead, hanging out for as long as possible before moving on to the next segment.

Option 2: Arm Flexion

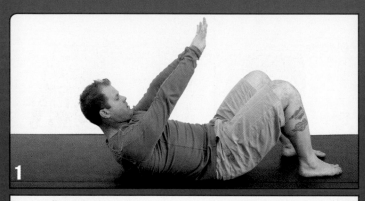

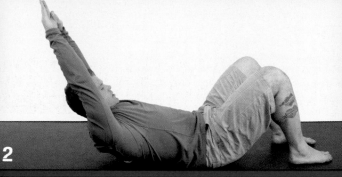

Starting at the base of my ribcage, I block the motion segment of the vertebrae with the thoracic-spine mobility tool and extend my arms.

I bring my arms overhead as I extend backward.

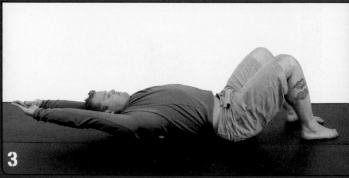

Keeping my butt glued to the ground, I extend backward and pull my arms overhead. Just as in the previous technique, I will hang out for 1 to 2 minutes before progressing to the next segment.

OVERHEAD RIB MOBILIZATION

If the shoulder blades are stiff, you're not going to be able get them into a good position. And if you can't, raising your arms overhead—which is necessary for swimming and strength-and-conditioning exercises like the press—puts you at risk for an overtension injury. To prevent such a situation, restore suppleness to the area using the technique below. If you glance at the photos, you'll notice that I place the ball on my first rib where it meets my scapula. The goal is to drive the ball into your ribs between the scapula and your spine and bring your arm overhead, which will allow you to open the shoulder and restore suppleness to the joint and surrounding tissue. When this mobilization is done correctly, the test/retest offers dramatic results. For an accurate comparison, mobilize one of your shoulders, stand up, and then raise both of your arms overhead. I suspect that you will be pleasantly surprised: the discrepancy in range of motion between the two sides will be shocking.

Target Area

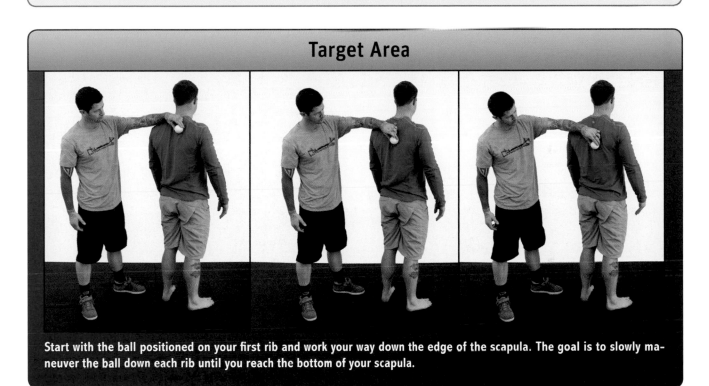

Start with the ball positioned on your first rib and work your way down the edge of the scapula. The goal is to slowly maneuver the ball down each rib until you reach the bottom of your scapula.

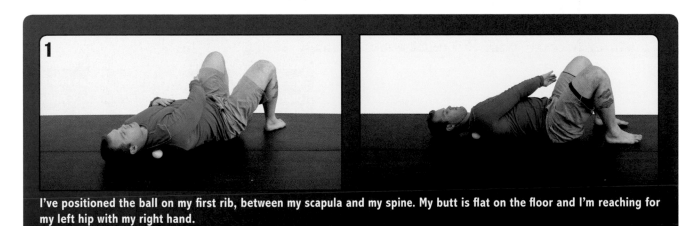

1

I've positioned the ball on my first rib, between my scapula and my spine. My butt is flat on the floor and I'm reaching for my left hip with my right hand.

2

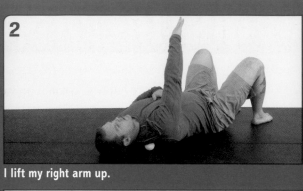 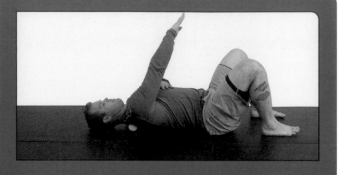

I lift my right arm up.

3

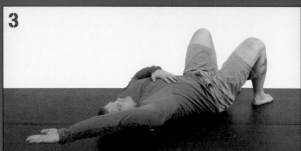 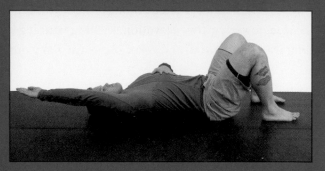

I extend my right arm completely overhead.

4

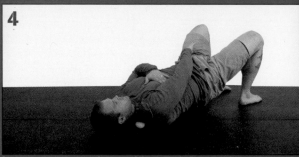 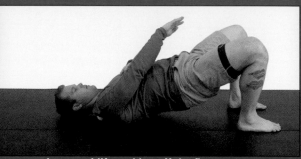

I return to my starting position. To increase the pressure, I engage my glutes and lift my hips off the floor.

5

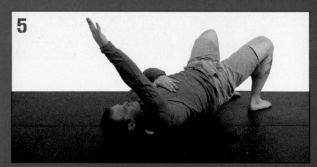 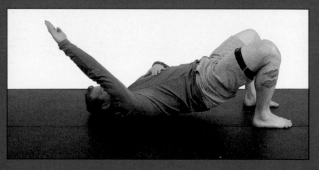

Keeping my hips elevated, I begin to raise my arm overhead.

6

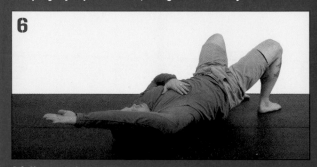 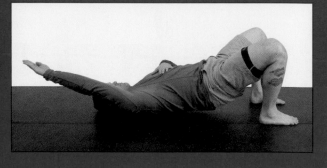

I fully extend my right arm overhead.

BANDED OVERHEAD DISTRACTION

In this sequence, I demonstrate an arm distraction overhead, which will restore external rotation and flexion range of motion to the shoulder. Think about pressing something overhead, the entry and catch phase of the swim stroke, and the ideal running stance. To correctly execute this technique, hook your wrist through a resistance band, step back to create tension, and then externally rotate your hand by reaching your palm toward the ceiling. If you're unable to do this by rotating your arm, you can use your opposite hand to manually rotate the other arm. The key is to get your armpit facing forward so that you can bias the lat and shoulder. Once accomplished, you can start hunting for sensitive areas by sweeping from side to side, lowering your elevation, kicking your leg back, etc. Like all the tissue-lengthening mobilizations, you want to contract and relax and really hang out in positions that bias stiff areas.

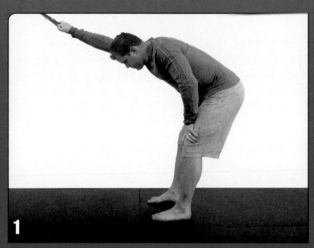

1 I've hooked my right wrist through the resistance band and created tension by sinking my hips back.

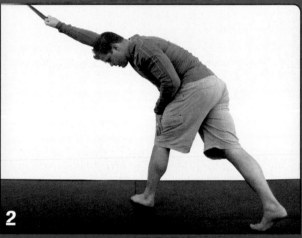

2 Keeping my back flat, I slide my right foot back and toward my left side.

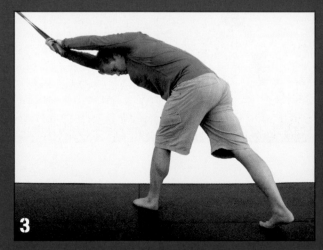

3 To achieve the ideal position, I need to externally rotate my right arm with my palm facing the ceiling. To accomplish this, I grab the top of my right hand with my left hand and move my hand into external rotation.

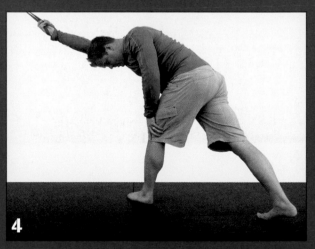

4 With my right palm facing the ceiling and my right armpit facing forward, I can start hunting for tight areas by bending my knees, sweeping my body from side to side, reversing my stance, etc.

BANDED BULLY

In the sequence below, I demonstrate a highly effective technique for opening the shoulder and restoring internal rotation. The key is to distract the shoulder into a good position using a band. A lot of people make the mistake of rolling the shoulder forward when they execute this technique, or similar stretches that bias internal rotation. Hooking a resistance band around the front of the shoulder and creating tension by walking forward prevents this from happening.

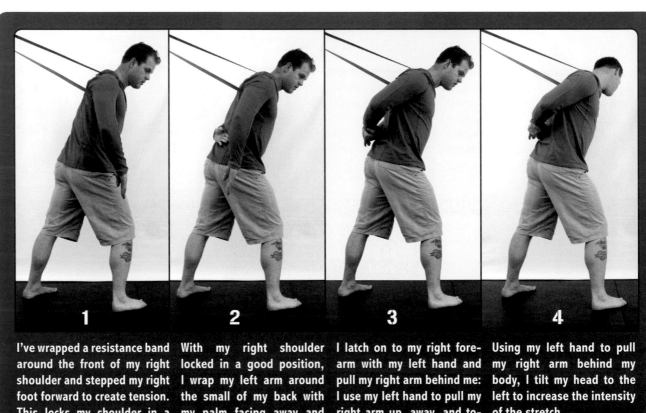

1

I've wrapped a resistance band around the front of my right shoulder and stepped my right foot forward to create tension. This locks my shoulder in a good position and keeps me from rolling my shoulder forward as I initiate the stretch.

2

With my right shoulder locked in a good position, I wrap my left arm around the small of my back with my palm facing away and pull my right arm behind my body.

3

I latch on to my right forearm with my left hand and pull my right arm behind me: I use my left hand to pull my right arm up, away, and toward my left.

4

Using my left hand to pull my right arm behind my body, I tilt my head to the left to increase the intensity of the stretch.

SUPER-FRIEND INTERNAL-ROTATION BIAS

The biggest mistake you can make when you can't get into an ideal position due to a lack of mobility is to buffer the movement using faulty mechanics. Although this problem is not limited to shoulder issues, compensating for missing range of motion is very common among athletes who have limited internal rotation in the shoulders. For example, if you notice that your shoulder rolls forward—whether you're swinging your arm back when you run, dropping down to do a push-up, or transitioning into the recovery phase of the swimming stroke—you have to restore normal range of motion to the joint before the problem becomes an injury that is difficult to get rid of.

To execute the mobilization technique demonstrated below, you're going to have to recruit a super-friend. His role is to simply anchor your shoulders to the ground so that you can mobilize from an optimized position. If you don't have access to a super-friend and you attempt this technique on your own, chances are that your shoulders will roll forward the moment you initiate the stretch, which reduces its effectiveness. In such a situation, implementing the previous mobilization is your best bet. Although this mobilization technique requires the assistance of a super-friend, it is an easy way to restore internal rotation to the shoulders.

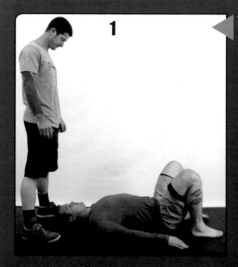

1. Brian is standing above me. I'm trying my best not to look up his shorts and make things weird.

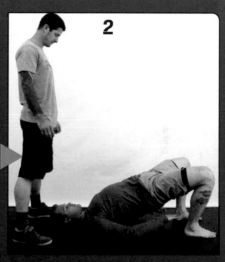

2. I lift my butt off the ground and maneuver both of my hands (palms down) under the small of my back.

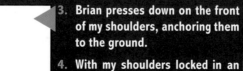

3. Brian presses down on the front of my shoulders, anchoring them to the ground.

4. With my shoulders locked in an ideal position, I lower my butt to the ground. It's important to note that as you lower your butt down, you should feel an enormous mobilization force. The key with this technique is to stop lowering your butt the moment you feel your shoulders trying to come off the ground.

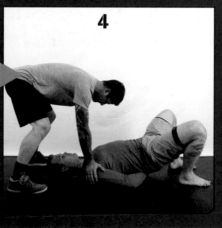

FUELING PROTOCOL

A desiccating wind howls across a great bowl of desert, lower than the sea, hotter, it would seem, than hell. For the ultra runners competing in Badwater, an event so extreme that it may be less a race than it is a crucible, the point of preparation is not so much to win, but to finish, and survive.

The race is held in the middle of July with temperatures reaching a blistering 120 degrees at head height, which means that inches off the desert floor it's hot enough to melt a pair of trainers. While racers perspire copiously, their sweat quickly vanishes into the hot, dry air. Their skin dries as they lose moisture to sweat, their tongues grow swollen, nausea and dizziness set in as they struggle to remain hydrated and fight off heatstroke.

These are the conditions for the infamous Badwater Ultramarathon, where elite runners push themselves to, and beyond the edge of, failure in a 135-mile race through Death Valley National Park in California. Athletes repetitively mention training, heart, skill, and physique as the means to legendary sports achievements, but the smart coach knows that any physical gift is rendered meaningless out here. What matters most doesn't grab the headlines, but it will save your life; that missing component is hydration nutrition.

It's not only in Death Valley where diet, hydration, electrolyte management, and nutrition count; whether you're running at altitude in the dead of winter, at sea level in the Mojave, or simply training on the beach, if you push yourself hard, you can and will fall prey to nutritive deficiency. You can be the most technically skilled athlete on the planet, but unless you understand smart race planning and follow intelligent fueling protocol, performing at your potential—whether it's in training or competition—is impossible.

It's like this: You can run with lousy form and the worst that's going to happen is that you'll get tired faster and wind up with some kind of injury, but if you eat poorly, don't drink enough water, or fail to manage electrolyte balance, you can literally die. Among high school athletes, heat-related illnesses are the third most common cause of death. If you're racing the Badwater Ultra, death by heatstroke might take only an hour.

In this book, we've provided blueprints for the Pose Method of running, swimming, and cycling mechanics; CrossFit; and Starrett's Movement and Mobility Method—all of which are tools to make you a more efficient, less-injury-prone, endurance athlete. Up to now we've been looking at the body from the outside in, meaning we've addressed performance using the language of movement and programming principles. To conclude this conversation we have to address the flip side of the performance coin, which means talking about nutrition, hydration, and electrolyte balance.

It should come as no big surprise that what you put into your body has a direct effect on how you look, feel, and perform. So it follows that you would want to put the most efficient fuel into your tank to optimize those three fitness parameters. It's like this: Your body operates just like any other machine that metabolizes fuel into usable energy. If the fuel runs out, the machine stops working. And if you put something in the machine that it isn't designed to process, it either compromises the machine's ability to function at optimal levels or it breaks down. The human machine—although infinitely more complex—operates in much the same manner, in that it needs a certain level and quality of fuel to function optimally.

Which is to say: If you don't eat properly, hydrate well, and keep your electrolytes in balance, it doesn't matter how technically proficient you are—your performance is going to suffer.

Before I delve into each fueling component, I have to mention that this chapter is not meant to be an exhaustive scientific analysis of diet and hydration. Rather, my goal is to outline the general principles advocated for all CrossFit Endurance athletes. Performance is the driving factor. However, just as each person's training program is individualized, hydration and nutrition needs are different from person to person. Finding the right balance requires a ton of personal experimentation and patience. My advice is to use the guidelines here to get started. If, after reading this chapter, you're hungry for more elaborate and comprehensive explanations, check out the resources in the back of the book.

To make this chapter easier to navigate, I've broken it up into three parts:

1) hydration

2) electrolyte balance

3) nutrition

HYDRATION

Drinking half your body weight in ounces of water has long been the general prescription for athletes: if you weigh 150 pounds, you would drink 75 ounces of water everyday. Although this is not a bad start to dealing with hydration, it's not entirely comprehensive. It doesn't address the energy demands of the athlete (calories burned), the environment (temperature), or more important, the individual. For example, what if you sweat twice as much as someone who weighs the same amount as you do? Or what if you hardly sweat at all? So, drinking half your body weight in water, drinking seven to eight glasses of water a day, or drinking 18 ounces of water for every hour of training are not rules that can be applied to everyone.

Hydration, like every other aspect of training, is a skill that is part science and part self-experimentation. To fine-tune your own personal hydration protocol and understand how to apply it before, during, and after a race or training session, you first have to know what it means to be fully hydrated.

For tangible evidence of whether you're drinking enough water, simply examine the color of your urine. If your urine is clear, and your trips to the bathroom are recurrent (three to five times a day), chances are you're fully hydrated. On the other hand, if your urine is dark yellow, has an odor, and your trips to the bathroom are infrequent, chances are you're not fully hydrated. Note that vitamin supplements can cause urine to darken, so it's important to monitor frequently to ensure that you're hydrated if this is your experience.

Knowing when you're dehydrated is a little trickier because of the lag time. Thirst is the first indication that you need to hydrate, but that sensation comes too late when you're training or competing. In other words, the feeling of being thirsty is usually a sign that you're already fairly dehydrated. It takes time for your body to process water and hydrate cells, so if you start a training session or race dehydrated, chances are your performance is going to be affected.

Remember, you're constantly losing water through respiration, urination, and perspiration, making it extremely important that you constantly drink water throughout the day. In fact, it's not uncommon to lose up to a pint of water between the time you go to bed and the time you wake up. To help you appreciate the significance of dehydration as it relates to performance, you first have to understand that the human body is about 70 percent water. Furthermore, muscle cells hold up to seven times more water than fat cells, which means that water will account for a larger percentage of a lean, muscular athlete's body weight than for an overweight couch potato's. So if you're a lean athlete with little body fat and you get dehydrated, your body will start to burn muscle because you don't have enough fat to burn, resulting in depleted muscle power and endurance.

Dehydration can start to become a major problem with as little as a 3 percent loss of fluid. At this point, research indicates that we lose about 10 percent of our performance potential. So if you're a 150-pound athlete, and you lose 4.5 pounds of water before a race, you can perform only at a max of 90 percent of your potential. A study conducted at Ball State University showed a 7 percent drop in speed over 10 kilometers by runners who were dehydrated by just 2 to 3 percent. With that in mind, there should be no question of the importance of being hydrated at the start of a training session or event. But what about staying hydrated during an event? As it turns out, speed, time, and distance affect water intake during training or a race.

Here's an example: Say you're running a 10K race or doing a 60-minute training session. If you're working at maximum capacity for that entire 60 minutes, consuming enough water to compensate for your sweat loss is difficult. Not only that, consuming water within that window can slow you down and negatively impact your performance. Think of trying to down water while running a sub-six-minute-mile pace. As long as you're hydrated going into the race or training session, if it's less than 60 minutes (assuming it's a max-effort affair) you won't experience a noticeable impact on your performance. However, in such a situation it's important to know how much water was lost so that you can refuel and recover immediately after your race or workout. The best way to address your personal hydration needs is to perform the sweat-rate test.

Sweat-Rate Test

1) Make sure you're fully hydrated.

2) Weigh in right before you train or race.
   Note: Weighing in without clothes is recommended to ensure accuracy.

3) Perform a time-trial effort at race pace.

4) Weigh in immediately after you train. Again: Weigh yourself without clothes to ensure accuracy.

5) For every pound lost you need to drink at least 16 ounces of water. So if you weighed in at 150 pounds before the time trial and 145 pounds after, you need to drink 80 ounces of water. And to that total, add the amount of water you consumed during your effort.

NOTE: *You should do a weigh-in before you go to bed and when you wake up to show you how much water is lost through respiration and sweat during the night.*

Hydration protocol for efforts longer than 60 minutes becomes increasingly difficult and is largely dependent on the individual. However, as a general rule, for athlete's training/racing longer than 60 minutes, if the temperature is 72 to 76 degrees, 16 to 20 ounces per hour is an adequate target. Again, this is subjective to the individual and should be tested prior to competition in climate-controlled environments. (To confirm targets for higher temperatures, please visit the consumption calculator at www.gssiweb.com/FluidLoss.aspx).

In summary, the best way to address your hydration needs is to make sure you're drinking enough water throughout the day, experiment and test your hydration levels using the sweat-rate test, pay attention to urine color and frequency, and train in an environment that simulates race conditions.

Hydration Highlights

✳ Make sure you're drinking water frequently throughout the day. Carry a water bottle with you wherever you go and drink from it often. Staying hydrated is not only important for your performance, but also prevents grogginess, headaches, and midday crashes that compromise energy and productivity.

✳ Don't wait until you're thirsty to start drinking water. If you're thirsty, you're probably already moderately dehydrated so grab a bottle of water and start guzzling!

✱ Take in an ample amount of fluids a couple of hours before training or a race to ensure adequate hydration. Taking in additional electrolytes in the form of food or supplementation is also highly recommended during the two-hour window before training or a race.

✱ To address your personal hydration needs, perform the sweat-rate test before and after training. You should also do a weigh-in just before bed and when you wake up in the morning.

✱ Water intake during training/racing depends on time and speed. For athletes training/racing longer than an hour, the minimum requirement for hydration is generally 16 to 20 ounces (or more) per hour, and can be as much as 35 to 40 ounces in extreme conditions.

✱ The key is to drink water steadily throughout the day rather than pound a gallon in one sitting. This is especially important during long races. If the target is 20 ounces of water an hour, drink 5 ounces every 20 minutes.

✱ Hydration and water loss (dehydration) varies from person to person. Find out what your personal hydration needs are. Catalog and experiment using the aforementioned methods, and test yourself in the appropriate conditions.

✱ To start your day off right, drink 16 to 20 ounces of water (or more) the moment you wake up (before your morning coffee) to replenish water lost during the night.

Dehydration Levels

☐ **Less than 3 percent:** manageable loss (performance is affected).

☐ **4 to 6 percent:** sleepiness, headaches, nausea, tingling in arms (performance and reaction time are affected).

☐ **10 to 15 percent:** muscles lose control, hearing impairment, dim vision (central nervous system and motor skills are affected).

☐ **15 percent:** death.

CARDIAC DRIFT by Dr. Brian Austin-Hicke

Cardiac drift is a physiological phenomenon that can occur in conjunction with dehydration. In this condition, heart rate increases as you become dehydrated because blood volume decreases and less blood is pumped with each heartbeat. Blood volume is defined as the amount of fluid in the circulatory system. Blood is approximately 50 percent water (Kraemer, Fleck, and Deschenes, 2012).

In hot, humid environments, cardiac drift can begin after 20 minutes of moderate-intensity steady-state training (Coyle and Gonzalez-Alonzo, 2001), which means that given a constant pace, heart rate increases as you become dehydrated. Coyle and Gonzales-Alonzo found that heart rate increases seven beats per minute for each 1 percent loss in body weight from dehydration. A steady-state, or constant-pace, hour run in 70-degree heat can result in a water loss of 1.5 to 3 pounds. For a 150-pound athlete, this translates to a body-weight loss of 1 to 2 percent. This, in turn, will increase heart rate by approximately 7 to 14 beats per minute. If this athlete maintains an 8-minute-mile pace for an hour run, and his starting heart rate is 150 beats per minute, at the end of the run his heart rate will be 157 to 164bpm.

In summary, dehydration increases the strain on an already taxed cardiovascular system, which will ultimately compromise performance.

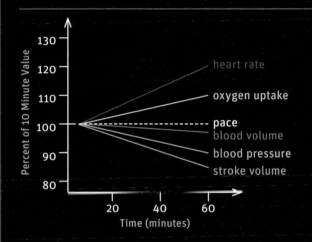

The Effect of Cardiac Drift in a Hydrated State on Key Physiological Measures

Adapted from Coyle & Gonzales-Alonso (2001)

Contributing Factors Decreasing Aerobic Performance Associated with Dehydration

(Kraemer, Fleck, and Deschenes, 2012)

Metabolic

- Decreased peak VO2
+ Increased blood-lactate levels
- Decreased lactate threshold
+ Increased glycogen use

Cardiovascular

- Decreased blood volume
- Decreased blood pressure
+ Increased heart rate (HR)
- Decreased stroke volume (SV)
- Decreased cardiac output (HR x SV)

Thermoregulation

+ Increased core temperature
- Decreased sweat rate
- Decreased skin blood flow

References

Coyle, E.F., and Gonzalez-Alonzo, J. 2001. "Cardiovascular Drift During Prolonged Exercise: New Perspectives." *Exercise and Sports Sciences Review*, 29(2): 88-92.

Kraemer, W.J.; Fleck, S.J.; and Deschenes, M.R. 2012. *Exercise Physiology*. Philadelphia: Wolters Kluwer.

ELECTROLYTES

Electrolytes—which include sodium (Na), chloride (Cl), potassium (K), magnesium (Mg), and calcium (Ca)—are minerals that are not only responsible for water retention, but also allow nerve transmission, muscle contraction, muscle relaxation, glycogen formation, ATP production, bone health, and more. Put simply, electrolytes are the glue for your hydration strategy. In order for your body to function properly and absorb the fluid you take in, you have to maintain a healthy electrolyte balance either through the food you eat or supplementation. However, just as with water, which can be dangerous when over- or underconsumed, you need to understand how to manage electrolytes in endurance efforts based on your exertion, sweat loss, and water intake. If electrolyte levels become too low or too high, your performance will suffer, and you may also suffer from more severe conditions, such as hypernatremia and hyponatremia.

- ☐ **Hypernatremia** is caused when sodium in the blood reaches extremely high levels. While overconsumption of sodium can be the main factor in this condition, it is usually associated with dehydration. As water leaves the body, sodium levels increase, causing dehydration. Hypernatremia can also be a result of eating something extremely high in salt or ingesting massive quantities of electrolytes, which is why you get thirsty after eating salty food—your body is instinctively seeking balance.

- ☐ **Hyponatremia** is caused by sodium loss in the blood from underconsumption of electrolytes, usually as a result of drinking too much water. Put simply, if you haven't maintained a healthy electrolyte balance, your body has a tough time absorbing water. This is characterized by what is commonly referred to as "slosh gut," which is when your stomach is full of water but your body can't absorb the fluid as fast as you're taking it in. This sodium-free blood travels to the brain, saturates brain cells, causing the brain to swell. In extreme cases, this can be fatal. Although this condition is rare and limited to novice endurance athletes, you still have to be careful. To prevent this from happening, be sure to add salts to your real food diet and supplement with electrolytes/salts for any effort longer than an hour.

While a blood test will give you an instantaneous snapshot of electrolyte levels, it's not very practical for day-to-day management. If you're eating a healthy diet—meaning you're consuming lean meats, vegetables, and some fruit—you don't cramp during extended efforts, and you're meeting your hydration needs, chances are your electrolytes are in balance. Conversely, if you cramp up during training sessions or at night after workouts, you could be deficient in electrolytes. This can also be a conditioning issue, meaning that your body has not quite adapted to the stress of the high-intensity or stamina-based training. In such a situation, you either need to lower the training volume or up your electrolyte intake.

To gauge how to replace electrolytes after a training session or race, use the sweat-rate test outlined in the hydration section of this chapter. Once you have confirmed your total weight loss, you can then correlate each pound lost with the following loss in electrolytes. Again, this is a general guideline and varies for everyone.

- 220 mg of sodium
- 63 mg of potassium
- 8 mg of magnesium
- 16 mg of calcium

The best way to replace these levels is through the consumption of real foods, such as lean meats, vegetables, fruits, and tubers, which have appropriate levels of nutrients and minerals. It's important to note, however, that when training intensifies or during extended efforts, you'll have to take supplements. When exploring this option, be sure to avoid supplements with an electrolyte replacement that has sugar or high-glycemic-index carbohydrates (simple sugars). Experiment with various products and stick with what works best for you.

Electrolyte Highlights

✳ Electrolyte balance is critical for performance and proper body functions. These minerals help retain water throughout your body, including in your muscles.

✳ Electrolyte management can be very personal and can vary dramatically from athlete to athlete. However, as a general guideline, drinking just water during the first hour of training or a race is fine. After that, you need to start supplementing with electrolytes. This will prevent hypernatremia, nausea, and cramping.

✳ The best way to confirm your electrolyte needs is to perform a sweat-rate test.

✳ Electrolytes can be taken in through food, liquid, or supplementation. Be sure to include salts in your diet, especially before/after training or a race. In terms of supplements, we have found SaltStick to work very well. It can be purchased at CrossFit Endurance's online store (http://www.crossfitendurance.com) or on SaltStick's Website (http://www.saltstick.com/), which has an incredible amount of information on electrolyte supplementation.

GENERAL FUELING PROTOCOLS

EVENT: 1 TO 2 HOURS

- Primary fuel is glycogen (depending on intensity of event for the individual).
- Hydration goal should be 16 to 20 ounces per hour with temperatures under 80 degrees Fahrenheit.

EVENT: 2 TO 4 HOURS

- Glycogen is depleted (this is a clue that nutrition planning needs to happen long before this point).
- Fueling transitions from glycogen to glucose and fat.
- Electrolytes take a larger role and must be used in the form of supplementation if salt is not added to the food.
- Have a target of specific fuels that work for YOU and stick to it.
  1. Fats: good fat vs. bad fat, medium-chain triglycerides?
  2. Protein: What sources are optimal for you: chicken breast, whey, casein?
  3. SaltSticks, gels, etc.

EVENT: 4 HOURS+

- Intensity trends lower.
- Fat becomes primary source of fuel.
- Carbohydrate consumption must continue if you already started.
- Electrolytes must be replaced by 500 to 2,000 mg per hour.

EVENT: 12 TO 18 HOURS+

- Carbohydrate burning contributes less at lower, more intense levels.
- Protein is a necessity.
- Fat produces most of the energy.
- Electrolytes and hydration guidelines remain the same as 4 to 12-hour markers, meaning electrolyte management does not typically change during these time frames.

NUTRITION

As I have mentioned, nutrition is the foundation on which your athletic potential is built. In other words, how you look, feel, and perform is predicated not only on an intelligently-structured training program, but also on an intelligently-structured eating, drinking, and supplementing regime. However, finding a plan that accelerates performance while improving overall health can be challenging, especially because nutrition is a complicated and hotly debated topic and everyone is different and has different needs. Fortunately, my recommendations are really simple—perhaps difficult to follow for some, but simple. Here they are:

Eat This:

- ☐ Grass-fed meat

- ☐ Free-range chicken (fowl)

- ☐ Wild-caught fish

- ☐ Seasonal/local and organic vegetables

- ☐ Seasonal/local and organic fruits

- ☐ Seasonal/local and organic seeds and nuts

- ☐ Seasonal/local and organic tubers (sweet potatoes)

- ☐ Medium-chain fats (coconut oil, olive oil, avocados)

Don't Eat This:

- **X** Industrialized meat products (grain-fed)

- **X** Processed, refined, genetically modified products (generally anything packaged in a bag or box)

- **X** Grains (wheat, oats, barley, corn, rice, and rye)

- **X** Dairy (milk, cheese, yogurt)

- **X** Legumes (beans, soy, and lentils)

- **X** Vegetable oils

- **X** Sugar and sugar substitutes

The **bottom line:** Eat real food in its most natural state and avoid anything that is manufactured, processed, or refined. Although there are several diets that revolve around eating "real food," the Paleo diet—which was founded by Dr. Loren Cordain and popularized with the help of *New York Times* best-selling author Robb Wolf—encompasses my recommendations to endurance athletes looking to optimize performance and health. Moreover, the Paleo diet dovetails nicely with my overall philosophy of working with the laws of nature—moving in biomechanically efficient positions, eating food that our bodies are evolutionarily designed to digest.

Most people are aware that eating clean, whole food from organic sources is a step toward better health and longevity, as well as increased performance and recovery. But maybe the reason for cutting out grains, dairy, and legumes isn't as clear.

Gluten is a protein found in wheat and other grains. When ingested, gluten damages the lining of the small intestine, compromising one's ability to absorb vital nutrients, and has been found to cause a multitude of problems, which include but are not limited to: acid indigestion, abdominal pain, fatigue, and diarrhea. People with celiac disease, which is an autoimmune disorder, are highly sensitive to gluten and have severe reactions when exposed to it.

Lectins are proteins that are most commonly found in grains and legumes, and, like gluten, cause damage to the gut lining, leading to a host of problems. Lectins are the plant's defense mechanism against being eaten. Unfortunately, this has not deterred us. Lectins prevent our gut from healing, and in that state it can't absorb vital nutrients.

Dairy can also cause a number of problems, particularly in people who are lactose intolerant. While dairy products do contain some beneficial properties, they can cause an inflammatory response, similar to that of gluten, in some people. The easiest way to figure out if dairy is not your best friend, says Paleo guru Robb Wolf, is to completely cut it out of your diet for 30 days, allowing the gut to heal, and then slowly introduce it back in to your diet and pay attention to how your body responds: a negative reaction means you shouldn't be messing with that stuff.

Legumes have been shown to do what gluten and dairy do: cause irritation to the gut's lining, resulting in inflammation. Just like dairy, legumes are to be avoided if you're following the Paleo diet.

So why, aside from not being able to effectively process these foods, do I encourage cutting them out of your diet? It boils down to gut health and inflammation: If you eat something that wreaks havoc on your digestive system—whether it's in the form of gluten, dairy, or legumes—your ability to absorb nutrients and process food is severely compromised. So in addition to not getting all the nutrients your body needs to function at optimal levels, the damaged gut lining signals an inflammatory reaction, which causes a whole mess of performance-inhibiting issues, which include, but are not limited to: diarrhea, acid indigestion, sore joints, and fatigue. Not exactly ideal for training or racing.

It's important to note that this inflammatory reaction varies from person to person. For example, if a celiac is exposed to gluten, he or she will get extremely sick, while someone else may not feel anything. If you fall into the latter category and you're happy with how you look, feel, and perform, perhaps you don't need to make any dietary changes. However, if you think you can improve the way your body functions, I highly recommend sticking with real food and staying away from grains, dairy, and legumes.

Here's my point: There's no arguing that our bodies need clean protein, fat, and carbohydrates to function at optimal levels. Moreover, if you routinely expose yourself to processed foods on a daily basis, you'll never really know if your body is having a negative reaction to them or not. The only way to know for certain is to cut out all processed junk and give the Paleo diet a shot.

Robb Wolf recommends a 30-day complete buy-in, meaning no grains, legumes, and dairy and only real food for 30 days. Then assess how you look, feel, and perform. If want more scientific analysis, you can get a

INFLAMMATION AND PERFORMANCE

The body's inflammatory process, an amazing aspect of the immune system, is designed to protect us from invading microbes, chemicals, allergens, and physical trauma. Inflammation occurs at the peak of the immune response, when conditions like fever trigger the body to increase blood flow, and send specialized immune cells to help remove and repair damaged tissue.

Put simply, inflammation is the body's way of dealing with stress, which can come from training and competition, inadequate sleep, emotional issues, or nutrition. Regardless of the cause, when the tissue is attacked, the central nervous system becomes overloaded, and the body responds by sending signals (i.e., inflammation) to the areas of the body that are in jeopardy. So inflammation can be both a good and a bad thing, meaning that it can save your life or kill you, depending on the situation. To prevent the latter, you have to find a balance and limit the negative factors by managing sleep, not overtraining, reducing stress, and eating food that doesn't irritate you.

blood panel and run a diagnostic workout before you start the diet. After two to three months get another blood panel and run yourself through the same diagnostic workout to measure your results. If you're not loving the results, by all means go back to your previous routine. But in my experience, athletes generally see great results and stick with the program. Don't just take my word for it; try it out for yourself and see if it works for you.

THE PALEO DIET in 300 Words

The premise of the Paleo diet is to eat like Paleolithic man, who survived by hunting animals and foraging for plants and seasonal fruits. Why? Because research shows that Homo sapiens living before the dawn of agriculture (roughly 8,000 years ago) were much healthier than people living after the advent of agriculture. Once we figured out how to cultivate food, we relied less on hunting and gathering and more on grains (wheat, oats, barley, corn, rice, and rye), dairy (milk, cheese, yogurt), and legumes (beans, soy, and lentils). This allowed us to feed large populations of people and keep them in one place, which is how communities took hold. This consolidation of energy allowed us to focus on things that would ultimately help the human race evolve.

So why was agriculture such a bad thing? As it turns out, rather than getting stronger, bigger, faster, and healthier, which would be the logical progression, humans have been on the physical decline. Since we started eating farmed foods our health has gotten worse, not better. The experts theorize that while these cultivated foods were convenient and abundant, we weren't necessarily designed to eat them. Our genes haven't really changed since the time of Paleolithic man even though our diet has, and it turns out that we're not genetically equipped to process grains, dairy, or legumes. Although lifestyle factors such as stress, sleep, and exercise do contribute to our deteriorating health, the fact that we continue to grow fatter and more susceptible to disease suggests that our diet is at least partly responsible for the rapid rise of chronic and degenerative diseases in Western culture.

We can't say for certain what Paleolithic man ate, but we do know what he didn't eat, and that includes grains and processed food. That much is clear.

Nutrition Highlights

✱ Eat real food in its most natural state and eliminate all manufactured, processed, and refined foods from your diet.

✱ Grains, legumes, and dairy products can irritate the lining of the gut and compromise digestion and your ability to break down and absorb nutrients, leading to more problems than you want to know about. Even if you're not a celiac (allergic to gluten) or lactose intolerant (allergic to dairy), foods that contain these substances can still cause a mild allergic reaction, and thus an inflammatory response, which impedes performance and other lifestyle factors such as sleep and energy.

✱ To heal your gut lining and adapt to the new lifestyle, give the Paleo diet a 30-day solid go. After that, you can reintroduce suspicious foods like dairy to see if you get an inflammatory reaction. However, it's recommend that you stay away from gluten permanently because of its anti-nutrient properties and the processing involved in all foods containing this protein. For more information and strategies for this 30-day plan, I recommend *The Paleo Solution* by Robb Wolf and his blog at robbwolf.com.

✱ Although I always recommend real food over supplements, getting protein into your system is difficult during races. In such a situation, I suggest using a whey protein supplement or something that is easy to digest like eggs. And make sure you experiment with different products before race day to make sure they don't have undesirable effects. (Obviously, you want to make sure the product you are using is gluten free.)

CROSSFIT ENDURANCE PROGRAMMING

In the introduction to this book, I provided a general breakdown of the CrossFit Endurance system, which not only shed light on the efficacy of CrossFit's constantly varied model, but also explained how it can increase the sport-specific capacity of an endurance athlete through the utilization of all energy pathways. In addition, I outlined the CFE hierarchy, which is a progression through skill/technique, intensity, and volume. To reiterate, the goal of this program is to place skill and technique at the forefront of your training, and replace some of the steady-state endurance efforts with functional exercise and sport-specific high intensity training. This model serves two primary functions in that it increases the broad work capacity of the CrossFit athlete, and the sport specific capacity of the endurance athlete.

Having already laid the foundation for the CrossFit Endurance model, I will now focus on the practical application of the program. Using sample templates for both the single sport and multisport athlete, you will learn not only the fundamental blueprint of the CrossFit Endurance programs, but also how to effectively build a personalized program based on your specific goals. Additionally, to ensure your program design is tailored specifically to your limitations as an athlete, which as you should already know is essential to improving athletic performance, I've provided a target-based programming approach, which can be used to prioritize the areas of training that require the most attention.

If you're familiar with the CrossFit Endurance program, then feel free to skip ahead to the target-based-program approach in this chapter. This section will give you the tools to construct your own program using sample templates or to adapt the 12-week sample program to your individual fitness level or goals. If you're new to CrossFit Endurance, on the other hand, I suggest that you start your training with the 6-week introductory program, as well as familiarize yourself with the sample templates.

REVISITING CFE KEY CONCEPTS

CONSTANT VARIANCE

Most endurance athletes embody the patterns characteristic of their sport even when they're not training. Although this seems like the logical extension of one's sport, it runs contrary to the realities of life. For example, the typical endurance runner is proficient at running long distances at low intensity, but ask him to squat below parallel with his torso upright and shins vertical, press a load overhead with his arms locked out, pick up something from the ground without rounding his back, or simply move fast at a moment's notice, all of which are necessary in day-to-day activities, and chances are he won't be able to do it without compromising his form.

The point is, you have to train your body to be proficient in your sport of choice, but it shouldn't cost you ease of movement in your everyday life. By switching up the exercises, intensity, and duration of your workouts, you challenge your body's natural adaptation system, which not only prepares you to respond to the needs of your day-to-day life, but also ensures quality growth within your particular sport.

As you know, this rule of constant variance is at the core of the CrossFit Endurance program. You will see this in the strength-and-conditioning component of training, as well as in the sport-specific aspect of training, which is expressed through constantly varied interval, tempo, and time-trial efforts.

CFE HIERARCHY (Skill, Intensity, Volume)

To continue to improve in your sport, you have to follow the CFE hierarchy, which is a progression through skill, high-intensity training, and incorporating volume in the form of longer-distance efforts. The key to this progression is to gain competency and a fundamental understanding of proper movement mechanics not only for your sport, but also for all the functional exercises utilized by CrossFit. In addition, being able to identify and successfully correct movement faults through precise cueing, as well as provide mobility prescriptions for any area that is preventing you from carrying out an exercise correctly, is critical to success with this program. As you continue to gain proficiency with the skill-based movements, you can layer on high-intensity efforts while slowly adding longer-duration efforts to build stamina.

PRIORITIZE WEAKNESS

Nobody wants to work on his or her areas of weakness. It's frustrating, time-consuming, and at times embarrassing. However, if you want to improve as an athlete, which is the ultimate goal, you have to address what needs the most work. For most endurance athletes, that means working on sport-specific skill, reclaiming full ranges of motion, and developing strength and anaerobic capacity. For CrossFit athletes, that means doing some metabolic conditioning in the form of intervals, as well as tempo and time-trial stamina efforts.

UNIVERSAL LAW OF SCALABILITY

Whether you're following the sample programs outlined in this chapter or on the CrossFit Endurance Website, or working with a CFE coach, always remember that exercises, range of movements, and sport-specific prescriptions can be scaled down to suit your individual fitness base. For example, if you're unable to perform a pull-up on a day that calls for pull-ups, you can make it work using a resistance band or do supine body rows instead. Similarly, if a workout calls for eight 400-meter sprints, you can reduce the number of sets or the distance. Along these same lines, if you can't perform a movement to its end range because of a lack of mobility, you can adjust the exercise to ensure that it's executed safely and accurately (i.e., squatting down to a box instead of to full depth). The universal law of scalability ensures that everybody, regardless of age, body type, or fitness level, can perform CrossFit and sport-specific endurance workouts.

RECOVER, ADAPT, AND PROGRESS

To avoid overtraining and injury and to ensure continuous results, you have to pay attention to the feedback your body is giving you every single day, which entails considerable self-experimentation and solid coaching. For the best results, you have to allow for adequate recovery time, give your body a chance to adapt to the new training stimulus, and progress according to how you feel and perform. In other words, listening to your body and keeping it simple are the keys to your success. If you're exhausted and your numbers are dropping, take some time off. If you feel good and you're getting stronger and faster, continue progressing through the program.

TRADITIONAL CROSSFIT TEMPLATE

Before I delve into the single- and multisport programs, you need to understand the traditional CrossFit template. As I've previously discussed, the typical endurance athlete usually ends up broken at some point in his or her athletic career from the countless miles logged, the lack of functional strength-and-conditioning protocol, and disregard for sport-specific skill work. As a result, athletes who fall into this category usually have limited ranges of motion, multiple injuries, and the inability to perform fundamental feats of strength—like dead lifting their own body weight.

When the CrossFit template is used in conjunction with sport-specific endurance workouts, it has been shown to not only highlight weaknesses that can compromise performance, but to also increase strength, speed, power, and sport longevity, as well as improve overall quality of life.

The general CrossFit prescription is a three days on, one day off training model. This general work-to-rest ratio has proved to be the most effective workout cycle for the majority of athletes. However, it's important to note that while the CrossFit Endurance program uses this prescription to program CrossFit workouts, sustaining this cycle while competing in endurance events is not easy. As you will soon see, the CFE templates acknowledge the challenges of maintaining this schedule during race season and accommodates for events, which are usually held on the weekend.

The CrossFit program comprises a broad range of movements, which are lumped into three general modalities: gymnastics, weightlifting, and monostructural movements.

Gymnastics (G):
Gymnastics refers to body-weight movements like push-ups, pull-ups, air squats, lunges, etc.

Weightlifting (W):
Weightlifting refers to movements performed with an external object. This includes, but is not limited to, power lifts (e.g., squat, dead lift, bench press), Olympic lifts (e.g., snatch, clean and jerk), dumbbell variants, kettlebell variants, etc.

Monostructural (M):
Monostructural refers to movements that promote metabolic conditioning like running, cycling, and rowing.

On the next page, I have included a list of exercises that fall into each category. You can use this list to build your own personalized workouts using the sample templates provided later in the book. You can also get more exercises for each category on CrossFit.com or CrossFitEndurance.com.

Here is a list of exercises that fall into the three CrossFit movement categories:

W Weightlifting	G Gymnastics	M Monostructural
Wide Stance Back Squat pg. 214	Push-Up pg. 240	Run pg. 22
Narrow Stance Back Squat pg. 215	Incline Push-Up pg. 241	Bike pg. 70
Box Squat pg. 217	Clapping Push-Up pg. 242	Swim pg. 150
Good Morning pg. 218	Ring Push-Up pg. 243	Row pg. 277
Front Squat pg. 219	Dip pg. 245	
Dead Lift pg. 221	Handstand Push-Up (HSPU) pg. 246	
Sumo Dead Lift pg. 223	Dead Hang Pull-Up pg. 248	
Bench Press pg. 225	Supine Row (Body Row) pg. 249	
Floor Press pg. 225	Kipping Pull-Up pg. 251	
Strict Press (Shoulder Press) pg. 226	Chin-Up pg. 251	
Push-Press pg. 228	L-Sit Pull-Up pg. 252	
Power Clean pg. 230	Rope Climb pg. 252	
Power Hang Clean pg. 232	Muscle Up pg. 254	
Clean pg.233	Air Squat pg. 257	
Push-Jerk pg. 234	Jump Squat pg. 258	
Split-Jerk pg. 235	Pistol pg. 259	
Power Snatch pg. 236	Lunge pg. 260	
Overhead Squat pg. 238	Box Step-Ups pg. 261	
Snatch pg. 238	Box Jumps pg. 261	
D-Ball Slam pg. 264	Burpee pg. 263	
Kettlebell Swing pg. 265	Hollow Rock pg. 281	
Thruster pg. 267	Plank pg. 282	
Dumbbell Power Clean pg. 270	Plank Push-Up pg. 283	
One-Arm Dumbbell Snatch pg. 271	L-Sit pg. 285	
Sumo Dead Lift High Pull pg. 272	Dragon Flies pg. 286	
Stone Clean pg. 274	Sit-Up pg. 287	
Tire Flips pg. 276	V-Up pg. 288	
Sled Drags pg. 279	Glute-Hamstring Sit-Up pg. 288	
	Back Extension pg. 290	
	Hip Extension pg. 290	
	Glute-Hamstring Raise pg. 291	

Here's How It Works:

The CrossFit workouts are generally structured in one of four ways:

Rounds for time:	As many rounds as possible (AMRAP) for time:	Reps for time / Distance for time	Max Effort
EXAMPLE: 3 rounds for time 400-meter run 21 kettlebell swings 9 pull-ups	*EXAMPLE:* AMRAP in 20-minutes 5 pull-ups 10 push-ups 15 squats	*EXAMPLE:* Reps for time Perform 100-burpees Or Run 5K	*EXAMPLE:* 1 Rep Max: Dead Lift Or Max rep: Pull-ups
Do a set amount of rounds as quickly as possible.	In a set amount of time, do as many rounds as possible.	Do a set amount of repetitions as quickly as possible...or cover a set distance as quickly as possible.	1 REP MAX: Lift a weight that you can only perform one time. MAX REP: Perform a movement until failure.

When looking over the program, you'll notice that the two-week template respects the constantly varied principle, in that workouts are structured into isolated modalities (G) or into a combination of modalities (WG, MGW).

CrossFit's General Weekly Prescription

☐ 5 to 6 CrossFit workouts

Sample Two-Week Template

Week 1

Day	Mon	Tues	Wed	Thurs	Fri	Sat	Sun
CrossFit	M	GW	MGW	OFF	G	WM	GWM

Week 2

Day	Mon	Tues	Wed	Thurs	Fri	Sat	Sun
CrossFit	OFF	W	MG	G	OFF	M	GW

To get the most out of your workouts, you should not only switch up the exercises you perform each day, but also switch up how you perform them (reps for time, ASRAP, max reps).

I provided the list of exercises for each of the three categories so that you can build your own workouts. However, CrossFit.com and CrossFitEndurance.com post workouts daily, so feel free to draw from these resources. If you choose to visit the CrossFit websites, you will find that they have named a lot of their workouts, commonly referred to as the CrossFit girls (Fran, Helen). If you look at the ones I've listed below, you will notice that they are not only a blend of gymnastics, weightlifting, and monostructural movements, but they also often blend the various workout structures—reps for time, AMRAP, ect. These benchmark workouts (again, a mix of gymnastics, weightlifting, and monostructural movements) are typically used as a diagnostic tool to monitor progress. For instance, say you perform Fran (see below) at the beginning of the month and then again at the end of the month. If you improve your time—meaning that you completed the workout in a shorter span of time—you can assume that you're getting fitter, stronger, faster, and more technical with the movements.

WG: weightlifting + gymnastics

Example: "Fran"

21-15-9 reps for time

(W) Thrusters (Female 65-pounds, Male 95-pounds)

(G) Pull-ups

Description: Perform 21 thrusters, 21 pull-ups, 15 thrusters, 15 pull-ups, and then finish with 9 thrusters and 9 pull-ups. Complete the workout in the shortest amount of time possible. Record your time after completing the last pull-up.

MWG: monostructural + weightlifting + gymnastics

Example: "Helen"

3 Rounds for time:

(M) 400-meter run

(W) 21-kettlebell swings

(G) 9-pull-ups

Description: Run 400-meters, perform 21-kettlebell swings, and then 9-pull-ups. Complete three rounds and record your time.

MG: monostructural + weightlifting

Example: "Nicole"

AMRAP in 20 min.

(M) 400-meter run

(G) Max rep pull-ups

Description: Run 400-meters and then perform as many pull-ups as possible without coming off the bar. Record the number of pull-ups completed for each round.

M: Monostructural

Example: Run 5K

Description: Run 5K as fast as possible

NOTE: As you will see in the subsequent templates, when M is scheduled on a CrossFit workout day, it will say, "see endurance" underneath. Translation: instead of performing a 5K run as well as the programmed sport-specific workout, you only implement the sport-specific workout.

SINGLE-SPORT CROSSFIT ENDURANCE PROGRAM

The goal for the single-sport athlete is to complete four to six CrossFit workouts per week while supplementing with two to three sport-specific endurance workouts per week. As you examine the template, you'll notice that the sport-specific workouts are divided into two categories: interval and stamina.

☐ **Interval:** The interval workouts are in the form of short intervals (SI) or long intervals (LI). A short interval can be anything from 50- to 400-meter sprints and helps develop shorter-range energy systems, speed, and anaerobic capacity. A long interval can be anything from 800 meters to a mile and helps build lactate and aerobic systems, as well as plays a key roll in anaerobic-threshold development.

☐ **Stamina:** The stamina workouts are in the form of a tempo (T) or time trial (TT). A tempo is running, swimming, or biking at a set pace for a set time or distance. A time trial is running, swimming, or biking as fast as possible for a set time or distance.

As you can see from the template, the interval workouts are usually performed on the same day as the CrossFit workouts. However, keep in mind that progressing according to your individual ability is paramount. That could mean starting out with the sport-specific workouts and then supplementing with CrossFit only after you've recovered from the endurance session, or vice versa. Despite the fact that overall training time is cut in half when compared with traditional endurance programs, building the capacity to do two high-intensity workouts in a day takes time. The key is to let your body adjust to the new stimulus and move forward accordingly.

Unlike the interval sessions, the stamina workouts are always performed on a CrossFit rest day. The reason for this is not only to test the capacity of what you can or can't handle, but also to ensure adequate recovery leading into the next training day. In addition, being well rested on stamina days is crucial because time trials and tempos are your diagnostic tools, a way of tracking sport-specific progress as you dial in your program from week to week.

I have to point out that your goal determines how hard you train in your stamina workouts. For example, if the workout calls for a 10K tempo pace, conventional endurance programs generally recommend anywhere from 50 percent to 85 percent effort. If your goal is to simply finish a marathon, running at low intensity (or race pace) is not going to prevent you from achieving that goal. However, if you want to place, or finish with a sub-3:30 marathon, you have to run at 80 percent effort or greater on stamina days. This ensures that your body knows what it is like to run harder and faster than the actual race pace.

As a quick recap, this template is designed to build strength and develop capacity in the shorter-range energy pathways for the single-sport endurance athlete, while giving the CrossFit athlete an extra dose of sport-specific metabolic conditioning. As you can see from the generally prescribed program, CrossFit is heavily emphasized over sport-specific training to develop broad-range capacity. Once you develop a base level of strength and competency in all metabolic pathways, as well as sport-specific skill (i.e. Pose running), you can start to increase the amount of sport-specific CrossFit Endurance workouts as well as add a strength bias into the program.

Note: CrossFit monostructural workouts are swapped out with sport-specific endurance intervals. So, if you're a runner, all you would do on a day that calls for a monostrucutal workout is short- or long-interval sprints.

CrossFit Endurance Single-Sport General Weekly Prescription

- ☐ 4 to 6 CrossFit workouts
- ☐ 2 interval
- ☐ 1 stamina

Two-Week Traditional CrossFit Endurance Program 3:1 CF

Week 1

Day	Mon	Tues	Wed	Thurs	Fri	Sat	Sun
CrossFit	M (see Endurance)	GW	MGW		G	WM	GWM
Endurance SS	SI			T/TT		LI	

Week 2

Day	Mon	Tues	Wed	Thurs	Fri	Sat	Sun
CrossFit		W	MG	WMG		M (see Endurance)	GW
Endurance SS	SI		LI				T/TT

- ☐ **G** Gymnastics
- ☐ **M** Monostructural
- ☐ **W** Weightlifting
- ☐ **SI** Short Interval
- ☐ **LI** Long Interval
- ☐ **T/TT** Tempo or Time Trial
- ☐ **S** Swim
- ☐ **B** Bike
- ☐ **R** Run
- ☐ **SS** Single Sport
- ☐ **3S** 3 Sports

MULTISPORT CROSSFIT ENDURANCE PROGRAM

The multisport CrossFit Endurance program is very similar to the single-sport program, in that there are four to six CrossFit workouts per week. But instead of also doing two to three sport-specific workouts per week, you do two sport-specific workouts per sport. If you're a triathlete, that would mean two run-based workouts, two cycling-based workouts, and two swim-based workouts per week. The general recommendation is four CrossFit workouts, and two or three sport-specific interval-based workouts in the first four to five days of the week. That leaves the rest of the week for one more interval-based workout and two stamina-based workouts. The general weekly recommendation for the vast majority of multisport athletes is to perform four CrossFit workouts, one interval workout per sport, and one stamina workout per sport per week.

As you can see from the template, the stamina-based workouts are deliberately scheduled during the weekend, which not only promotes recovery entering the next week of CrossFit and interval-based training, but also simulates endurance events, which are typically held on a Saturday or Sunday. The majority of multisport athletes need only one or two stamina sessions per week. Even at the elite level, three to four stamina sessions can be performed only periodically on a weekly basis. Athletes who stubbornly try to do that much stamina work on a regular basis inevitably break down.

At first glance, you will look at this template and say to yourself, "Damn, that is a lot of volume!" However, this is when it becomes extremely important for you understand your personal limitations or the limitations of the athlete you're coaching. To ensure continual results and avoid overtraining, you have to understand what you can and can't handle on a day-to-day basis. Not only that, you have to be smart with your schedule and manage intensity and recovery. For example, if you are exhausted at the beginning of another training day or workout session, take the day off and give yourself an opportunity to recover or dial back the intensity. Remember, you're not going to get stronger or faster or build stamina with more training. Pushing your body past its limits is one of the biggest mistakes athletes make with this program. This is no different than going out and running a hundred miles a week without building up to it. Give yourself time to adapt to the training load and allow for ample recovery.

Another key concept that is particularly important to the multisport athlete is to prioritize sport-specific weaknesses. With so many skills to train, athletes will often focus on what they're best at and give short shrift to the areas that need the most improvement, which limits growth and overall performance. For example, if you're a strong runner with good form but you suck at swimming, running once every cycle is probably not necessary. Instead, you may want to consider swapping out the running intervals or stamina work with swimming, or use that time to rest and recover. Here's an example:

Sample Stamina Prescription: 1 Stamina Workout Per Week

Standard Cycle		Biased Cycle	
Week 1	Run	Week 1	Swim
Week 2	Bike	Week 2	Bike
Week 3	Swim	Week 3	Swim
Week 4	Run (Repeat Cycle)	Week 4	Run

CrossFit Endurance Multisport General Weekly Prescription

- ☐ 4 to 6 CrossFit workouts (4 is the general prescription)
- ☐ 1 to 2 interval workouts per sport (1 is the general prescription)
- ☐ 1 to 2 stamina workouts (1 is the general prescription)

Two-Week Traditional CrossFit Endurance Program: Triathlete/3 Sport

Week 1

Day	Mon	Tues	Wed	Thurs	Fri	Sat	Sun
CrossFit	M (see Endurance)	GW	MGW	G			
Endurance 3S	SIS	SIR		LIB	LIS	T/TT B	T/TT R

Week 2

Day	Mon	Tues	Wed	Thurs	Fri	Sat	Sun
CrossFit	WM	GWM	W	MG			
Endurance 3S	SIB	LIR	LIS		SIS	T/TT R	T/TT B

BRICK TRAINING

Brick training is a model used to get multisport endurance athletes used to transitioning from one element to the next (i.e., transitioning from the bike to the run) without slowing down. For example, when you hop off the bike and transition to the run, you're legs may feel like bricks. Although CrossFit does a good job of conditioning athletes to handle this transition through constantly varied movement, I recommend adding brick training to your program one to two months before race day for sport-specificity purposes. It might look something like this: Run 5K at race pace or better, then bike 20 miles at 90 percent. A more complex example might look something like this: 3 rounds of swim 400 meters, then bike 5 miles, then run 1.5 miles.

LINEAR-STRENGTH-BIAS CROSSFIT ENDURANCE PROGRAM

The linear-strength-bias program incorporates an additional strength element into the traditional CrossFit Endurance program. This template is typically used on endurance athletes who need to prioritize strength development. Remember, you need a solid strength base before incorporating CrossFit workouts. Depending on your fitness level, you can either replace the CrossFit workouts with the strength-bias element or do a short CrossFit workout—less than 10 minutes—after completing the strength circuit. Once again, this takes a keen understanding of what you can or can't handle.

As you can see from the template, the linear progression follows a simple formula of five sets of five repetitions, focusing on power lifts in the form of a squat, dead lift, and press. The goal is to add 5 to 10 pounds each week until you can't go any further. Once you can no longer add additional weight, you can repeat the cycle or adjust the set and rep scheme. For example, you can decrease the number of reps and keep the set scheme the same, or decrease the sets and increase the number of reps. The former strategy requires you to add more weight, while the latter can be performed using the same weight as the five-by-five model. Regardless of your method, the goal is to break the barrier previously reached at the end of each cycle.

Single-Sport Linear-Strength-Bias General Weekly Prescription

- ☐ 3 strength workouts (1 squat, 1 dead lift, 1 press)
- ☐ 3 to 4 CrossFit workouts (short workouts, generally under 10 minutes)
- ☐ 2 interval
- ☐ 1 stamina

Multisport Linear-Strength-Bias General Weekly Prescription

- ☐ 3 strength workouts (1 squat, 1 dead lift, 1 press)
- ☐ 3 to 4 CrossFit workouts (short workouts, generally under 10 minutes)
- ☐ 3 to 4 intervals per sport
- ☐ 1 to 2 stamina

Linear-Strength-Bias CrossFit Endurance Program

Single-Sport Week 1

Day	Mon	Tues	Wed	Thurs	Fri	Sat	Sun
Strength	Squat 5 x 5		Dead Lift 5 x 5		Press 5 x 5	OFF	
CrossFit		MG	MGW	GW	M (see Endurance)	OFF	
Endurance SS		SI			LI	OFF	T/TT

Single-Sport Week 2

Day	Mon	Tues	Wed	Thurs	Fri	Sat	Sun
Strength	Squat 5 x 5 add 5 lbs.		Dead Lift 5 x 5 add 5 lbs.		Press 5 x 5 add 5 lbs.	OFF	
CrossFit	G	GW	GWM	WM		OFF	
Endurance SS		SI		LI		OFF	T/TT

Three-Sport Week 1

Day	Mon	Tues	Wed	Thurs	Fri	Sat	Sun
Strength	Squat 5 x 5		Dead Lift 5 x 5		Press 5 x 5		
CrossFit		MG	MGW	GW	M		
Endurance 3S	SIS	SIR		LIB	LIS	T/TT B	T/TT R

Three-Sport Week 2

Day	Mon	Tues	Wed	Thurs	Fri	Sat	Sun
Strength	Squat 5 x 5 add 5 lbs.		Dead Lift 5 x 5 add 5 lbs.		Press 5 x 5 add 5 lbs.		
CrossFit	G	GW	GWM	WM			
Endurance 3S	SIB	LIR	SIS		LIS	T/TT R	T/TT B

CONJUGATE-STRENGTH-BIAS CROSSFIT ENDURANCE PROGRAM

The conjugate system was developed in Russia and then successfully implemented and made popular by Louie Simmons, a world-renowned power-lifting coach and the founder of Westside Barbell. It is a constantly varied strength-bias model for increasing strength, power, and speed. The conjugate-strength-bias program follows the same parameters as the linear-strength-bias program, in that it's used as a supplement to, or in place of, a CrossFit workout to emphasize strength. But unlike the linear progression, which generally follows the same set and rep scheme throughout the entire cycle, the conjugate model is constantly varied template that focuses on two modalities: max-effort (ME) and dynamic-effort (DE) lifts. The general prescription is two max-effort days followed by two dynamic-effort days.

Max Effort (ME):

Maximum effort refers to maxing out each set for as many repetitions as possible. The goal is to lift 90 to 95 percent of your one-rep max for the prescribed lift. If you don't know your one-rep max, work up to a heavy double (two repetitions) and stick with that weight for that day. For the best results, shoot for four sets with each lift, making sure to maintain good form as you complete the set. The moment you start to default into bad positions stop or reduce the weight.

Dynamic Effort (DE):

Dynamic effort refers to moving the bar with as much speed as possible. The goal is to complete two reps every 30 to 90 seconds for 8 to 12 sets. If you slow down during the contraction phase of the prescribed movement (usually three-quarters of a second or slower) or form is compromised, reduce the weight.

ME	Max Effort, working to a 2-rep max effort for 4 to 5 sets
DE	Dynamic Effort, 50 to 60 percent of 1RM. Usually 2 reps every 30 to 90 seconds for 8 to 12 sets

Single-Sport Conjugate-Strength-Bias General Weekly Prescription

- ☐ 3 strength workouts (1 squat, 1 dead lift, 1 press)
- ☐ 3 to 4 CrossFit workouts (short workouts, generally less than 10 minutes)
- ☐ 2 interval
- ☐ 1 stamina

Multisport Conjugate-Strength-Bias General Weekly Prescription

- ☐ 3 strength workouts (1 squat, 1 dead lift, 1 press)
- ☐ 3 to 4 CrossFit workouts (short workouts, generally less than 10 minutes)
- ☐ 3 to 4 intervals per sport
- ☐ 1 to 2 stamina

Conjugate Three-Day Strength-Bias CrossFit Endurance Program

Single-Sport Week 1

Day	Mon	Tues	Wed	Thurs	Fri	Sat	Sun
Strength	ME Squat		ME Press		DE Dead Lift	OFF	
CrossFit		MG	MGW	GW	M (see Endurance)	OFF	
Endurance SS		SI		LI	LI	OFF	T/TT

Single-Sport Week 2

Day	Mon	Tues	Wed	Thurs	Fri	Sat	Sun
Strength	DE Squat		ME Press		ME Dead Lift	OFF	
CrossFit	G	GW	GWM	WM		OFF	
Endurance SS		SI		SI		OFF	T/TT

Three-Sport Week 1

Day	Mon	Tues	Wed	Thurs	Fri	Sat	Sun
Strength	ME Squat		ME Press		DE Dead Lift		
CrossFit		MG	MGW	GW	M		
Endurance 3S	SIS	SIR		LIB	LIS	T/TT B	T/TT R

Three-Sport Week 2

Day	Mon	Tues	Wed	Thurs	Fri	Sat	Sun
Strength	DE Squat		ME Press		ME Dead Lift		
CrossFit	G	GW	GWM	WM			
Endurance 3S	SIB	LIR	SIS			T/TT R	T/TT B

POST-EVENT RECOVERY CIRCUIT

As a general rule, you should always do a simple functional movement circuit after a long endurance race. Remember, whatever you do right after a race dictates the rate at which you will recover. Think of it like this: Your body has been cycling through limited ranges thousands of times, causing your tissues to get extremely tight, short, and overworked. One of the best ways to restore motion, flush out toxins, and accelerate recovery is to get into the gym as quickly as possible (immediately following the race) and run through a body-weight or light- to medium-weight strength-and-conditioning circuit. It's important to note that this is just one piece of the recovery process and should be used in conjunction with proper post-race nutrition, hydration, mobility, ice baths, etc.

Sample Post-Race Strength-and-Conditioning Circuit

- ☐ **3 rounds**

- ☐ **5 to 15 reps of each exercise with adequate rest between stations**

1. **Glute-hamstring developer sit-ups**
2. **Glute-hamstring developer hip extensions and/or back extensions**
3. **Kettlebell or dumbbell swings**
4. **Bench press or push-ups**
5. **Pull-ups or squats**

TARGET-BASED PROGRAMMING APPROACH

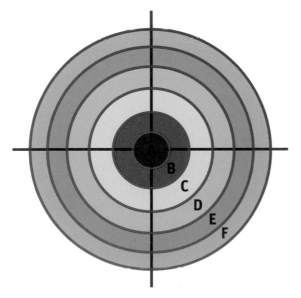

A) POSE Running technique

B) Strength development

C) CrossFit, etc.

D) POSE Running technique

E) Strength development

F) CrossFit, etc.

As I've repeatedly stated, an intelligently constructed training program should always revolve around an athlete's greatest weaknesses. It is human nature to choose the path of least resistance, so you have to make a conscious effort to focus on the attributes that require the most attention. The purpose of the target-based programming approach is to give you a clear idea of how to prioritize your training so that you can create a personalized program using the CrossFit Endurance templates or adapt the sample programs to cater to your individual goals and limitations.

Here is how it works: In the center of the target you have the bull's-eye. This represents the area of your body (or aspect of your training) that requires the most attention. Each concentric circle expanding outward represents another category in your athletic profile. The further out you go, the less time and attention you need to spend in or on that area. It's important to note that this approach to programming can be used in a very broad sense, encompassing your entire athletic profile, or specifically for certain aspects of your training. For example, Kelly Starrett uses the target-based approach by having athletes place their biggest mobility issue in the bull's-eye, and then working progressively outward, pinpointing areas that require less attention.

To help you understand how this approach can be used to design a personalized CFE program, let's take a hypothetical athlete, assess his strengths and weaknesses, and then use that information to construct a foundation for his target-based program template.

As you study the athlete's profile, be sure to keep the following points in mind:

- ☐ The CrossFit Endurance progression: Prioritize skill/technique, add intensity, and then see how much volume you or the person you are training can handle. Using this model, you can create three targets expanding over an imaginary timeline, which encompass all three of these categories. It's important to remember that this timeline will be different for everyone.

- ☐ Because mobility is something that should be practiced everyday—remember Starrett's no-days-off rule—the mobility target is separate from the CrossFit Endurance targets. For that reason, there is a separate mobility target created for our hypothetical athlete. However, this target works in conjunction with the other primary targets, in that it deals with issues that affect the athlete's performance and capacity for movement. As we progress through skill, intensity, and then volume, we will continue to use the mobility target as a way to deal with missing range, muscle stiffness, and pain. It's important to note that this target may change as the athlete progresses through the three CrossFit Endurance targets.

The strengths and weaknesses identified in this hypothetical athlete highlight general issues within that particular paradigm. In other words, the strengths and weaknesses outlined are the most common and generalized attributes associated with a typical endurance runner. Of course, there could be a multitude of other limiting factors or strengths, but to keep things simple, we're sticking with the broad characteristics.

ENDURANCE RUNNER

Description: Our hypothetical athlete is an endurance runner who follows a traditional long, slow distance program. He's had no exposure to proper running mechanics and doesn't take mobility protocol seriously. As a result, he typically runs with his shoulders and back rolled forward, heel-strikes, and doesn't keep his midline engaged. Because he's got limited range of motion in his hamstrings, anterior hips, and ankles/calves, he can't squat below parallel without his knees caving inward and has recurring pain in his lower back and knees. He is proficient with body weight exercises, meaning that he's strong enough to execute the movement, but because of his lack of mobility and attention to technique, he doesn't perform exercises correctly or to end range.

Although he can handle longer-duration runs, he can't run 100-, 200-, or 400-meter sprints faster than his long-distance pace. He's had zero exposure to compound movements like Olympic weightlifting, and because he has no plyometric training, he can't jump higher than 12 inches off the ground. In addition, he often suffers from knee and lower-back pain.

Data Points

- ☐ Male
- ☐ Age: 36
- ☐ Half-marathon time: 1:33
- ☐ 10K: 42 min.
- ☐ 5K: 20 min.
- ☐ 1M: 6:05
- ☐ 800 m: 2:55
- ☐ 400 m: 1:26
- ☐ 200 m: 41 sec.
- ☐ Back squat: 135 lbs.
- ☐ Dead lift: 200 lbs.
- ☐ Press: 95 lbs.

Primary Weaknesses

- ☐ Lacks skill/technique in both running and body-weight exercises.
- ☐ Limited range of motion.
- ☐ Inability to perform or recover from high-intensity exercise.

Primary Strengths

- ☐ Incredible ability in aerobic/oxidative state and longer-range anaerobic activity.
- ☐ Proficient with body-weight movements.

Data Points

It should be a no-brainer that this athlete needs to prioritize skill by addressing running mechanics and learn how to correctly perform functional movements. In addition, he needs to focus on his positions of restriction by focusing on his mobility. In this particular case, we can assume that his lack of technique as it relates to functional body-weight exercise is a combination of two things: 1) he's never been taught how to correctly perform the movement and 2) he doesn't have the range of motion to get into the correct positions. To get this athlete moving in the right direction, he has to progress through three targets, which follow the CrossFit Endurance progression through skill, intensity, and volume. In conjunction with this, he also has to create a mobility target so that he can increase his range and fix his areas of restriction. This target will be used throughout every progression and adapt to the areas that need the most attention.

Target 1: Skill

During this stage of development, we take his biggest weakness and place that in the bull's-eye. In this particular case, because he's a runner, we obviously need to teach him how to run using proper mechanics. Working our way out, we also need to teach him how to correctly perform basic gymnastics/body-weight exercises. We also need to add some serious mobility practice to restore normal range to his tissues and alleviate some of the pain and discomfort he is currently experiencing.

A	Running Mechanics	B	Gymnastics/Body-Weight Mechanics	C	Weightlifting
a)	Heel Strike	a)	Squat	a)	Squat
b)	Shoulder/Posture	b)	Push-ups	b)	Press
c)	Other Mechanical Faults	c)	Pull-up	c)	Clean

Mobility Target

A	Upper Back (posture)	B	Hip	C	Lower Leg	D	Upper Leg
a)	Thoracic Spine	a)	Anterior Hip (hip extension/posture)	a)	Foot (restore sliding surface)	a)	Hamstrings (lower-back pain, knee pain, restore range)
b)	Shoulders	b)	Glutes (lower-back pain, external/internal rotation)	b)	Ankle (restore range)	b)	Quads (hip extension, knee pain)
				c)	Calf (relieve stiffness/knee pain)		

Target 2: Strength / Intensity

After making some progress in the skill/technique department—meaning he knows how to move correctly, he's restored some range to his stiff muscles, and he's no longer in serious pain—we can start focusing on strength, which for this athlete is a huge limiting factor. In addition, we will also start incorporating higher-intensity workouts into his regimen to build up his anaerobic capacity.

A	Strength (3-day split) 5 x 3 progressing to 5 x 5	B	CrossFit	C	Running (progress if athlete shows competency in each)
a)	Squat	a)	Combine all other issues pertaining to movement (other than sport) as they relate to functional movements used in CrossFit.	a)	100 m efforts
b)	Press			b)	400 m efforts
c)	Dead Lift			c)	1M TT

D	Olympic Lifts	E	Jumping (jump rope, box jumps, etc.)

Target 3: Volume

Having tested his skill with some high-intensity training, we can test his limits and see how much volume he can handle. Based on how he feels and performs, we can adjust the program accordingly.

A	Strength	B	CrossFit	C	Running
	a) Squat (5 to 7 sets of 3 to 5 reps) b) Press (same as squat) c) Dead Lift (same as squat)		a) Short (less than) 15 to 10-minute WODS after strength-day workouts, or skip strength and just use CrossFit as a 3-on 1-off model. b) 1 to 2 more days of CrossFit if you follow the CFE template.		a) 10 to 20 x 100s with 3 to 5 minutes recovery between intervals. b) 2 to 4 x 400s with 3 minutes recovery between intervals. c) 1 x 1M

WORKOUT LEGEND

ENDURANCE WODS

SS = Single Sport

3S = Three Sports / Triathlon / Multisport

m = Meter

M = Miles

y = Yards

m/y = Meters or Yards

10" = 10-second rest

90" = 90-second rest

C2 = Concept 2 rower

TT = Time Trial: A measurement of maximum work capacity/power output over a set amount of time or distance. The time trial is often called the race of truth. It is done alone and should be retested under similar conditions and the same distance/time.

Tempo = Reduced but consistent pace for time or distance. 100 percent is all-out effort. Range between 85 percent and 95 percent.

Tabata = 8 rounds of 20 seconds on, 10 seconds rest, maximum effort.

On the Minute = Start each set at the beginning of a new minute.

On :45 seconds = You have 45 seconds to perform the distance and rest. You start each set on :45 second interval.

AMRAP = As many rounds as possible

AFAP = As fast as possible

Rx = As prescribed

Unbroken = If you come off the bar, you start that element again, until completion

Pood = A Russian unit of weight equivalent to about 16.4 kilograms (36.1 pounds): 1 pood, 1.5 pood, 2 pood are common.

Accommodating Resistance = Use of bands and/or chains

OHS = Overhead squat

Lifts are listed as number of sets then reps: 3x5 means 3 sets of 5 reps.

1RM = 1 rep max

% (percentage) of weight will be listed for personal and individual strength programming.

ME = Max Effort: Typically working to a 2-rep max for 5 sets but not limited to that example. If 1RM PR is there take it, if not don't.

DE = Dynamic Effort: Typically taking 50 to 70 percent of 1RM for that exercise and moving through exercise with maximal speed (controlled!). Usually 2 to 3 reps on 90-sec to 30-sec interval.

Ground to Overhead = The weight starts on the ground and you get it overhead, however you like. Could be a snatch, a clean and push-press, or a clean and jerk.

SAMPLE PROGRAMS

6-Week Progression into the Program

If you're new to the CrossFit Endurance program and you haven't been exposed to the exercises outlined in the strength-and-conditioning chapter, I suggest that you start with the 6-week progression outlined below. This preparatory cycle introduces fundamental movements that play a key role in the CFE program as well as build an anaerobic base for the more challenging 12-week cycles presented at the end of the chapter.

Like all the programs presented in this chapter, progress at your own pace. For some athletes, that could mean going through the 6-week program and then immediately jumping into a 12-week cycle (or individualized program). For others, that could mean repeating the 6-week cycle (or specific weeks) until competency with the movements and capacity is developed. Remember, this is a guide, not a program etched in stone.

It's important to mention that the majority of CrossFit affiliate gyms have a similar program, which introduces the athlete to fundamental movements used in the CrossFit program as well as develops a base level of strength-and-conditioning. As I've stated before, having a coach assess and cue your movement is the quickest and most efficient way to progress through the CrossFit Endurance program.

6-week progression into the program

Week 1

	Day 1	Day 2	Day 3
CFE Prep	3 rounds (no time limit): 5 pull ups/supine rows, 10 push ups, 15 squats, 20 sit ups. 1 min of hollow rock holds total	3 rounds (no time limit): 5 pull ups/supine rows, 10 push ups, 15 lunges, 20 sit ups. 1 min of hollow rock holds total	5 rounds (no time limit): 5 pull ups/supine rows, 10 push ups, 15 squats, 20 sit ups. 1 min of hollow rock holds total
Run Prep	10 x 50 m walk 50 m back and repeat	N/A	10 x 100 m walk 100 m back and repeat

Week 2

	Day 1	Day 2	Day 3
CFE Prep	4 rounds for time: 5 pull ups/supine rows, 10 push ups, 15 lunges, 20 sit ups. 90 seconds of hollow rocks total	4 rounds for time: 5 pull ups/supine rows, 10 push ups, 15 squats, 20 sit ups. 90 seconds of hollow rocks total	5 rounds for time: 5 pull ups/supine rows, 10 push ups, 15 lunges, 20 sit ups. 90 seconds of hollow rocks total
Run Prep	15 x 50 m walk 50 m back and repeat	N/A	15 x 100 m walk 100 m back and repeat

Week 3

	Day 1	Day 2	Day 3
CFE Prep	10 min AMRAP (As Many Rounds As Possible): 5 pull ups/supine rows, 10 push ups, 15 squats, 20 sit ups. 2 min of hollow rock work total	25 pull ups/supine rows, 50 push ups, 75 lunges, 100 sit ups for time. 2 min of hollow rock work total	5 rounds for time: 5 pull ups/supine rows, 10 push ups, 15 squats, 20 sit ups. 2 min of hollow rocks total
Run Prep	20 x 50 m walk 50 m back and repeat	N/A	20 x 100 m walk 100 m back and repeat

6-week progression into the program

Week 4

	Day 1	Day 2	Day 3
CFE Prep	25 pull ups/supine rows, 50 push ups, 75 lunges, 100 sit ups for time. 2 min of hollow rock work total	10 rounds (no time limit): 5 pull ups/supine rows, 10 push ups, 15 squats, 20 sit ups. 2:30 min of hollow rock holds total	10 min "Cindy" AMRAP: 5 pull ups, 10 push ups, 15 squats
Run Prep	10 x 100 m on 1 min	N/A	20 x 50 m on :30

Week 5

	Day 1	Day 2	Day 3
CFE Prep	35 pull ups/supine rows, 65 push ups, 90 lunges, 115 sit ups for time. 2 min of hollow rock work total	15 min AMRAP: 5 pull ups/supine rows, 10 push ups, 15 squats, 20 sit ups. 2 min of hollow rock work total	5 rounds **add weighted vest or back pack if you have. Up to 10 lbs** (no time limit): 5 pull ups/supine rows, 10 push ups, 15 lunges, 20 sit ups. 2:30 min of hollow rock holds
Run Prep	8 min of 100 m on :45	10 min of 50 m on :20 - :30	4 x 200 m on 2 min

Week 6

	Day 1	Day 2	Day 3
CFE Prep	50 pull ups/supine rows, 75 push ups, 100 squats, 125 sit ups for time. 3 min of hollow rock work total	3 - 4 rounds (not for time): 25 pull ups/supine rows, 25 push ups, 25 Lunges, 25 sit ups	"Cindy" 20 min AMRAP: 5 pull ups/10 supine rows, 10 push ups, 15 squats
Run Prep	8 min of 100 m on :45 rest 4 min, 4 min of 100 m on :45	5 min of 50 m on :15 - :20	6 x 200 m on 2 min

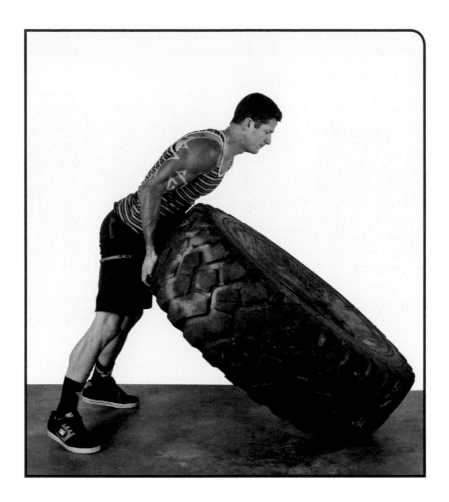

12-Week Sample Template:

After you've completed the 6-week progression into the program, you can either segue into online programming (CrossFitEndurance.com), start plugging workouts into a sample template based on your goals and fitness level, or start this 12-week sample program. As you will notice, the 12-week sample program introduces a linear strength bias and incorporates more challenging CrossFit workouts. As with the 6-week program, be sure to scale movements and weight to suit your skill set and fitness base. Most people can't handle training more than three or four days a week when first implementing the CFE model. For that reason, the 12-week program is broken up into three days. Tackle these workouts in a way that doesn't compromise progress.

My recommendation is this: Prioritize the strength element and try to complete three CrossFit WODs throughout the week. Note: generally athletes will do their strength and then complete the CrossFit workout right after. If you can recover that same day, implement one of the prescribed sport-specific workouts. If you're fatigued, take the rest of the day off and do your run, bike, or swim element on another day.

When you view the sample program, you will notice that when it comes to strength exercises, I only list the basic movement, such as squat, dead lift, or press. It is important to note that you are not limited to just the basic movements. For example, if the program calls for a squat, you can implement a back squat, box squat, front squat, or overhead squat. Similarly, if the program calls for a press, you can implement an overhead press (shoulder press, push-press, push-jerk) or a midrange press (bench press, floor press). Sticking with the CrossFit methodology, you want to constantly vary your movements, as well as perform exercises that suit your individual needs and abilities.

12-Week Program with Linear Strength Bias

week 1		Day 1	Day 2	Day 3
CrossFit	**Strength**	Squat 5x5	Press 5x5	Dead Lift 5x5
		3 rounds for time of: 5 power cleans, 10 box jumps, 15 supine ring rows	12-15-21-15-12 for time of: box jumps push-up (HSPU, ring push-up)	Max reps in: 0:30 Pull-ups, 0:15 rest, 0:30 burpess, 0:15 rest, 0:30 KB swings, Rest 1:00 min. Complete 7 rounds
Endurance	swim	10 x 50 m/y on 1 min	4 x 200 m/y w/ 90 sec rest	500 m/y TT
	bike	10 x 1/4 mile/400 m on 1 min	4 x 2M w/ 2 min spin/rest between	10M TT
	run	8 x 200 m w/ 2 min rest	2 x 800 m w/ 3 min rest	5k TT

week 2		Day 1	Day 2	Day 3
CrossFit	**Strength**	Squat 5x5	Press 5x5	Dead Lift 5x5
		AMRAP in 10:00 min: 7 push-press, 7 push-jerks, 5 pull-ups	5, 4, 3, 2, 1 for time: hang power clean, rope climb	4 rounds for time: 15 supine ring rows 10 knee to elbows, 5 front squats
Endurance	swim	15 x 50 m/y on 1 min	5 x 200 m/y on time from previous week	800 m/y @ 90% of 500 m pace
	bike	10 x 1/4 mile/400 m on 1 min	4 x 2M w/ 2 min spin/rest between	10M TT
	run	10 x 200 m w/ 2 min rest	3-4 x 800 m w/ 3 min rest	5k @ 85% of 5k TT pace

week 3		Day 1	Day 2	Day 3
CrossFit	**Strength**	Squat 5x5	Press 5x5	Dead Lift 5x5
		5 rounds for time: 10 pull-ups, 15 KB swings , 20 push-ups	4 rounds for time: 10 knee to elbows 15 box jumps, row 500 m	AMRAP in 12 min: 12 dips, 9 overhead squats, 12 burpees
Endurance	swim	10 x 75 m/y on 1:30	10 x 100 m/y on 2 min	800 m/y TT
	bike	6 x 1M repeats w/ 2 min spin/rest	4 x 4 min TT w/ 4 min spin/rest	12M TT
	run	10-12 x 200 m w/ 90 sec rest	4-5 x 800 m w/ 2:30 rest	5M @ last weeks 5k pace

12-Week Program with Linear Strength Bias

week 4

	Day 1	Day 2	Day 3
Strength	**Squat 5x5**	**Press 5x5**	**Dead Lift 5x5**
CrossFit	9-6-3 for time: push-jerk, dead hang pull-ups	400 m farmers walk with 50% of bodyweight. Every time you set down the weight, perform 10 burpees	AMRAP in 8 min: 3 Rope Climbs, 10 KB swings
Endurance swim	6 x 1M w/ 90 sec spin/rest	3 x 400 m/y TT with 3 min rest	1000 m/y @ 85% of 800 TT pace
bike	6 x 1M w/ 90 sec spin/rest	4 x 4 min w/ 4 min spin/rest holding avg watts or distance of last weeks TT's or better.	20M @ 85% of 12M TT pace
run	4 x 400 m w/ 2 min rest	3 x 1000 m with 3 min rest	10k TT

week 5

	Day 1	Day 2	Day 3
Strength	**Squat 5x5**	**Press 5x5**	**Dead Lift 5x5**
CrossFit	"Annie" 50-40-30-20-10 for time of: double unders sit-ups	4 rounds for time: 10 thrusters, 50 m of walking lunges - use dumbbells if appropriate	3 rounds for time: 300m row, 15 ball slams, 5 pull-ups
Endurance swim	20 x 25 m/y TT's on 1 min	6 x 200 m on 3 min	500 m/y TT
bike	8 x 1k on 2 min spin between	3 x 5 min at 4 min avg -5% from last week w/ 4 min spin/rest	20M TT
run	6 x 400 m w/ 2 min rest	3 x 800 m TT with 5 min rest between	5k @ 10k TT pace

week 6

	Day 1	Day 2	Day 3
Strength	**Squat 5x5**	**Press 5x5**	**Deadlift 5x5**
CrossFit	"Cindy" AMRAP in 20 min: 5 pull-ups 10 push-ups, 15 squats	5-4-3-2-1 for time of: hang power clean, broad jumps for distance	AMRAP in 10 min: 1-arm DB snatch, 10 pull-ups, 20 double unders
Endurance swim	15 x 50 m/y on :45 sec	2 x 500 m on 95% of 500 TT	1000 m/y of last 1000 m/y
bike	5 x 1k on 90% of 1k's last week w/ 2 min spin, then 1k TT	4 x 4 min w/ 4 min spin/rest	10M TT
run	6 x 400 m w/ 90 sec rest	2 x 200 m w/ 90 sec rest, 2 x 400 m w/ 2 min rest, 2 x 1000 m w/ 3 min rest	7M @ 95% of 10k TT pace

12-Week Program with Linear Strength Bias

week 7		Day 1	Day 2	Day 3
CrossFit	Strength	Squat 5x5	Press 5x5	Dead Lift 5x5
	CrossFit	1 Round for time: row 500 m, 50 air squats, 40 push-ups, 30 KB swings, 20 burpees, 10 pull-ups, row 500 m	AMRAP in 12 min: 15 jump squats, 15 box jumps, 15 knee to elbow	"Fran" 21-15-9 for time of: thrusters 95/65, pull-ups
Endurance	swim	20 x 50 on :45-1 min	5 x 200 m TT's on 2-3 min recoveries	1000 @ 95% of last 800 TT
	bike	3 x 1k w/ 90 sec spin, 3 x 2k w/ 2 min spins	5 x 2M w/ 3 min spins	20M @ 85% of 10M TT pace
	run	6 x 400 m w/ 90 sec rest	4 x 1000 m w/ 2-3 min rest	10M TT

week 8		Day 1	Day 2	Day 3
CrossFit	Strength	Squat 5x5	Press 5x5	Dead Lift 5x5
	CrossFit	3 Rounds for time: 100 m sled drag, 15 supine rows, 10 dips	For Time: 30 box jumps, 40 walking lunges, 50 pull-ups, 60 push-ups, 70 sit-ups, 80 air squats	10! (10,9,8,7....3,2,1) for time of: 1-arm DB snatch burpees
Endurance	swim	4 x (3 x 75) as 1. 80%, 2. 90%, 3. 100% all on 1:30 or less	3 x 400 on 7 min or less	500 TT
	bike	5 x 2k w/ 2 min spin	3 x 5k TT w/ 5 min spins	25M TT
	run	4 x 200 m w/ 60 sec rest 4 x 400 m w/ 90 sec rest	4 x 4 min w/ 3 min rest	5k @ last weeks 10M TT pace

week 9		Day 1	Day 2	Day 3
CrossFit	Strength	Squat 5x5	Press 5x5	Dead Lift 5x5
	CrossFit	3 Rounds for time of: 9 hang power clean, 12 box jumps, 15 KB swings	AMRAP in 10 min: 1 rope climb, 3 dead lifts, 5 pull-ups	3 Rounds for time rest 2 min between each round: 15 GHD sit-ups, 15 GHD glute hamstring raises, 50m sled pull
Endurance	swim	20 x 50 (1. 25 sec rest, 2. 20 sec rest, 3. 15 sec rest, 4. 10 sec rest, 5. 5 sec rest)	10 x 100 on 1:45 or :15 sec less rest	800 m/y TT
	bike	5 x 2k repeats w/ 90 sec spin/ rest	4 x 5 min w/ 3-4 min spin between	15M @ 85%
	run	6 x 400 m TT's w/ 3-4 min recoveries	5 x 4 min w/ 3 min rest between	2 x 5k @ 90% of 5k TT time... Rest 5-10 min between

12-Week Program with Linear Strength Bias

week 10	Day 1	Day 2	Day 3
Strength	**Squat 5x5**	**Press 5x5**	**Dead Lift 5x5**
CrossFit	4 Rounds for time: 10 dips, 20 weighted walking lunges, 500m row	2 hang power cleans @ 75% of 1 RM on the minute for 10 minutes.	AMRAP in 8 mins: 7 back squats, 7 pull-ups
Endurance swim	10 x 75 all out w/ 25 easy	5 x 200 m on 2:45 or :15 sec less recovery	1000 m/y @ 85% of 800 TT pace
bike	8 x 1M w/ 60 sec spin/rest	5 x 5 min w/ 3-4 min spin/rest	2 x 10M @ 12M TT pace spin 5-10 min between
run	8 x 300 m w/ 60 sec rest	3 x 1200 m w/ 2-3 min rest	10k TT

week 11	Day 1	Day 2	Day 3
Strength	**Squat 5x5**	**Press 5x5**	**Dead Lift 5x5**
CrossFit	Max reps in 1 min of: KB swings, pull-ups, box Jumps, ball slams, rest 2 mins, 3 rounds	100 m of walking lunges, 60 sit-ups, 50 supine rows, 40 step-ups (20 each leg), 30 jump squats, 20 knee to elbows, 10 broad jumps	7 rounds for time: 7 overhead squats, 7 burpees
Endurance swim	20 x 25 TT's w/ easy 50 between	6 x 200 on 2:45 or :15 sec less recovery	500 m/y TT
bike	20 x 25 TT's w/ easy 50 between	5 x 5 min w/ 3-4 min spin rest	3 x 10M @ last weeks pace for 2... w/ 5-10 min spins between
run	5 x 400 m w/ 60 sec rest	2 x 1M with 5 min rest between	3 x 5k @ 10k TT pace w/ 5-10 min rest

week 12	Day 1	Day 2	Day 3
Strength	**Squat 5x5**	**Press 5x5**	**Dead Lift 5x5**
CrossFit	2 push jerks on the minute for 10 mins	100m row sprint, 12 ball slams, rest 1 min, complete 5 rounds, time each round	Rounds in 20 mins: 5 chin-ups, 10 dips, 10 pistols (5 each leg)
Endurance swim	20 x 50 on :45	6 x 200 on 2:45 or :15 sec less recovery	800 @ 5 sec slower per 100 than 500 TT pace
bike	6 x 1k TT's w/ 2M spin between	3 x 5k w/ 1M spin between	10M - 30M TT
run	6 x 400 m w/ 60 sec rest	3 x 1M with 5 min rest between	5k - 15k TT

SAMPLE WODS

NAMED ENDURANCE WODS

San Francisco Crippler

- ☐ 30 Back Squats body weight
- ☐ 1,000 Meter Row

Option 2:

- ☐ 30 Back Squats 135/225
- ☐ 1,000 Meter Row

Newport Crippler

- ☐ 30 Back Squats body weight
- ☐ 1 Mile Run

Option 2:

- ☐ 30 Back Squats 135/225
- ☐ 1 Mile Run

Peterson's Ghost
Run WOD Only.

- ☐ 2 x 1 mile
  Recover 3 min
- ☐ 2 x 800 m
  Recover 2 min
- ☐ 2 x 400 m
  Recover 90 seconds
- ☐ Res/recover 3-5 min
- ☐ 1 mile TT
  Recover 3 min
- ☐ 2 x 800 holding 5 seconds faster than 1 mile TT pace
  Recover 2 min
- ☐ 2 x 400 m holding 5 seconds faster than 1 mile TT pace
  Recover 90 seconds

Tosh

Choose one of the following sports:

- ☐ **Swim:** 3 x (50 m/y + 100 m/y + 200 m/y)
- ☐ **Bike:** 3 x (1/2 mile + 1 mile + 2 mile)
- ☐ **Run:** 3 x (200 m + 400 m+ 600 m)
- ☐ **C2:** 3 x (250 m +500 m+ 750 m)

Rest the exact time it takes you to do each interval in each set.

EX: 200 m run in 35 seconds rest 35 seconds, 400 m run, rest 400 m time, run 600 m, rest 600 m time, run 200 m, etc. No extra rest between rounds.

Short Tosh

Choose one of the following sports:

- ☐ **Swim:** 3 rounds (25 m/y+ 50 m/y+ 100 m/y)
- ☐ **Bike:** 3 rounds (1/4 mile+ 1/2 mile+ 1 mile)
- ☐ **Run:** 3 rounds (100 m+ 200 m+ 400 m)
- ☐ **C2:** 3 rounds (125 m+ 250 m+ 500 m)

Rest the exact time it takes you to do each interval in each set.

EX: 200 m run in 35 seconds, rest 35 seconds then 400 m run, rest 400 m time, run 600 m, rest 600 m time, run 200 m, etc. No extra rest between rounds.

Heavy Tosh

Choose one of the following sports: Use a weighted vest or ruck.

- ☐ **Swim:** 10 lbs vest or add cut t-shirt for drag, 3 rounds (50 m/y + 100 m/y + 200 m/y)
- ☐ **Bike:** 30 lbs vest 3 rounds (1/2 mile + 1 mile+ 2 mile)
- ☐ **Run:** 20 lbs vest 3 rounds (200 m + 400 m+ 600 m)
- ☐ **C2:** 20 lbs vest 3 rounds (250 m +500 m+ 750 m)

Rest the exact time it takes you to do each interval in each set.

EX: 200 m run in 35 sec. Rest 35 sec then 400 m run, rest 400 m time, run 600 m, rest 600 m time, run 200 m, etc. No extra rest between rounds. Scale weight as needed.

NAMED ENDURANCE WODS

Mack's 20:10

Choose one of the following sports:

Do 20:10 (Tabata) x Distance until completion. 20 seconds on, 10 seconds recovery.

- ☐ **Swim: 800 m**
- ☐ **Bike: 5 miles**
- ☐ **Run: 2 miles**
- ☐ **C2: 3K**

Lactate Shuttle

Choose one of the following sports:

- ☐ **Swim**
- ☐ **Bike**
- ☐ **Run**
- ☐ **C2**

5 min on,
2:30 min recovery
6 min on, 3 min recovery
7 min on. Done.
All out max efforts!

24 min Pyramid

Choose one of the following sports:

- ☐ **Swim**
- ☐ **Bike**
- ☐ **Run**
- ☐ **C2**

4 min on, 2 min recovery
5 min on, 2 min recovery
6 min on, 2 min recovery
5 min on, 2 min recovery
4 min on, Done!

20 min AMRAP

Choose one of the following sports:

20 minute AMRAP "As Many Rounds As Possible"

- ☐ **Swim: 50 m**
  Recover 30 seconds
- ☐ **Bike: 1/4 mile**
  Recover 30 seconds
- ☐ **Run: 200 m**
  Recover 30 seconds
- ☐ **C2: 200 m**
  Recover 30 seconds

Complete as many rounds as possible in the 20 minute time frame. Rest is included as part of the 20 minutes.

10 x Max Wattage

Choose one of the following sports: Bike and C2 ONLY!

If you normally Run or Swim, Choose C2.

- ☐ **Bike: 10 Rounds:**
  Ride your body weight in watts for 1 min. When the 1 min expires, sprint in the saddle for 10 seconds to reach maximal wattage. Recover 2 min between rounds. Use a Computrainer or Power Tap to measure for accurate readings.

- ☐ **C2: 10 Rounds:**
  Row your body weight in watts for 1 min. When the 1 min expires, pull 8 strokes as hard as possible to attain maximal wattage. Recover 2 min between rounds. Use an Erg to measure for accurate readings.

THOM

Choose one of the following sports:

- ☐ **Swim**
- ☐ **Bike**
- ☐ **Run**
- ☐ **C2**

18 rounds: 60 seconds on, 20 seconds recovery After completing 18 rounds, perform 50 burpees.

Fastest pace possible!
Bike can be done using an ERG stationary bike with a distance measure, or bike in large chain ring with an odometer.

JERRY

One sport only:

- ☐ **Run: 4 x 5k TT**

Recover 5-15 min between efforts. Deviate less than 2 min from fastest 5k.

RUN WODS / 2 SET WODS

2 x 10 min + 2 x 2 min

2 x 10 min
Recover 5 min between intervals.

Next interval scheme starts after the 5 min recovery.

2 x 2 min
Recover 1 min between intervals.

Work for max distance/speed on each interval. Remain consistent and try to best the previous distance/speed traveled with each attempt.

2×5/5×1

2× 5 min
2 min recovery

Work for max distance/speed on each interval. Remain consistent and try to best the previous distance/speed traveled with each attempt.

Next interval scheme starts after the 2 min recovery.

5 x 1 min
30 sec recovery

Work for max distance/speed on each interval. Remain consistent and try to best the previous distance/speed traveled with each attempt.

5 x 2 min+4 x 1 min

5 x 2 min
3 min recovery between intervals.

Next interval scheme starts after the 2 min recovery.

4 x 1 min
1 min recovery between intervals.

Work for max distance/speed on each interval. Remain consistent and try to best the previous distance/speed traveled with each attempt.

2 rounds of 5 x 1 min on, 2 min off

2 Rounds of:

5 x 1 min on
2 min recovery

5 min rest between each set of 5.

RUN WODS / REPEATS BY MINUTES

3×8 min

3× 8 min intervals
4 min recovery between intervals.

Work for max distance/speed on each interval. Remain consistent and try to best the previous distance/speed traveled with each attempt.

3×7 min

3× 7 min intervals
3 min recovery between intervals.

Work for max distance/speed on each interval. Remain consistent and try to best the previous distance/speed traveled with each attempt.

4×5 min

4× 5 min intervals
3 min recovery between intervals.

Work for max distance/speed on each interval. Remain consistent and try to best the previous distance/speed traveled with each attempt.

5×3 min

5× 3 min intervals
3 min recovery between intervals.

Work for max distance/speed on each interval. Remain consistent and try to best the previous distance/speed traveled with each attempt.

RUN WODS / REPEATS BY MINUTES

3 x 3 min

3× 3 min
3 min recovery between intervals.

Work for max distance/speed on each interval. Remain consistent and try to best the previous distance/speed traveled with each attempt.

6 x 2 min

6× 2 min
1 min recovery between intervals.

Work for max distance/speed on each interval. Remain consistent and try to best the previous distance/speed traveled with each attempt.

12 x 1 min

12 × 1 min
Recover 30 seconds between intervals.

Work for max distance/speed on each interval. Remain consistent and try to best the previous distance/speed traveled with each attempt.

5 x 1 min

5 x 1 min
Recover 3 min between intervals.

Work for max distance/speed on each interval. Remain consistent and try to best the previous distance/speed traveled with each attempt.

4.2.1 Intervals

4 min on, 3 min recovery

2 min on, 30 sec recovery

1 min on, 3 min recovery

2 min on, 30 sec recovery

4 min on, Done!

Work for max distance on each interval. Remain consistent and try to best the previous distance/speed traveled with each attempt.

Intervals By Time

Choose the duration based on the length of your event.

SC:	LC:	Advanced:
1 x 8 min, recover 3 min	1 x 10 min, recover 6 min	1 x 15 min, recover 8 min
1 x 3 min, recover 2 min	1 x 8 min, recover 3 min	1 x 8 min, recover 3 min
2 x 1 min, recover 1 min	1 x 3 min, recover 2 min	1 x 3 min, recover 2 min
3 x 30 sec, recover 15 sec	2 x 1 min, recover 1 min	2 x 1 min, recover 1 min

SC: Work for max distance/speed on each interval. Remain consistent and try to best the previous distance/speed traveled with each attempt.

LC: Work for max distance/speed on each interval.

Advanced: Work for max distance/speed on each interval. Remain consistent and try to best the previous distance/speed traveled with each attempt.

RUN WODS / LADDER

1 min Ladder

All out efforts.

1 min on, 1 min recovery

1 min on, 50 sec recovery

1 min on, 40 sec recovery

1 min on, 30 sec recovery

1 min on, 20 sec recovery

1 min on, 10 sec recovery

Go back up the ladder until you finish with 1 min on, 50 sec off, 1 min on.

90 sec Ladder

All out efforts.

90 sec on, 1 min recovery

90 sec on, 45 sec recovery

90 sec on, 30 sec recovery

90 sec on, 15 sec recovery

90 sec on, 30 sec recovery

90 sec on, 45 sec recovery

90 sec on, Done!

10 x Intervals 5 x Rest

All out efforts.

10 x 200 m with 5 times the recovery (if it takes 40 sec to run the 200 m then you recover 3:20)

10 x Sprints

10 x 100 m

All out sprint , 90 sec recovery.

10 x 1:1

10 x 400 m

Recovery is the exact time it took to complete the interval. 1:1 ratio

6 x Intervals

6 x 400 m

2 min recoveries.

5 x Intervals

5 x 800 m holding fastest possible pace without slowing more than 5 sec per fastest 800.

90 second recoveries.

2 x Intervals

2 x 12 min

Recover 2 min between each interval.

Work for max distance/speed on each interval. Remain consistent and try to best the previous distance/speed traveled with each attempt.

Tabata

20:10 x 8 rounds

20 seconds on, 10 seconds recovery.

All out efforts.

Use a treadmill, set at 12% grade at 0-30 sec slower pace per mile than best 5k pace. Do not reduce the speed!

120:60×6

2 min on, 1 recovery, x 6

Work for max distance/speed on each interval. Remain consistent and try to best the previous distance/speed traveled with each attempt.

30:60×10

30:60 x 10 rounds
30 seconds on, 60 seconds recovery for 10 rounds.

All out efforts.

Use a treadmill, set at 12% grade at 0-30 sec slower pace per mile than best 5k pace. Do not reduce the speed!

30:20×12

30:20 x 12 rounds
30 seconds on, 20 seconds recovery.

All out efforts.

Use a treadmill, set at 12% grade at 0-30 seconds slower pace per mile than best 5k pace. Do not reduce the speed!

30:20×8

30:20 x 8 rounds
30 seconds on, 20 seconds recovery.

All out efforts.

Use a treadmill, set at 12% grade at 0-30 seconds slower pace per mile than best 5k pace. Do not reduce the speed!

RUN WODS / LADDER

Long Intervals

SC: 3 x 1 mile

Recover 1-3 min
Hold within 5-10 seconds.

LC: 2 x 5k

Recover 5-10 min.
Hold within 1-2 min.

Advanced: 3 x 5k

Recover 5-15 min
Hold within 2-3 min

Long Intervals

SC: 3 x 1 mile

Recover 2 min.
Hold within 10 seconds of best 1 mile.

LC: 3 x 2k

Recover 4 min.
Hold within 20 seconds of best 2 mile

Advanced: 3 x 5k

Recover 5 – 10 min.
Hold within 2 min of best 5k

The 30s

All out efforts!

3 Rounds, 2 minute rest between rounds.

30 sec on, 30 sec recovery

30 sec on, 25 sec recovery

30 sec on, 20 sec recovery

30 sec on, 15 sec recovery

30 sec on, 10 sec recovery

30 sec on, 5 sec recovery

30 sec on, rest!

20 sec Sprints

Sprint/Recover:

3 rounds of:

20 sec/60 sec

20 sec/50 sec

20 sec/40 sec

20 sec/30 sec

20 sec/20 sec

20 sec/10 sec

Start next round after 10 sec rest.

RUN WODS / HILL WORK

10 x 30 sec Hill Sprints

10 x 30 sec hill sprints

All out efforts.

30 sec rest at top before descending hill easy, "walk if needed". Rest 1 min at the bottom of the hill before the next sprint.

Treadmill use 7-10% grade.

2 min recovery between sprints.

Hill Repeats

10 x 30 sec hill sprints

Recover 1 min before descending hill easy.

1 min recovery at bottom of hill before next repeat.

Treadmill use 7% grade.

2 min recovery between sprints.

Hill Climb Time Trial

1 mile hill climb

Incline between 6-15%

Tempo 80-85% RPE 15-17

25 min hill climb

4-8% avg grade

Weighted Hill Time Trial

1 mile hill climb

Incline between 6-12%.

Add 10-20 lb weighted vest.

RUN WODS / TIME TRIAL BY DISTANCE

Time Trial D 1
1.5 mile TT

Time Trial D 7
5k

Time Trial D 9
SC: 5k

LC: 10k or 10 mile TT (choice)

Advanced: 13.1 mile TT

Time Trial D 10
SC: 10 mile

LC: 18 mile

Advanced: 25 mile

Time Trial D 13
SC: 2 mile TT

LC: 10k TT

Advanced: 13.1M TT

Time Trial D 15
SC: 5k TT

LC: 10k

Advanced: 10k TT

RUN WODS / TIME TRIAL BY TIME

Time Trial T 1
9 minute
All out Effort

Time Trial T 10
35 min TT

Time Trial T 15
60 min TT

Time Trial T 16
90 min TT

Time Trial T 17
20 min TT

RUN WODS / TEMPO BY DISTANCE

Tempo 85-95%
10k total:

85% for first 5k then pick it up to 95% on the last 5k.

Tempo 80-90%
80% for the first half, 90% for the last half. Choose distance based on your event.

SC: 1.5 mile

LC: 5 miles

Advanced: 10 miles

RUN WODS / TEMPO BY TIME

Tempo 80-90%
SC: 20 min

LC: 60 min

Advanced: 90 min

Tempo 80-85%
SC: 25 min

LC: 60 min

Advanced: 75 min

Tempo 80-85% RPE 15-16
SC: 20 min

LC: 30 min

Advanced: 60 min

Tempo 80-85%
SC: 35 min

LC: 1 hrs

Advanced: 2 hrs

Tempo 85% RPE 16
SC: 20 min

LC: 30 min

Advanced: 60 min

Tempo 80-85% RPE 15-17
25 min hill climb 4-8% avg grade.

BIKE WODS / 2 SET WODS

2 x 10 min+2 x 2 min

2x10 min
Recover 5 min between intervals.

Next interval scheme starts after the 5 min recovery.

2x 2 min
Recover 1 min.

Work for max distance on each interval. Remain consistent and try to best the previous distance traveled with each attempt.

5 x 2 min+4 x 1 min

5x2 min
Recover 3 min between intervals.

Next interval scheme starts after the 3 min recovery.

4x 1 min
Recover 1 min between intervals.

Work for max distance/watts on each interval. Remain consistent and try to best the previous distance traveled with each attempt.

2×5/5×1

2× 5 min
Recover 2 min between intervals.

Next interval scheme starts after the 2 min recovery.

5x1 min
Recover 30 seconds between intervals.

Work for max distance on each interval. Remain consistent and try to best the previous distance traveled with each attempt.

2 rounds of 5 x 1 min on, 2 min off

2 Rounds of:

5 x 1 min on
Recover 2 min between intervals.

5 min easy between each set of 5 intervals.

Work for max distance/watts on each interval. Remain consistent and try to best the previous distance traveled with each attempt.

BIKE WODS / REPEATS BY MINUTES

3×8 min

3× 8 min intervals
Recover 4 min between intervals.

Work for max distance/watts on each 8 min rounds. Remain consistent and try to best the previous distance traveled with each attempt.

3×7 min

3× 7 min intervals
Recover 3 min between intervals.

Work for max distance/watts on each of the 7 min rounds. Remain consistent and try to best the previous distance traveled with each attempt.

4×5 min

4× 5 min intervals
Recover 3 min between intervals.

Work for max distance/watts on each 5 min round. Remain consistent and try to best the previous distance traveled with each attempt.

5×3 min

5× 3 min intervals
Recover 3 min between intervals.

Work for max distance/watts on each 3 min round. Remain consistent and try to best the previous distance traveled with each attempt.

BIKE WODS / REPEATS BY MINUTES

3 x 3 min

3 × 3 min
Recover 3 min between intervals.

Work for max distance/watts on each 3 min round. Remain consistent and try to best the previous distance traveled with each attempt.

6 x 2 min

6 × 2 min
Recover 1 min between intervals.

Work for max distance/watts on each 3 min round. Remain consistent and try to best the previous distance traveled with each attempt.

12x1 min

12 × 1 min
Recover 30 seconds between intervals.

Hold maximal distance/watts as consistent as possible.

5 x 1min

5 x 1 min
Recover 3 min between intervals.

Work for max distance/watts on each 1 min round. Remain consistent and try to best the previous distance traveled with each attempt.

4.2.1 Intervals

4 min on,
3 min recovery

2 min on,
30 sec recovery

1 min on,
3 min recovery

2 min on,
30 sec recovery

4 min on, Done!

Intervals By Time

Choose duration based on the length of your event.

SC:	LC:	Advanced:
1 x 8 min, recover 3 min	1 x 10 min, recover 6 min	1 x 15 min, recover 8 min
1 x 3 min, recover 2 min	1 x 8 min, recover 3 min	1 x 8 min, recover 3 min
2 x 1 min, recover 1 min	1 x 3 min, recover 2 min	1 x 3 min, recover 2 min
3 x 30 sec, recover 15 sec	2 x 1 min, recover 1 min	2 x 1 min, recover 1 min

BIKE WODS / LADDER

1 min Ladder

All out efforts.

1 min on, 1 min recovery

1 min on, 50 sec recovery

1 min on, 40 sec recovery

1 min on, 30 sec recovery

1 min on, 20 sec recovery

1 min on, 10 sec recovery

Go back up the ladder until you finish with 1 min on, 50 sec recovery, 1 min on.

Work for max distance/watts on each interval. Remain consistent and try to best the previous distance traveled with each attempt.

90 sec Ladder

All out efforts.

90 sec on, 1 min recovery

90 sec on, 45 sec recovery

90 sec on, 30 sec recovery

90 sec on, 15 sec recovery

90 sec on, 30 sec recovery

90 sec on, 45 sec recovery

90 sec on, Done!

Work for max distance/watts on each interval. Remain consistent and try to best the previous distance traveled with each attempt.

10 x Intervals
5 x Rest

All out efforts.

10 x 1/4 mile
with 5 times the recovery.

If it takes 30 seconds to bike the 1/4 mile then recover 2:30

Work for max distance/watts on each interval. Remain consistent and try to best the previous distance traveled with each attempt.

8 x Sprints

After a solid warm up.

8 x 1K
2 min recovery between intervals. All out sprints.

Work for max distance/watts on each interval. Remain consistent and try to best the previous distance traveled with each attempt.

10x 1:1

10 x 1 mile
Recover the exact time it took to complete the 1 mile. 1:1 work:rest ratio.

Work for max distance/watts on each interval. Remain consistent and try to best the previous distance traveled with each attempt.

4 x Intervals

4 x 2 miles
2 min recovery after each mile.

Work for max distance/watts on each interval. Remain consistent and try to best the previous distance traveled with each attempt. Slowing less than 5 sec per fastest 2 mile.

5 x Intervals

5 x 2k
90 second recovery after each mile.

Work for max distance/watts on each interval. Remain consistent and try to best the previous distance traveled with each attempt. Slowing less than 5 sec per fastest 2k.

2 x Intervals

2×15 min
Recover 2 min

Work for max distance/watts on each interval. Remain consistent and try to best the previous distance traveled with each attempt.

Tabata

20:10 x 8 rounds
20 seconds on, 10 seconds recovery.

All out efforts.

Use a Monarch ERG, stationary bike with wattage tool or something similar that can hold a load of 200+ watts.

120:60 × 6

6 x 2 min
on, recover 1 min.

Work for max distance/watts on each interval. Remain consistent and try to best the previous distance traveled with each attempt.

30:60×10

30:60 x 10 rounds
30 sec on 60 sec recovery for 10 rounds.

All out efforts.

Use an ERG, stationary bike with wattage tool or something similar that can hold a load of 200+ watts.

30:20×12

30:20 x 12 rounds
30 sec on, 20 sec recovery

All out efforts.

Use a Monarch ERG, stationary bike with wattage tool or something similar that can hold a load of 200+ watts

30:20×8

30:20 x 8 rounds
30 sec on, 20 sec recovery.

All out efforts.

Use a Monarch ERG, stationary bike with wattage tool or something similar that can hold a load of 200+ watts.

BIKE WODS / LADDER

Long Intervals

SC: 3 × 5 mile
Recover 30-60 seconds. Hold within 30-60 seconds.

LC: 2 x 10 mile
Recover 2-3 min. Hold within 1-2 min.

Advanced: 3 x 10 mile
Recover 4-8 min Hold within 1-2 min.

Long Intervals

SC: 3 x 4 miles
Recover 1 min.

LC: 3 x 6 miles
Recover 2 min.

Advanced: 3 x 10 mile
Recover 5 min.

20 sec Sprints

Sprint/Recover, 3 rounds of:

20 sec/60 sec	20 sec/40 sec	20 sec/20 sec	Start next round after 10 sec rest.
20 sec/50 sec	20 sec/30 sec	20 sec/10 sec	

The 30s

All out efforts.

3 Rounds, 2 minute rest between rounds.

30 sec on, 30 sec recovery

30 sec on, 25 sec recovery

30 sec on, 20 sec recovery

30 sec on, 15 sec recovery

30 sec on, 10 sec recovery

30 sec on, 5 sec recovery

30 sec on, Done!

Work for max distance/watts on each interval. Remain consistent and try to best the previous distance traveled with each attempt.

BIKE WODS / HILL WORK

10 x 30 sec Hill Sprints

10 x 30 sec hill sprints
2 min recovery. All out efforts.

Come into the hill at speed to maximize the 30 second sprint. If you do not have a hill, use tension on a trainer or ergometer with steady/heavy tension.

Hill Repeats

4 x 1 mile hill repeats
Hold fastest pace/watts on each 1 mile.

Recovery is how long it takes you to come down the hill. If you do not have a hill, use tension on a trainer or ergometer with steady/heavy tension.

BIKE WODS / HILL CLIMB TEMPO

Tempo 80-85%

25 min hill climb

30 min hill climb 4-8% avg grade.

Hill Climb Time Trial

2 mile hill climb

Incline 6-15%. Maximal effort.

Weighted Hill Time Trial

2 mile hill climb

Remain in the saddle, push as big of a gear as possible.

Cadence 60+ RPM. Incline 6-12%.

BIKE WODS / TIME TRIAL

Time Trial D 1
8 mile TT

Time Trial D 7
12 mile TT

Time Trial D 9
SC: 12 mile TT
LC: 25 mile TT
Advanced: 30 mile TT

Time Trial D 10
SC: 10 mile
LC: 18 mile
Advanced: 25 mile

Time Trial D 13
SC: 12 mile TT
LC: 20 mile TT
Advanced: 30 mile TT

Time Trial D 15
SC: 12 mile TT
LC: 18 mile TT
Advanced: 22 mile TT

BIKE WODS / TIME TRIAL BY TIME

Time Trial T 1
9 minute
All out effort.

Time Trial T 10
35 min TT

Time Trial T 15
20 min TT

Time Trial T 16
90 min TT

Time Trial T 17
24 min TT

BIKE WODS / TEMPO BY DISTANCE

Tempo 85-95%
20 miles total:
85% for first 10 miles then pick it up to 95% on the last 10 miles.

Tempo 80-90%
80% for the first half, 90% for the last half. Choose distance based on your event.
SC: 10 mile
LC: 18 miles
Advanced: 25 miles

BIKE WODS / TEMPO BY TIME

Tempo 80-90%
SC: 20 min
LC: 60 min
Advanced: 90 min

Tempo 80-85%
SC: 60 min
LC: 75 min
Advanced: 90 min

Tempo 80-85%
SC: 60 min
LC: 60 min
Advanced: 80 min

Tempo 80-85%
SC: 35 min
LC: 1 hrs
Advanced: 2 hrs

Tempo 85% RPE 16
SC: 60 min
LC: 60 min
Advanced: 80 min

Tempo 80-85% RPE 15-17
30 min hill climb 4-8% avg grade.

SWIM WODS / 2 SET WODS

2 x 10 min+2 x 2 min

2 x 10 min
Recover 5 min between intervals.

Next interval scheme starts after the 5 min recovery.

2 x 2 min
Recover 1 min between intervals.

Work for max distance/speed on each interval. Remain consistent and try to best the previous distance/speed traveled with each attempt.

2 × 5 / 5 × 1

2 × 5 min
Recover 2 min between intervals.

Next interval scheme starts after the 2 min recovery.

5 x 1 min
30 sec recovery between intervals.

Work for max distance/speed on each interval. Remain consistent and try to best the previous distance/speed traveled with each attempt.

5 x 2 min+4 x 1 min

5 x 2 min
3 min recovery between intervals.

Then:

4 x 1 min
1 min recovery between intervals.

Work for max distance/speed on each interval. Remain consistent and try to best the previous distance/speed traveled with each attempt.

2 rounds of 5 x 1 min on, 2 min off

2 Rounds of:

5 x 1 min on
2 min recovery.

5 min easy between each set of 5.

SWIM WODS / REPEATS BY MINUTES

3×8 min

3× 8 min intervals
4 min recovery between intervals.

Work for max distance/speed on each interval. Remain consistent and try to best the previous distance/speed traveled with each attempt.

3×7 min

3× 7 min intervals
3 min recovery between intervals.

Work for max distance/speed on each interval. Remain consistent and try to best the previous distance/speed traveled with each attempt.

4×5 min

4× 5 min intervals
3 min recovery between intervals.

Work for max distance/speed on each interval. Remain consistent and try to best the previous distance/speed traveled with each attempt.

5×3 min

5× 3 min intervals
3 min recovery between intervals.

Hold highest avg pace.

SWIM WODS / REPEATS BY MINUTES

3 x 3 min

3 × 3 min
3 min recovery between intervals. Hold highest avg pace.

6 x 2 min

2 min on, 1 min off x 6
Cover as much distance as possible on each 2 min round.

12 x 1 min

12 × 1 min
Recover 30 seconds between intervals.

Work for max distance/speed on each 1 min interval. Remain consistent and try to best the previous distance/speed traveled with each attempt.

5 x 1 min

5 x 1 min
Recover 3 min between intervals.

Work for max distance/speed on each interval. Remain consistent and try to best the previous distance/speed traveled with each attempt.

4.2.1 Intervals

4 min on,
3 min recovery

2 min on,
30 sec recovery

1 min on,
3 min recovery

2 min on,
30 sec recovery

4 min on, Done!

Intervals By Time

Choose the duration based on the length of your event.

SC:	LC:	Advanced:
1 x 8 min, recover 3 min	1 x 10 min, recover 6 min	1 x 15 min, recover 8 min
1 x 3 min, recover 2 min	1 x 8 min, recover 3 min	1 x 8 min, recover 3 min
2 x 1 min, recover 1 min	1 x 3 min, recover 2 min	1 x 3 min, recover 2 min
3 x 30 sec, recover 15 sec	2 x 1 min, recover 1 min	2 x 1 min, recover 1 min

Work for max distance/speed on each interval. Remain consistent and try to best the previous distance/speed traveled with each attempt.

SWIM WODS / LADDER

1 min Ladder

All out efforts.

1 min on, 1 min recovery

1 min on, 50 sec recovery

1 min on, 40 sec recovery

1 min on, 30 sec recovery

1 min on, 20 sec recovery

1 min on, 10 sec recovery

Go back up the ladder until you finish with 1 min on, 50 sec off, 1 min on.

Work for max distance/speed on each interval. Remain consistent and try to best the previous distance/speed traveled with each attempt.

90 sec Ladder

All out efforts.

90 sec on, 1 min recovery

90 sec on, 45 sec recovery

90 sec on, 30 sec recovery

90 sec on, 15 sec recovery

90 sec on, 30 sec recovery

90 sec on, 45 sec recovery

90 sec on, Done!

Work for max distance/speed on each interval. Remain consistent and try to best the previous distance/speed traveled with each attempt.

SWIM WODS/ LADDER

10 x Intervals 5 x Rest

All out efforts.

10 x 50 m/y

With 5 times the recovery (if it takes you 30 seconds to swim 50 m/y rest 2:30).

20 x Sprints

After a solid warm up.

20 x 25 m/y

mid pool start and finish. NO WALL STARTS.
1 min recovery.

All out sprints.

10 x 1:1

10 x 75 m/y

recovery is exact time it took to complete the interval. 1:1 Ratio.

2 x Intervals

2 × 8 min
Recover 2 min.

Work for max distance/ speed on each round. Remain consistent and try to best the previous distance/speed traveled with each attempt.

4x Intervals

4 x 100 m/y
30 second recovery.

Hold highest avg pace.

5x Intervals

5 x 200 m
30 seconds recovery.

Hold highest avg pace.

Tabata

20:10 x 8 rounds
20 seconds on, 10 seconds recovery.

All out efforts. Use pool or open water.

120:60×6

2 min on, 1 mi recovery x 6

Work for max distance/speed on each 2 min round. Remain consistent and try to best the previous distance/speed traveled with each attempt.

30:60×10

30:60 x 10 rounds
30 seconds on, 60 seconds recovery, for 10 rounds.

All out efforts. Use pool or open water.

30:20×12

30:20 x 12 rounds
30 seconds on, 20 seconds off.

All out efforts. Use pool or open water.

30:20×10

30:20 x 10 rounds
30 seconds on, 20 seconds off.

All out efforts. Use pool or open water.

30:20×8

30:20 x 8 rounds
30 seconds on, 20 seconds recovery.

All out efforts. Use pool or open water.

Long Intervals

SC: 3 x 300 m
Recover 45-60 sec.
LC: 2 x 700 m
Recover 60 sec.
Advanced: 3 x 700 m
Recover 1-2 min.

Long Intervals

SC: 3 x 300 m
Recover 1 min.

The 30s

All out efforts.

3 Rounds:

30 sec on,
30 sec recovery

30 sec on,
25 sec recovery

30 sec on,
20 sec recovery

30 sec on,
15 sec recovery

30 sec on,
10 sec recovery

30 sec on,
5 sec recovery

30 sec on, Done!
2 min rest between rounds.

20 sec Sprints

Sprint/Recover:

3 rounds of:

20 sec/60 sec

20 sec/50 sec

20 sec/40 sec

20 sec/30 sec

20 sec/20 sec

20 sec/10 sec

Start next round after 10 sec rest.

SWIM WODS / PULLING WODS (Using paddles and buoy)

10 x 30 sec Sprints

10 x 30 second sprints

2 min recovery.

All out effort using paddles and buoy.

10 X Repeats

10 x 100 m/y
Using paddles and buoy. 15 sec recovery.

Tempo 80-85%

20 min
Add cut T-shirt or drag shorts.

Weighted Time Trial

500m
Add a cut T-shirt, drag shorts, or parachute for drag.

SWIM WODS / TIME TRIAL BY DISTANCE

Time Trial D 1
400 m TT

Time Trial D 7
600 m TT

Time Trial D 9
SC: 500 m TT
LC: 500 m TT
Advanced: 500 m TT

Time Trial D 10
SC: 400 m TT
LC: 600 m TT
Advanced: 800 m TT

Time Trial D 13
SC: 800 m TT
LC: 1000 m TT
Advanced: 1200 m TT

Time Trial D 15
1000 m TT

SWIM WODS / TIME TRIAL BY TIME

Time Trial T 1
9 minute
All out effort. Cover as much distance as possible.

Time Trial T 10
15 min TT

Time Trial T 15
20 min TT

Time Trial T 16
30 min TT

Time Trial T 17
12 min TT

SWIM WODS / TEMPO BY DISTANCE

Tempo 85-95%

1000m/y total:
85% for first 500m/y then pick it up to 95% on the last 500m/y.

Tempo 80-90%

80% for the first half, 90% for the last half. Choose distance based on your event.

SC: 10 mile **LC:** 18 miles **Advanced:** 25 miles

SWIM WODS / TEMPO BY TIME

Tempo 80-90%	Tempo 80-85%	Tempo 80-85%	Tempo 80-85%	Tempo 85%	Tempo 80-85%
SC: 20 min	**SC:** 10 min	**SC:** 12 min	**SC:** 35 min	**SC:** 12 min	**20 min** add cut T-shirt or drag shorts.
LC: 60 min	**LC:** 15 min	**LC:** 15 min	**LC:** 1 hrs	**LC:** 15 min	
Advanced: 90 min	**Advanced:** 20 min	**Advanced:** 35 min	**Advanced:** 2 hrs	**Advanced:** 35 min	

ROW WODS / 2 SET WODS

2 x 10 min+2 x 2 min

2 x 10 min

Recover 5 min between intervals.

Next interval scheme starts after the 5 min recovery.

2 x 2 min

Recover 1 min.

Set the drag factor between 120-140. Work for max distance on each interval. Remain consistent and try to best the previous distance traveled with each attempt.

5x 2 min+4x 1 min

5 x 2 min

Recover 3 min between intervals.

Next interval scheme starts after the 3 min recovery

4 x 1 min

Recover 1 min between intervals.

Set the drag factor between 120-140. Work for max distance on each interval. Remain consistent and try to best the previous distance traveled with each attempt.

2×5/5×1

2 × 5 min

Recover 2 min between intervals.

Next interval scheme starts after the 2 min recovery.

5 x 1 min

Recover 30 seconds between intervals.

Set the drag factor between 120-140. Work for max distance on each interval. Remain consistent and try to best the previous distance traveled with each attempt.

2 rounds of 5x1 min on, 2 min off

2 Rounds of:

5 x 1 min on

Recover 2 min between intervals.

5 min of easy rowing between each set of 5.

Set the drag factor between 120-140. Work for max distance on each interval. Remain consistent and try to best the previous distance traveled with each attempt.

ROW WODS / REPEATS BY THE MINUTE

3×8 min

3× 8 min intervals
Recover 4 min between intervals.

Set the drag factor between 120-140. Work for max distance on each interval. Remain consistent and try to best the previous distance traveled with each attempt.

3×7 min

3× 7 min
Recover 3 min between intervals.

Set the drag factor between 120-140. Work for max distance on each interval. Remain consistent and try to best the previous distance traveled with each attempt.

4×5 min

4× 5 min
Recover 3 min between intervals.

Set the drag factor between 120-140. Work for max distance on each interval. Remain consistent and try to best the previous distance traveled with each attempt.

5×3 min

5× 3 min
Recover 3 min between intervals.

Set the drag factor between 120-140. Work for max distance on each interval. Remain consistent and try to best the previous distance traveled with each attempt.

3 x 3 min

3 × 3 min
Recover 3 min between intervals.

Set the drag factor between 120-140. Work for max distance on each interval. Remain consistent and try to best the previous distance traveled with each attempt.

6 x 2 min

6× 2 min
Recover 1 min between intervals.

Set the drag factor between 120-140. Work for max distance on each interval. Remain consistent and try to best the previous distance traveled with each attempt.

12 x 1 min

12 × 1 min
Recover 30 seconds between intervals.

Set the drag factor between 120-140. Work for max distance on each interval. Remain consistent and try to best the previous distance traveled with each attempt.

5 x 1min

5 x 1 min
Recover 3 min between intervals.

Set the drag factor between 120-140. Work for max distance on each interval. Remain consistent and try to best the previous distance traveled with each attempt.

4.2.1 Intervals

4 min on, 3 min recovery

2 min on, 30 sec recovery

1 min on, 3 min recovery

2 min on, 30 sec recovery

4 min on, Done!

Set the drag factor between 120-140. Work for max distance on each interval.

Intervals By Time

Choose the duration based on the length of your event.

SC:	LC:	Advanced:
1x8 min, recover 3 min	1x10 min, recover 6 min	1x 15 min, recover 8 min
1x3 min, recover 2 min	1x 8 min, recover 3 min	1x 8 min, recover 3 min
2x1 min, recover 1 min	1x 3 min, recover 2 min	1x 3 min, recover 2 min
3x30 sec, recover 15 sec	2x 1 min, recover 1 min	2x 1 min, recover 1min

Set the drag factor between 120-140.

ROW WODS / LADDER

1 min Ladder

All out efforts.

1 min on, 1 min recovery

1 min on, 50 sec recovery

1 min on, 40 sec recovery

1 min on, 30 sec recovery

1 min on, 20 sec recovery

1 min on, 10 sec recovery

Go back up the ladder until you finish with 1 min on, 50 sec off, 1 min on.

Set the drag factor between 120-140. Work for max distance on each interval. Remain consistent and try to best the previous distance traveled with each attempt.

90 sec Ladder

All out efforts.

90 sec on, 1 min recovery

90 sec on, 45 sec recovery

90 sec on, 30 sec recovery

90 sec on, 15 sec recovery

90 sec on, 30 sec recovery

90 sec on, 45 sec recovery

90 sec on, Done!

Set the drag factor between 120-140. Work for max distance on each interval. Remain consistent and try to best the previous distance traveled with each attempt.

10 x Intervals 5 x Rest

All out efforts.

10 x 250 m with 5 times the recovery (if it takes 45 seconds to row 250 m then you recover 3:45).

Set the drag factor between 120-140. Work for max speed on each interval.

10 x Sprints

10 x 125 m

All out sprint , recover 1 min.

Set the drag factor between 120-140. Work for max speed on each interval.

10 x 1:1

10 x 40 cals

Recovery is exact time it took to complete the interval. 1:1 ratio.

Set the drag factor between 120-140. Work for max distance on each interval.

6 x Intervals

6 x 500 m

Recover 2 min after each interval.

Set the drag factor between 120-140. Work for max speed on each interval. Remain consistent and try to best the previous pace with each attempt.

5 x Intervals

5 x 1000 m

Recover 90 sec between each interval.

Set the drag factor between 120-140. Work for max speed on each interval. Remain consistent and try to best the previous pace with each attempt.

2 x Intervals

2 x 8 min

Recover 2 min between each interval.

Set the drag factor between 120-140. Work for max distance on each interval. Remain consistent and try to best the previous distance traveled with each attempt.

Tabata

20:10 x 8 rounds

20 seconds on, 10 seconds recovery.

All out efforts.

120:60 × 6

2 min on, 1 recovery x 6

Set the drag factor between 120-140. Work for max distance on each 2 min round. Remain consistent and try to best the previous distance traveled with each attempt.

30:60 × 10

30:60 x 10 rounds

30 seconds on, 60 seconds recovery for 10 rounds.

All out efforts.

Set the drag factor between 120-140.

30:20 × 12

30:20 x 12 rounds

30 seconds on, 20 seconds recovery.

All out efforts.

Set the drag factor between 120-140.

ROW WODS / LADDER

30:20 × 8

30:20 x 8 rounds
30 seconds on, 20 seconds recovery.

All out efforts.
Set the drag factor between 120-140.

Long Intervals

SC: 3 x 1000 m
hold within 3-5 sec recover 20-40 sec.

LC: 2 x 1800 m
hold within 5-10 sec recover 30-60 sec.

Advanced: 3 x 1800 m
hold within 10-15 sec rest 1-2 min.

Set the drag factor between 120-140.

Long Intervals

SC: 3 x 600 m
Hold within 5 scc of best 600 m.
Recover 1 min.

LC: 3 x 1000 m
Hold within 10 scc of best 1000m.
Recover 2 min.

Advanced: 4 x 1250 m
Hold within 20 scc of best 1250 m.
Recover 3 min.

Set the drag factor between 120-140.

The 30s

All out efforts. **3 Rounds:**

30 sec on, 30 sec recovery

30 sec on, 25 sec recovery

30 sec on, 20 sec recovery

30 sec on, 15 sec recovery

30 sec on, 10 sec recovery

30 sec on, 5 sec recovery

30 sec on, Done!

2 min recovery between rounds.

Set the drag factor between 120-140. Work for max distance on each interval. Remain consistent and try to best the previous distance traveled with each attempt.

10 x 30 sec Sprints

10 x 30 sec Sprints

All out efforts.

2 min recovery between sprints

Set the drag factor between 120-140.

Come into each sprint at speed to maximize the 30 sec sprint.

Work for max distance on each interval. Remain consistent and try to best the previous distance traveled with each attempt.

20 sec Sprints

Sprint/Recover:

3 rounds of:

20 sec/60 sec

20 sec/50 sec

20 sec/40 sec

20 sec/30 sec

20 sec/20 sec

20 sec/10 sec

Start next round after 10 sec rest.

Set the drag factor between 120-140. Work for max speed/distance on each interval. Remain consistent and try to best the previous speed/distance traveled with each attempt.

3 X Repeats

3 x 1k repeats
2 min recovery
Set the drag factor between 120-140.

Tempo 80-85% RPE 15-17

20 min
Set the drag factor between 110-130.

ROW WODS / TIME TRIAL BY DISTANCE

Time Trial

1500 m
Set the drag factor between 110-130.

Time Trial

2000 m
Set the drag factor between 110-130.

Time Trial D 1

2 k TT
Set the drag factor between 110-130.

Time Trial D 7

4000 m
Set the drag factor between 110-130.

ROW WODS / TIME TRIAL BY DISTANCE

Time Trial D 9

8k TT

Set the drag factor between 110-130.

Time Trial D 10

SC: 2k **LC:** 5k

Advanced: 8k

Set the drag factor between 110-130.

Time Trial D 13

SC: 2k TT **LC:** 3k TT

Advanced: 6k TT

Set the drag factor between 110-130.

Time Trial D 15

5k TT

Set the drag factor between 110-130.

ROW WODS / TIME TRIAL BY TIME

Time Trial T 1

9 min

All out effort. Set the drag factor between 110-130.

Time Trial T 7

12 min

Set the drag factor between 110-130.

Time Trial T 10

15 min

Set the drag factor between 110-130.

Time Trial T 15

20 min

Set the drag factor between 110-130.

Time Trial T 16

30 min

Set the drag factor between 110-130.

ROW WODS / TEMPO BY DISTANCE

Tempo 85-95%

3000 m total:
85% first 1500 m recover 1 min, then 95% for second 1500 m.

Set the drag factor between 110-130.

Tempo 80-90%

80% for the first half, 90% for the last half. Choose distance based on your event.

SC: 2k **LC:** 5k **Advanced:** 8k

Set the drag factor between 110-130.

ROW WODS / TEMPO BY TIME

Tempo 80-90%

SC: 20 min
LC: 60 min
Advanced: 90 min

Set the drag factor between 110-130.

Tempo 80-85% RPE 15-17

SC: 15 min
LC: 20 min
Advanced: 25 min

Set the drag factor between 110-130.

Tempo 80-85% RPE 15-16

25 min

Set the drag factor between 110-130.

Tempo 80-85%

SC: 35 min
LC: 1 hrs
Advanced: 2 hrs

Set the drag factor between 110-130.

Tempo 85%

25 min

Set the drag factor between 110-130.

Tempo 80-85%

20 min

Set the drag factor between 110-130.

RESOURCES

Recommended Books:

4-Hour Body: An Uncommon Guide to Rapid Fat-Loss, Incredible Sex, and Becoming a Superhuman by Tim Ferriss

Dr. Nicholas Romanov's Pose Method of Running by Dr. Nicolas Romanov

Pose Method of Triathlon Techniques by Dr. Nicolas Romanov

Sport and Exercise Biomechanics, Paul Grimshaw, Adrian Lees, Neil Fowler, Adrian Burden

Andy Pruitt's Complete Medical Guide for Cyclists by Dr. Andy L. Pruitt Ed.C., Chris Carmichael, and Fred Matheny

Bicycling Science by David Gordon Wilson

Fit by Lon Kilgore

Paleo Diet for Athletes: A Nutritional Formula for Peak Athletic Performance by Dr. Loren Cordain and Joe Friel

The Paleo Solution: The Original Human Diet by Robb Wolf

Recommended Websites:

Crossfitendurance.com

Crossfit.com

Endurancewod.com

Mobilitywod.com

Zone5endurance.com

Posetech.com

BikeCalculator.com

Robbwolf.com

ABOUT THE AUTHORS AND CONTRIBUTORS

Brian MacKenzie

Brian MacKenzie is a world-renowned strength and conditioning coach and the creator of CrossFit Endurance (www.crossfitendurance.com), which specializes in movement with an emphasis in running, cycling, and swimming mechanics. MacKenzie and his program have been featured in *Competitor Magazine*, *Runners World*, *Triathlete Magazine*, *Men's Journal*, *ESPN Rise*, *The Economist*, Tim Ferriss' *New York Times* bestseller *The 4-Hour Body*, *Men's Running UK*, *LA Sport & Fitness*, and *Rivera Magazine*. He has consulted with several teams, including the 2012 Western Athletic Conference Champions San Jose State Women's Swim Team.

Glen Cordoza

Glen Cordoza is one of the most published authors in the world on the topics of MMA, Brazilian Jiu-jitsu, Muay Thai kick-boxing, and fitness with over seventeen books to his credit. These works include co-authorship with such marital art luminaries as Randy Couture, BJ Penn, Anderson Silva, Fedor Emelianenko, Lyoto Machida, Eddie Bravo, Cung Le, Antonio Nogueira, and Marcelo Garcia. He is also the co-author of *Becoming a Supple Leopard* by Kelly Starrett. In addition to Glen's accomplishments as an author, he is a strength-and-conditioning coach and has competed as a professional mixed martial artist (MMA) and Muay Thai boxer.

Doug Katona

Doug Katona is managing partner and head coach of CrossFit Endurance. He is an internationally recognized presenter, educator, and highly sought-after strength-and-conditioning coach for endurance sports and CrossFit. He is a Cat. 2 cyclist, duathlete, as well as a master level POSE instructor.

Chris Michelmore

Chris Michelmore is the Head National Coach at De Anza Cupertino Aquatics in Cupertino, CA. Chris has produced multiple National Junior Team Members, Senior National, World Trial, and Olympic Trial qualifiers. Having taught everyone from children to collegiate champions, he has a unique understanding of how to coach and train people of all ages and ability levels.

Kelly Starrett

Dr. Kelly Starrett, DPT is the innovator of the Movement and Mobility Method, a highly effective system used to resolve pain, prevent injuries, and optimize athletic performance. Dr. Starrett's revolutionary human performance model uses strength-and-conditioning movements to predict, prioritize, and resolve inefficiencies in movement that lead to loss of performance and injury. Kelly is the founder of the acclaimed MobilityWod.com website, author of *Becoming a Supple Leopard*, and co-founder of San Francisco CrossFit, where he continues to work with some of the world's best athletes.